THE PRACTICE AND THEORY
OF INDIVIDUAL
PSYCHOLOGY

Founded by C. K. Ogden

The International Library of Psychology

INDIVIDUAL DIFFERENCES
In 21 Volumes

THE PRACTICE AND THEORY OF INDIVIDUAL PSYCHOLOGY

ALFRED ADLER

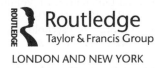
Routledge
Taylor & Francis Group

LONDON AND NEW YORK

First published in 1924 by
Routledge, Trench, Trubner & Co., Ltd.
2 Park Square, Milton Park, Abingdon, Oxfordshire OX14 4RN
711 Third Avenue, New York, NY 10017

First issued in paperback 2014

Routledge is an imprint of the Taylor and Francis Group, an informa business

© 1924 Alfred Adler, Translated by P Radin

British Library Cataloguing in Publication Data
A CIP catalogue record for this book
is available from the British Library

The Practice and Theory of Individual Psychology
ISBN 0415-21051-8
Individual Differences: 21 Volumes
ISBN 0415-21130-1
The International Library of Psychology: 204 Volumes
ISBN 0415-19132-7

ISBN 13: 978-1-138-87536-4 (pbk)
ISBN 13: 978-0-415-21051-5 (hbk)

PREFACE TO THE ENGLISH TRANSLATION

INDIVIDUAL PSYCHOLOGY is now a definite science with a limited subject-matter, and no compromise can be admitted. This intransigence arises not from the attitude or intention of its founder but from the inexorable logic of a treatment of phenomena as mutually related. We shall never agree to change the fundamentals of human psychology which it has established and to adopt others in their stead. And we shall also never be under the necessity of undertaking a special enquiry into sexual factors long after the other aspects of psychic life have been investigated. Individual psychology covers the whole range of psychology in one survey, and as a result it is able to mirror the indivisible unity of the personality.

We entertain the highest respect and admiration for our predecessors and regard our own achievements only as the development into a science of their brilliant intuitions. At the same time we may modestly lay claim to the formulation of fundamental principles which have hitherto never found expression in psychological literature.

This by no means implies that we do not envisage the further progress of our science. We are concerned at present to establish convincing proofs of the unity of the personality on evidence which will leave no room for doubt. We also succeed more quickly in tracing the strangest aberrations of the human mind to the sense of some personal peculiarity which gives rise to a failure to cope with reality. The Unconscious of the text-books, in which current attempts to elucidate its meaning have already distinguished several levels, each able to serve as an *asylum ignorantiae*, resolves itself for us chiefly into the patient's failure to understand his impulses in relation to his social environment. In consonance with our earliest conclusions, dreams are seen with increasing clearness to be a preparation for confronting some problem which has presented itself, in accordance with the desire for superiority, and by means of an analogy. As one of the most important safeguards we have the *elimination* of the customary modes of life, whereby neurotic or perverse behaviour is rendered possible. This shows the worthlessness of pleasure and pain as causes and justification for unsocial behaviour. They can always be modified and take the form of further safeguards when once a wrong course is to be adopted. The effects of suggestion and auto-suggestion are revealed ever more clearly as partial phenomena which can never be rationally explained except in relation to a total setting.

Our contention, too, that all forms of neurosis and developmental failure are expressions of inferiority and disappointment rests on a firm basis. And if success in treating these maladies—even in their gravest forms—is a criterion, then its practical application has shown that Individual psychology comes well out of the test. To encourage the student I would further add that we Individual psychologists are in a position, if a proper procedure is observed, to get a clear conception of the fundamental psychic error of the patient at the first consultation. And the way to a cure is thus opened.

ALFRED ADLER.

VIENNA, 23rd October 1923.

CONTENTS

vii

INDIVIDUAL PSYCHOLOGY

THE PRACTICE AND THEORY OF INDIVIDUAL PSYCHOLOGY

I

Individual Psychology, its Assumptions and its Results

(1914)

A SURVEY of the views and theories of most psychologists indicates a peculiar limitation both in the nature of their field of investigation and in their methods of inquiry. They act as if experience and knowledge of mankind were, with conscious intent, to be excluded from our investigations and all value and importance denied to artistic and creative vision as well as to intuition itself. While the experimental psychologists collect and devise phenomena in order to determine types of reaction—that is, are concerned with the physiology of the psychical life properly speaking — other psychologists arrange all forms of expression and manifestations in old customary, or at best slightly altered, systems. By this procedure they naturally rediscover the interdependence and connection in individual expressions, implied from the very beginning in their schematic attitude toward the psyche.

Either the foregoing method is employed or an attempt is made by means of small, if possible measurable individual phenomena of a physiological nature, to construct psychical states and thought by means of an equation. The fact that all subjective thinking and subjective immersion on the part of the investigator are excluded—although in reality they dominate the very nature of these connections—is from this viewpoint regarded as an advantage.

The method employed, and the very importance it seems to possess as a preparation for the human mind, reminds us of the type of natural science completely

1

antiquated to-day, with its rigid systems, replaced everywhere now by views that attempt to grasp living phenomena and their variations as connected wholes, biologically, philosophically, and psychologically. This is also the purpose of that movement in psychology that I have called "*comparative individual-psychology*". By starting with the assumption of the *unity of the individual*, an attempt is made to obtain a picture of this unified personality regarded as a variant of individual life-manifestations and forms of expression. The individual traits are then compared with one another, brought into a common plane, and finally fused together to form a composite portrait that is, in turn, individualized.[1]

It may have been noticed that this method of looking upon man's psychic life is by no means either unusual or even particularly daring. This type of approach is particularly noticeable in the study of child-psychology, in spite of other lines of inquiry also used there. It is the essence and the nature above all of the work of the artist, be he painter, sculptor, musician, or particularly poet, so to present the minute traits of his creations that the observer is able to obtain from them the general principles of personality. He is thus in a position to reconstruct those very things that the artist when thinking of his *finale* had previously hidden therein. Since life in any given society, life without any of the preconceptions of science, has always been under the ban of the question "whither?", we are warranted in definitely stating that, scientific views to the contrary notwithstanding, no man has ever made a judgment about an event without endeavouring to strain toward the point which seems to bind together all the psychic manifestations of an individual; even to an *imagined goal* if necessary.

When I hurry home, I am certain to exhibit to any observer the carriage, expression, the gait, and the gestures that are to be expected of a person returning home. My reflexes indeed might be different from those anticipated, the causes might vary. The essential point to be grasped psychologically and the one which interests us exclusively and practically and psychologically more than all others, *is the path followed*.

[1] William Stern has come to the same conclusions starting from a different method of approach.

Let me observe that if I know the goal of a person I know in a general way what will happen. I am in a position to bring into their proper order each of the successive movements made, to view them in their connections, to correct them and to make, where necessary, the required adaptations for my approximate psychological knowledge of these associations. If I am acquainted only with the causes, know only the reflexes, the reaction-times, the ability to repeat and such facts, I am aware of nothing that actually takes place in the soul of the man.

We must remember that the person under observation would not know what to do with himself were he not orientated toward some goal. As long as we are not acquainted with the objective which determines his "life-line", the whole system of his recognized reflexes, together with all their causal conditions, can give us no certainty as to his next series of movements. They might be brought into harmony with practically any psychic resultant. This deficiency is most clearly felt in association-tests. I would never expect a man suffering from some great disappointment to associate "tree" with "rope". The moment I knew his objective, however, namely suicide, then I might very well expect that particular sequence of thoughts—expect it with such certainty that I would remove knives, poison, and weapons from his immediate vicinity.

If we look at the matter more closely, we shall find the following law holding in the development of all psychic happenings: *we cannot think, feel, will, or act without the perception of some goal.* For all the causalities in the world would not suffice to conquer the chaos of the future nor obviate the planlessness to which we would be bound to fall a victim. All activity would persist in the stage of uncontrolled gropings; the economy visible in our psychic life unattained; we should be unintegrated and in every aspect of our physiognomy, in every personal touch, similar to organisms of the rank of the amœba.

No one will deny that by assuming an objective for our psychic life we accommodate ourselves better to reality. This can be easily demonstrated. For its truth in individual examples, where phenomena are torn from their proper connections, no doubt exists. Only watch, from this point of view, the attempts at walking made by a small child or a woman recovering from a confinement. Naturally he who approaches this whole matter without any theory is likely to find its deeper significance escape him. Yet it is a fact that before the first step has been taken the objective of the person's movement has already been determined.

In the same way it can be demonstrated that all psychic activities are given a direction by means of a previously determined goal. All the temporary and partially visible objectives, after the short period of psychic development of childhood, are under the domination of an imagined terminal goal, of a final point felt and conceived of as definitely fixed. In other words the psychic life of man is made to fit into the fifth act like a character drawn by a good dramatist.

The conclusion thus to be drawn from the unbiased study of any personality viewed from the standpoint of individual-psychology leads us to the following important proposition : *every psychic phenomenon, if it is to give us any understanding of a person, can only be grasped and understood if regarded as a preparation for some goal.*

To what an extent this conception promotes our psychological understanding, is clearly apparent as soon as we become aware of the *multiplicity of meaning of those psychical processes that have been torn from their proper context.* Take for example the case of a man with a " bad memory ". Assume that he is quite conscious of this fact and that an examination discloses an inferior capacity for the repetition of meaningless syllables. According to present usage in psychology, which we might more properly call an abuse, we would have to make the following inference : the man is suffering, from hereditary or pathological causes, from a deficient capacity for repetition. Incidentally, let me add, that in this type of investigation we generally find the inference already stated in different words in the premises. In this case *e.g.* we have the following proposition : if a man has a bad memory, or if he only remembers a few words—then he has an inferior capacity for repetition.

The procedure in individual - psychology is completely different. After excluding the possibility of all organic causes, we would ask ourselves what is the objective of this weakness of memory? This we could only determine if we were in possession of an intimate knowledge of the whole individual, so that an understanding of one part becomes possible only after we have understood the whole. And we should probably find the following to hold true in a large number of cases: this man is attempting to prove to himself and to others that for certain reasons of a fundamental nature, that are either not to be named or have remained unconscious, *but which can most effectively be represented by poorness of memory*, he must not permit himself to perform some particular act or to come to a given decision (change of profession, studies, examination, marriage). We should then have unmasked this weakness of memory as tendencious and could understand its importance as a weapon against a contemplated undertaking. In every test of ability to repeat we should then expect to find the deficiency due to the secret life-plan of an individual. The question then to be asked is how such deficiencies or evils arise. They may be simply " arranged " by purposely underlining general physiological weaknesses and interpreting them as personal sufferings. Others may succeed either by subjective absorption into an abnormal condition or by pre-occupation with dangerous pessimistic anticipations, in so weakening their faith in their own capacities, that their strength, attention or will-power are only partially at their disposal.

A similar observation may be made in the case of affects. To give one more example, take the case of a woman subject to outbreaks of anxiety recurring at certain intervals. As long as nothing of greater significance than this was discernible, the assumption of some hereditary degeneration, some disease of the vaso-motor system, of the vagus nerve, etc., sufficed. It is also possible that we might have regarded ourselves as having arrived at a fuller understanding of the case, if we had discovered in the previous history of the patient, some frightful experience, or traumatic condition and attributed the disease to it. As soon, however, as we examined the personality of this individual and inquired into her directive-lines we discovered an excess of will-to-power, with which anxiety as a weapon of aggression had associated itself, an anxiety which was to become operative as soon as the force of the will-power had abated and the desired resonance was absent, a situation occurring, for example, when the patient's husband left the house without her consent.

Our science demands a markedly individualizing procedure and is consequently not much given to generalizations. For general guidance I would like to propound the following rule: *as soon as the goal of a psychic movement or its life-plan has been recognized, then we are to assume that all the movements of its constituent parts will coincide with both the goal and the life-plan.*

This formulation, with some minor provisos, is to be maintained in the widest sense. It retains its value even if inverted : *the properly understood part-movements must when combined, give the picture of an integrated life-plan and final goal.* Consequently we insist that, without worrying about the *tendencies, milieu and experiences,* all psychical powers are under the control of a directive idea and all expressions of emotion, feeling, thinking, willing, acting, dreaming as well as psycho-pathological phenomena, are permeated by one unified life-plan. Let me, by a slight suggestion, prove and yet soften down these heretical propositions : more important than tendencies, objective experience and milieu is *the subjective evaluation,* an evaluation which stands furthermore in a certain, often strange, relation to realities. Out of this evaluation however, which generally results in the development of a permanent mood *of the nature of a feeling of inferiority* there arises, depending upon the unconscious technique of our thought-apparatus, an imagined goal, an attempt at a planned final compensation and a life-plan.

I have so far spoken a good deal of men who have "grasped the situation". My discussion has been as irritating as that of the theorists of the "psychology of understanding" or of the psychology of personality, who always break off just when they are about to show us what exactly it is they have understood, as for instance, Jaspers. The danger of discussing briefly this aspect of our investigations namely, *the results of individual-psychology,* is sufficiently great. To do so we should be compelled to force the dynamics of life into static words and pictures, overlook differences in order to obtain unified formulas, and have, in short, in our description

to make that very mistake that in practice is strictly pro-
hibited : of approaching the psychic life of the individual
with a dry formula, as the Freudian school attempt.

This then being my assumption, I shall in the following present to you the most important results of our
study of psychic life. Let me emphasize the fact that
the dynamics of psychic life that I am about to describe
hold equally for healthy and diseased. What distinguishes the nervous from the healthy individual is
the stronger safeguarding tendency with which the
former's life - plan is filled. With regard to the
"positing of a goal" and the life-plan adjusted to
it there are no fundamental differences.

I shall consequently speak of a general goal of man.
A thorough-going study has taught us that we can
best understand the manifold and diverse movements
of the psyche as soon as our *most general pre-supposition*,
that the psyche has as its objective the *goal of superiority*,
is recognized. Great thinkers have given expression to
much of this ; in part everyone knows it, but in the
main it is hidden in mysterious darkness and comes
definitely to the front only in insanity or in ecstatic
conditions. Whether a person desires to be an artist,
the first in his profession, or a tyrant in his home, to
hold converse with God or humiliate other people ;
whether he regards his suffering as the most important
thing in the world to which everyone must show
obeisance, whether he is chasing after unattainable
ideals or old deities, over-stepping all limits and norms,
at every part of his way he is guided and spurred on
by his longing for superiority, the thought of his
godlikeness, the belief in his special magical power.
In his love he desires to experience his power over his
partner. In his purely optional choice of profession the
goal floating before his mind manifests itself in all sorts
of exaggerated anticipations and fears, and thirsting
for revenge, he experiences in suicide a triumph over
all obstacles. In order to gain control over an object
or over a person, he is capable of proceeding along a
straight line, bravely, proudly, overbearing, obstinate,
cruel ; or he may on the other hand prefer, forced by
experience, to resort to by-paths and circuitous routes, to
gain his victory by obedience, submission, mildness and
modesty. Nor have traits of character an independent

existence, for they are also adjusted to the individual life-plan, really representing the most important preparations for conflict possessed by the latter.

This goal of complete superiority, with its strange appearance at times, does not come from the world of reality. Inherently we must place it under "fictions" and "imaginations". Of these Vaihinger (*The Philosophy of 'As If'*) rightly says that their importance lies in the fact that whereas in themselves without meaning, they nevertheless possess in practice the greatest importance. For our case this coincides to such an extent that we may say *that this fiction of a goal of superiority so ridiculous from the view-point of reality, has become the principal conditioning factor of our life as hitherto known.* It is this that teaches us to differentiate, gives us poise and security, moulds and guides our deeds and activities and forces our spirit to look ahead and to perfect itself. There is of course also an obverse side, for *this goal introduces into our life a hostile and fighting tendency,* robs us of the simplicity of our feelings and is always the cause for an estrangement from reality since it puts near to our hearts the idea of attempting to over-power reality. Whoever takes this goal of godlikeness seriously or literally, will soon be compelled to flee from real life and compromise, by seeking a life within life ; if fortunate in art, but more generally in pietism, neurosis or crime.[1]

I cannot give you particulars here. A clear indication of this super-mundane goal is to be found in every individual. Sometimes this is to be gathered from a man's carriage, sometimes it is disclosed only in his demands and expectations. Occasionally one comes upon its track in obscure memories, phantasies and dreams. If purposely sought it is rarely obtained. However, every bodily or mental attitude indicates clearly its origin in a striving for power and carries within itself the ideal of a kind of perfection and infallibility. In those cases that lie on the confines of neurosis there is always to be discovered a reinforced pitting of oneself against the environment, against the dead or heroes of the past.

A test of the correctness of our interpretation can be easily made. If everyone possesses within himself an ideal of superiority, such as we find to an exaggerated

[1] *Cf.* also "The Problem of Distance", in this volume.

degree among the nervous, then we ought to encounter phenomena whose purpose is the oppression, the minimizing and undervaluation of others. Traits of character such as intolerance, dogmatism, envy, pleasure at the misfortune of others, conceit, boastfulness, mistrust, avarice,—in short all those attitudes that are the substitutes for a struggle, force their way through to a far greater extent, in fact, than self-preservation demands.

Similarly, either simultaneously or interchangingly, depending upon the zeal and the self-confidence with which the final goal is sought, we see emerging indications of pride, emulation, courage, the attitudes of saving, bestowing and directing. A psychological investigation demands so much objectivity that a moral evaluation will not disturb the survey. In fact *the different levels of character-traits* actually neutralize our good-will and our disapproval. Finally we must remember that these hostile traits, particularly in the case of the nervous, are often so concealed that their possessor is justifiably astonished and irritated when attention is drawn to them. For example, the elder of two children can create quite an uncomfortable situation in trying to arrogate to himself through defiance and obstinacy, all authority in the family. The younger child pursues a wiser course, poses as a model of obedience and succeeds in this manner in becoming the idol of the family and in having all wishes gratified. As ambition spurs him on, all willingness to obey becomes destroyed and pathological-compulsion phenomena develop, by means of which every parental order is nullified even when the parents notice that the child is making efforts to remain obedient. Thus we have an act of obedience immediately nullified by means of a compulsion-thought. We get an idea of the circuitous path taken here in order to arrive at the same objective as that of the other child.

The whole weight of the personal striving for power and superiority passes, at a very early age in the case of the child, into the form and the content of its striving, its thought being able to absorb for the time being only so much as the eternal, real and physiologically rooted *community-feeling* permits. Out of the latter are developed tenderness, love of neighbour, friendship and love, the desire for power unfolding itself in a veiled manner and seeking secretly to push its way along the path of group consciousness.

At this place let me go out of my way to endorse an old fundamental conception of all who know human nature. Every marked attitude of a man can be traced back to an origin in childhood. In the nursery are formed and prepared all of man's future attitudes. Fundamental changes are produced only by means of an exceedingly high degree of introspection or among neurotics by means of the physician's individual psychological analysis.

Let me, on the basis of another case, one which must have happened innumerable times, discuss in even greater detail the positing of goals by nervous people. A remarkably gifted man who by his amiability and refined behaviour had gained the love of a girl of high character, became engaged to her. He then forced upon her his ideal of education which made severe demands upon her. For a time she endured these unbearable orders but finally put an end to all further ordeals by breaking off relations. The man then broke down and became a prey to nervous attacks. The individual-psychological examination of the case showed that the superiority-goal in the case of this patient—as his domineering demands upon his bride indicated— had long ago pushed from his mind all thought of marriage, and that his object really was to secretly work toward a break, secretly because he did not feel himself equal to the open struggle in which he imagined marriage to consist. *This disbelief in himself* itself dated from his earliest childhood, to a time during which he, an only son, lived with an early widowed mother somewhat cut off from the world. During this period, spent in continuous family quarrels he had received the ineradicable impression, one he had never openly admitted to himself, that he was not sufficiently virile, and would never be able to cope with a woman. These psychical attitudes are comparable to a permanent inferiority-feeling and it is easily understood how they had decisively interfered in his life and compelled him to obtain prestige along other lines than those obtainable through the fulfilment of the demands of reality.

It is clear that the patient attained just what his concealed preparations for bachelordom aimed at, and what his fear of a life-partner, with the quarrels and restless relationship this implied, had awakened in him. Nor can it be denied that he took the same attitude toward both his bride and his mother, namely the wish to conquer. This attitude induced by a longing for victory has been magnificently misinterpreted by the Freudian school as the permanently incestuous condition of being enamoured of the mother. As a matter of fact this reinforced childhood-feeling of inferiority occasioned by the patient's painful relation to his mother, spurred this man on to prevent any struggle in later life with a wife by providing himself with all kinds of safeguards. Whatever it is we understand by love, in this particular case it is simply *a means to an end* and that end is the final securing of a triumph over some suitable woman. Here we have the reason for the continual tests and orders and for the cancelling of the engagement. This solution had not just "happened", but had on the contrary been artistically prepared and arranged with the old weapons of experience employed previously in the case of his mother. A defeat in marriage was out of the question because marriage was prevented.

Although we consequently realize nothing puzzling in the behaviour of this man and should recognize in his domineering attitude simply aggression *posing as love*, some words of explanation are necessary to clear up the less intelligible nervous break-down. We are here entering upon the real domain of the psychology of neuroses. As in the nursery so here our patient has been worsted by a woman. The neurotic individual is led in such cases to strengthen his protections and to retire to a fairly great distance from danger.[1] Our patient is utilizing his break-down in order to feed an evil reminiscence, to bring up the question of guilt again, to solve it in an unfavourable sense for the woman, so that in future he may either proceed with even greater caution or take final leave of love and matrimony! This man is thirty years old now. Let us assume that he is going to carry his pain along with him for another ten or twenty years and that he is going to mourn for his lost ideal for the same length of time. He has thereby protected himself against every love-affair and permanently saved himself from new defeat.

[1] Cf. "The Problem of Distance" in this volume.

He interprets his nervous break-down by means of old, now strengthened, weapons of experience, just as he had as a child refused to eat, sleep or to do anything and played the rôle of a dying person. His fortunes ebb and *his beloved carries all the stigma*, he himself rises superior to her in both culture and character, and lo and behold : he has attained that for which he longed, for he is the superior person, becomes the better man and his partner like all girls is the guilty one. Girls cannot cope with the man in him. In this manner he has consummated what as a child he had already felt, the duty of demonstrating his superiority over the female sex.

We can now understand that this nervous reaction can never be sufficiently definite or adequate. *He is to wander through the world as a living reproach against women.*[1]

Were he aware of his secret plans he would realize how ill-natured and evil-intentioned all his actions have been. However he would, in that case, not succeed in attaining his object of elevating himself above women. He would see himself just as we see him, falsifying the weights and how everything he has done has only led to a goal previously set. His success could not be described as due to "fate" nor assuredly would it represent any increased prestige. But his goal, his life-plan and his life-falsehood demand this prestige ! In consequence it so "happens" that the *life-plan remains in the unconscious*, so that the patient may believe that an *implacable fate* and not a long prepared and long meditated plan for which he alone is responsible, is at work.

I cannot go into a detailed description of what I call the "distance" that the neurotic individual places between himself and the final issue, which in this case is marriage. The discussion of the manner in which he accomplishes it I must also postpone to my chapter on nervous "arrangements". I should like to point out here however that the "distance" expresses itself clearly in the "hesitating attitudes," the principles, the point of view and the life-falsehood. In its evolution neurosis and psychosis play leading rôles. The appro-

---

[1] The paranoidal trait is recognizable. Cf. "Life-lie and Responsibility in Neurosis and Psychosis ", in this volume.

priation for this purpose of perversions and every type of impotence arising from the latter is quite frequent. Such a man concludes his account and reconciles himself with life by constructing one or a number of "if-clauses". "If conditions had been different. . . ."

The importance of the educational questions that arise and upon which our school lays the greatest stress (*Heilen und Bilden*, Munich, 1913) follows from what has been discussed.

From the method of presentation of the present work it is to be inferred that as in the case of a psycho-therapeutic cure, our analysis proceeds backwards ; examining first the *superiority-goal*, explaining by means of it the type of *conflict-attitude*[1] adopted particularly by nervous patients and only then attempting to investigate the sources of the vital psychic mechanism. One of the bases of the psychical dynamics we have already mentioned, the presumably unavoidable artistic trait of the psychical apparatus which, by means of the *artistic artifice of the creation of a fiction and the setting of a goal*, adjusts itself to and extends itself into the world of possible reality. I shall now proceed to explain briefly how the goal of godlikeness transforms the relation of the individual to his environment into hostility and how the struggle drives an individual towards a goal either along a direct path such as aggressiveness or along by-ways suggested by precaution. If we trace the history of this aggressive attitude back to childhood we always come upon the outstanding fact that *throughout the whole period of development, the child possesses a feeling of inferiority in its relations both to parents and the world at large*. Because of the immaturity of his organs, his uncertainty and lack of independence, because of his need for dependence upon stronger natures and his frequent and painful feeling of subordination to others, a sensation of inadequacy develops that betrays itself throughout life. This feeling of inferiority is the cause of his continual restlessness as a child, his craving for action, his playing of rôles, the pitting of his strength against that of others, his anticipatory pictures of the future and his physical as well as mental preparations. The whole potential educability of the child depends

[1] The "struggle for existence", the "struggle of all against all", etc., are merely other perspectives of the same kind.

upon this feeling of insufficiency. In this way the future becomes transformed into the land that will bring him compensations. His conflict - attitude is again reflected in his feeling of inferiority ; and only conflict does he regard as a compensation which will do away permanently with his present inadequate condition and will enable him to picture himself as elevated above others. Thus the child arrives at the positing of a goal, an imagined goal of superiority, whereby his poverty is transformed into wealth, his subordination into domination, his suffering into happiness and pleasure, his ignorance into omniscience and his incapacity into artistic creation. The longer and more definitely the child feels his insecurity, the more he suffers either from physical or marked mental weakness, the more he is aware of life's neglect, the higher will this goal be placed and the more faithfully will it be adhered to. He who wishes to recognize the nature of this goal, should watch a child at play, at optionally selected occupations or when phantasying about his future profession. The apparent change in these phenomena is purely external for in every new goal the child imagines a predetermined triumph. A variant of this weaving of plans, one frequently found among weakly aggressive children, among girls and sickly individuals, might be mentioned here. This consists of so misusing their frailties that they compel others to become subordinate to them. They will later on pursue the same method until their life-plan and life-falsehood have been clearly unmasked.

The attentive observer will find the nature of the *compensatory dynamics* presenting a quite extraordinary aspect as soon as he permits the sexual rôle to be relegated to one of minor importance and realizes that it is the former that is impelling the individual toward superhuman goals. In our present civilization both the girl and the youth will feel themselves forced to extraordinary exertions and manoeuvres. A large number of these are admittedly of a distinctively progressive nature. To preserve this progressive nature but to ferret out those by-paths that lead us astray and cause illness, to make these harmless, that is our object and one that takes us far beyond the limits of medical art. It is to this aspect of our subject that society, child-

education and folk-education may look for germs of a
far-reaching kind. *For the aim of this point-of-view
is to gain a reinforced sense of reality, the development
of a feeling of responsibility and a substitution for latent
hatred of a feeling of mutual goodwill, all of which
can be gained only by the conscious evolution of a feeling
for the common weal and the conscious destruction of the
will-to-power.*

He who is looking for the power-phantasies of the
child will find them drawn with a master hand by
Dostoevsky in his novel entitled *A Raw Youth*.
I found them blatantly apparent in one of my patients.
In the dreams and thoughts of this individual the following wish recurred repeatedly : others should die so that
he might have enough room in which to live, others
should suffer privations so that he might obtain more
favourable opportunities. This attitude reminds one of
the inconsiderateness and heartlessness of many men
who trace all evil back to the fact that there are already
too many people in the world ; impulses that have
unquestionably made the world-war more palatable.
The feeling of certainty, in fictions of this kind, has
been taken over in the above-mentioned case from the
basic facts of capitalistic trade, where admittedly, the
better the condition of one individual the worse that
of another. "I want to be a grave-digger", said a
four-year-old boy to me ; "I want to be the person
who digs graves for others".

II

Psychical Hermaphrodism and the Masculine Protest—
The Cardinal Problem of Nervous Diseases

(1912)

A TREMENDOUS step in the direction of progress was taken when, in our doctrines concerning nervous diseases, that view-point came to the front which regarded all nervous disturbances as due to changes in the psyche, these to be treated by influences brought to bear upon the psyche itself. The issue was brought to a definite focus by the interposition of competent scientists like Struempel, Moebius and others. We must likewise add the experiences of the French in the domain of hypnotic experiment and hypnotic therapeutics, which proved the transformability of nervous symptoms and the possibility of influencing them by an approach through the psyche. In spite of the progress made, however, cures remained uncertain so that even well-known scientists, uninfluenced by theoretical considerations, continued to treat neurasthenia, hysteria, compulsion- and anxiety-neuroses by means of the old medicines and by the application of electricity and hydrotherapy. All that was gained by our increased knowledge consisted for many years in a heaping up of catch-words supposed to unlock and exhaust the meaning and the nature of complicated neurotic mechanisms. For some the key lay in "irritable weakness", for others, in "suggestibility", "shock", "hereditary stigma", "degeneration", "pathological reaction", "lability of psychical equilibrium", and other conceptions of the same type which were supposed to constitute the secret of nervous diseases. The gain that accrued to the patient was in the main merely an arid suggestion-therapy, fruitless attempts to dislodge from the patient's mind the idea of disease and the even more fruitless attempt to keep psychical injuries permanently away. Yet this therapeutic procedure did frequently develop into a useful "traitement moral", whenever the patient happened to be under the care of physicians with a knowledge of the world or gifted with intuition. Among laymen, however, there grew up a prejudice against this treatment, augmented by premature conclusions and the observation that accidental neuroses were increasing rapidly, thus giving the impression that the nervous individual was suffering from "auto-suggestions" and guilty of conscious exaggerations, as if it were possible for him by strengthening his energy, to overcome the symptoms of his illness.

Eventually Josef Breuer hit upon the idea of questioning the patient, first in the case of hysterical paralysis, concerning the meaning and development of his own disease. He, and Freud, used this method without any preconceptions and confirmed the outstanding presence of memory-lacunae preventing both the patient and the physician from obtaining a real insight into the causes and the history of the disease. The attempts to formulate inferences with regard to the forgotten material from the knowledge of the psyche, the pathological traits of character, the phantasies and the dream-life of the patient, were successful and led to the creation of the *psycho-analytical method and view-point*. Thanks to this method Freud was able to trace back to earliest childhood the roots of nervous diseases and to disclose a number of psychical phenomena, such as *repression* and *transference*. During treatment, formerly unconscious stirrings and desires of the patient were repeatedly brought to the surface by different investigators who, in identical ways and for the most manifold forms of nervousness, made use of the psycho-analytic method, frequently working quite independently of one another. Freud himself looked for the cause of nervous disease in the transformations and the specific constitution of the sexual instinct, a theory that has been frequently attacked and one which is not inseparably connected with the psychological method.

As the basic principle for the practice of the *individual-psychological method* I would like to emphasize the following: *the retracing of all the nervous symptoms occurring in an individual case back to their "lowest common denominator"*. That this reduction, made with the aid of the patient is correct, is proved by the fact

B

that the psychical picture gained in each case coincides with a real psychical situation that can be traced back to the patient's earliest childhood. In other words the psychic foundations of neurotic disease and its symptoms have been taken over unchanged from childhood. Upon this foundation, however, has been erected in the course of years, a widely ramifying super-structure, the individual neurosis, which is not amenable to treatment unless the basis itself is changed. Into this superstructure have been absorbed all the developmental tendencies, character-traits and personal experiences. Among these I would particularly like to emphasize the mood-residues which go back to a single or a repeated failure along the main line of human endeavour. This is the actual cause for the appearance of the neurotic disease. From that moment on, all the thoughts of the patient are centred upon the idea of making good his failure, of running greedily after useless triumphs and above all, of protecting himself against new failures and the trials of fortune. His manifesting neurosis, assuming the nature of a means of support, makes this possible. Nervous anxiety, pains, paralyses and nervous doubts prevent him from participating actively in life. In exchange the nervous compulsion bestows upon him, in his compulsion-thinking and his compulsion-acting, the semblance of his lost activity, giving him thus as his excuse for remaining passive, a legitimate disease.

I found myself compelled in the exercise of the individual - psychological method, to break up still further this infantile situation of pretending to be ill. In so doing I came upon sources arising out of the injurious influences of family life. Beyond that however a cause cropped up that helped in part to form this detrimental milieu, namely the *familial organic constitution*. Regularly and inexorably was it forced upon my attention that the possession of inherited inferior organs, organic systems and glands with internal secretions, created a situation, in the early stages of a child's development, *whereby a normal feeling of weakness and helplessness had been enormously intensified and had grown into a deeply-felt sense of inferiority*.[1] On account of the delayed and defective as well as inadequate

---

[1] S. Adler, *Studie über Minderwertigkeit der Organe* (1907), and its continuation : Adler, " Ueber neurotisch Disposition ", in *Heilen und Bilden*.

constitution of organic inferiority, conditions of the following nature were initially visible : weakness, sickliness, awkwardness, ugliness, (often caused by external degenerative symptoms), clumsiness and a large number of infantile defects, such as twitching of the eyes, cross-eyedness, left-handedness, deaf-and-dumbness, stuttering, speech defects, vomiting, bed-wetting and stool-anomalies for which the child was frequently subjected to humiliation, or made the object of ridicule, for which he was often punished and which rendered him socially unfit. The infantile psychic picture often shows striking intensification of traits otherwise normal, such as infantile helplessness, the need for cuddling, for tenderness ; and these then develop into anxiety, fear of being alone, timidity, shyness, fear of strangers and unknown people, hyper - sensitiveness to pain, prudishness, permanent fear of punishment and fear of the consequences of every act—in short into characteristics that impart *unmistakable feminine traits* to the boy.

It is not long before this *feeling of being pushed aside* comes to the front, markedly so in those children disposed to neurosis. Together with it there develops a *hyper-sensitiveness* which repeatedly disturbs the peaceful and even flow of the psyche. Children of this type desire to possess, eat, hear, see and know everything. They wish to surpass all others and accomplish everything alone. Their phantasy plays with all kinds of ideas of greatness. They wish to save other people, picture themselves as heroes, believe in an aristocratic origin and regard themselves as persecuted and hard-pressed, like Cinderella. The basis for a burning, insatiable ambition whose frustration can be foretold with certainty, has been laid. It is at this time that the evil instincts also develop and become strengthened. *Avarice* and *envy* grow to boundless limits *because the child is not able to wait for the gratification of his wishes. Greedily and restlessly* he chases after every triumph, becomes unteachable, irascible, despotic toward younger people, lies to his elders and watches everyone with tenacious mistrust. It is clear to what an extent a good teacher can improve such a developing egoism and a bad teacher aggravate it. Under favourable circumstances an unquenchable thirst for knowledge may arise or that hot-house growth, the precocious child. Under unfavourable conditions there grow up either criminal tendencies or the picture of an exhausted man trying to cover up his flight from the demands of life by a prepared neurosis.

The following is the final conclusion to be drawn from direct observations of the child's life : The infantile traits of submissiveness, lack of independence and obedience, in short, the passivity of the child are very soon and, in the case of individuals with neurotic disposition very abruptly, displaced by hidden traits of defiance and rebellion, *i.e.* by signs of resentment. An accurate insight discloses *a mixture of passive and active characteristics although there is always present likewise a tendency for a girlish kind of obedience to change into a boyish kind of defiance.* There are indeed sufficient reasons for coming to the belief that these traits of defiance are to be interpreted as a reaction, a protest against the synchronous stirrings of obedience or against an enforced submission ; that furthermore their purpose consists in obtaining for the child a more speedy gratification of his instincts, importance, attention and privileges. When the child has reached this fatal point in his development he feels himself threatened by an enforced submission and consequently obstructs all the arrangements of its everyday life—eating, drinking, falling asleep, washing, stool and urinary functions. The demands of the community-feeling are strangled. The craving for power expresses itself, in the main, in an arid inadequate sham-fight and an imaginary prestige.

Another, perhaps the most dangerous type of neurotically-disposed child, exhibits these contrasting tendencies of submissiveness and active protest wrought together into a closer union resembling that subsisting between means and end. These children have apparently guessed at a little of the dialectic of life and *wish to gratify their unlimited desires by the most complete kind of submission* (*masochism*). They are just the people who can least stand undervaluation, lack of success, compulsion, waiting, the delay in victory and they, just as those with different dispositions, are thoroughly frightened by actions, decisions, anything strange or new. They develop an alibi for the fatal weakness of which they are conscious, in order thereafter to avoid the demands of the community and to isolate themselves.

This apparent double-life, which in the case of normal children remains within definite limits, and which enters into the formation of the character of mature individuals, *does not permit the nervous person a single-minded pursuit of his goal and checks him in his decisions by means of constructions of his own making, anxiety and doubt.*

Other types take refuge from anxiety and doubt in a *compulsion* and unceasingly continue their pursuit of success. They are always suspecting attacks, belittlement, injustice; trying desperately to play the rôle of a saviour and hero, not infrequently exerting their powers upon unsuitable objects. (Don Quixotism.) Insatiable and lusting after the semblance of power, they demand proofs of love without ever feeling satisfied. (Don Juan, Messalina.) They never attain to any harmony in their strivings, for the twofold nature of their being, *the apparent double-life of the neurotic (" double vie ", "dissociation", "split-personality", of many authors), is definitely grounded in the fact that the psyche partakes of both feminine and masculine traits. Both appear to strive for unity* but purposely fail in their synthesis in order to rescue the personality from colliding with reality. It is at this point that individual-psychology can intervene to some purpose, and by means of an intensified introspection and an extension of consciousness, secure the domination of the intellect over divergent and hitherto unconscious stirrings.

The deep-rooted feeling that permeates the folk-soul and which has always awakened the interest of poets and thinkers, that evaluation and symbolizing of types of phenomena as " masculine " and " feminine ",[1] although seemingly arbitrary and yet coinciding with our social life, impresses itself early upon the infant mind. Thus the child, with occasional variations, regards the following as masculine: strength, greatness, riches, knowledge, victory, coarseness, cruelty, violence and activity as such, their opposites being feminine.

The normal craving of the child for nestling, the exaggerated submissiveness of the neurotically-disposed individual, the feeling of weakness, of inferiority pro-

---

[1] We have but to call to mind such proverbs as: "A man's word is his bond", expressions of poets (Schiller's " Dignity of Man "—"Frailty, thy name is woman ! ") or gifted writers like Moebius, Flies, Weininger, etc.

tected by hyper-sensitiveness, the realization of actual futility, the sense of being permanently pushed aside and of being at a disadvantage, all these are gathered together into a feeling of femininity. On the contrary, active strivings, both in the case of a girl as of a boy, the pursuit of self-gratification, the stirring up of instincts and passions are thrown challengingly forward as a masculine protest. On the basis of a false evaluation, but one which is extensively nourished by our social life, there thus develops *a psychical herma-phrodism of the child, "logically" dependent upon its inward opposition. From within itself is then unfolded that frequently unconscious urge toward a reinforced masculine protest which is to represent the solution for the disharmony.*

The unavoidable acquaintance with the sexual pro-blem intensifies, first and foremost, the masculine protest, feeds the disharmonic complex with sexual phantasies and sexual stirrings, leads to early sexual maturity and may, through mistakes, be the occasion for all perversions. If the rôle of sex either remains or is kept unclear to the child, the psychical herma-phrodism is deepened, thereby increasing the inward psychical tension.[1]

The natural uncertainty, the vacillation and doubt, become fixed and reinforcements are carried to both poles of the hermaphrodite nature. The difficulty of mastering this increased split in consciousness, is thus tremendously augmented and this mastery is only attained by the manœuvre of resorting to nervous symptoms, by psychic retreat and by isolation. The energy and effort of will of the physician, the patient, and the educator, founder on this problem. It is only the individual-psychological method that can then throw light upon these phenomena of the unconscious and that can attempt to correct a false development.

---

[1] Adler, "Der psychische Hermaphroditismus im Leben u. in der Neurose", in *Heilen und Bilden*, and *Problem der Homosexualität*, 2nd edition.

III

New Leading Principles for the Practice of Individual-Psychology

(1913)

I. EVERY neurosis can be understood as an attempt to free oneself from a feeling of inferiority in order to gain a feeling of superiority.

II. The path of the neurosis does not lead in the direction of social functioning, nor does it aim at solving given life-problems but finds an outlet for itself in the small family circle, thus achieving the isolation of the patient.

III. The larger unit of the social group is either completely or very extensively pushed aside by a mechanism consisting of hyper-sensitiveness and in-tolerance. Only a small group is left over for the manœuvres aiming at the various types of superiority to expend themselves upon. At the same time pro-tection and the withdrawal from the demands of the community and the decisions of life are made possible.

IV. Thus estranged from reality, the neurotic man lives a life of imagination and phantasy and employs a number of devices for enabling him to side-step the demands of reality and for reaching out toward an ideal situation which would free him from any service for the community and absolve him from responsibility.

V. These exemptions and the privileges of illness and suffering give him a substitute for his original hazardous goal of superiority.

VI. Thus the neurosis and the psyche represent an attempt to free oneself from all the constraints of the community by establishing a counter-compulsion. This latter is so constituted that it effectively faces the peculiar nature of the surroundings and their demands.

Both of these convincing inferences can be drawn from the manner in which this counter-compulsion manifests itself and from the neuroses selected.

VII. The counter-compulsion takes on the nature of a revolt, gathers its material either from favourable affective experiences or from observations. It permits thoughts and affects to become preoccupied either with the above-mentioned stirrings or with unimportant details, as long as they at least serve the purpose of directing the eye and the attention of the patient away from his life-problems. In this manner, depending upon the needs of the situation, he prepares anxiety- and compulsion-situations, sleeplessness, swooning, perversions, hallucinations, slightly pathological affects, neurasthenic and hypochondriacal complexes and psychotic pictures of his actual condition, all of which are to serve him as excuses.

VIII. Even logic falls under the domination of the counter-compulsion. As in psychosis this process may go as far as the actual nullification of logic.

IX. Logic, the will to live, love, human sympathy, co-operation and language, all arise out of the needs of human communal life. Against the latter are directed automatically all the plans of the neurotic individual striving for isolation and lusting for power.

X. To cure a neurosis and a psychosis it is necessary to change completely the whole up-bringing of the patient and turn him definitely and unconditionally back upon human society.

XI. All the volition and all the strivings of the neurotic are dictated by his prestige-seeking policy, which is continually looking for excuses which will enable him to leave the problems of life unsolved. He consequently automatically turns against allowing any community-feeling to develop.

XII. If therefore we may regard the demand for a complete and unified understanding of man and for a comprehension of his (undivided) individuality as justified—a view to which we are forced both by the nature of reason and the individual-psychological knowledge of the urge toward an integration of the personality—then the method of *comparison*, the main tool of our method, enables us to arrive at some conception of the power-lines along which an individual strives to attain superiority. The following will serve as the two contrasting-poles for comparison :

1. Our own attitude in a situation similar to that of a patient hard-pressed by some demand. In such a case it is essential for the practitioner to possess, in a considerable degree, the gift of *putting himself in the other person's place*.

2. The patient's attitudes and anomalies dating from early childhood. These can always be shown as dominated by the relation of the child to his environment, by his erroneous and in the main generalized evaluation (of himself), by his obstinate and deep-rooted feeling of inferiority and by his striving after power.

3. Other types of individuals, particularly those specifically neurotic. In these cases we shall come upon the patent discovery that what one type attains by means of neurasthenic troubles, another endeavours to obtain by means of fear, hysteria, neurotic - compulsion or psychosis. Traits of character, affects, principles and nervous symptoms, pointing toward the same goal and, when torn from their context, frequently giving a contrary significance, all these serve as a protection against the shock caused by the demands of the community.

4. Those very demands of the community which the nervous individual, in varying degrees, side-steps, such as co-operation, fellow-feeling, love, social adaptation and the responsibilities of the community.

By means of this individual-psychological investigation we realize that the neurotic individual, far more than the ordinary normal man, arranges his psychic-life in accordance with the desire for power over his fellow-men. His longing for superiority enables him continually and extensively to reject all outside compulsion,

the demands made upon him by others and the responsibilities imposed by Society. The realization of this
basic fact in the psychic-life of the neurotic, so lightens
the task of obtaining an insight into psychic inter-
connections that it is bound to become the most
useful working-hypothesis in the investigation and
curing of neurotic diseases, until a more profound
understanding of the individual enables us to dis-
entangle and grasp in their full significance, the real
factors involved in each case.

What irritates the healthy man in this type of
argument and the conclusions drawn therefrom, is the
suggestion that an imagined goal constructed by
an emotionally-conditioned superiority, can possess
greater force than rational deliberation. But we find
this inversion of an ideal frequently enough both in the
life of healthy individuals as in that of whole nations.
War, political abuses, crimes, suicide, ascetic penances,
provide us with similar surprises. A good many of
our sufferings and tortures we ourselves originate and
take upon ourselves under the influence of some idea.
That a cat should catch mice, that without ever
having been taught to do so, should be prepared for
it even in the first days of its existence, is no more
remarkable than that the neurotic individual, according to his nature and destiny, his position and his
self-evaluation, should evade and find unbearable
every form of compulsion ; that he should secretly or
openly, consciously or unconsciously look for excuses
to free himself, frequently originating them himself.
The reason for the intolerance of the neurotics toward
the constraints of society, as the history of their childhood shows, is to be sought in the continuous conflict-
attitude that has been practised for many years against
the environment. This is forced upon the child, without there being any real justification for its expressing
itself in just such a reaction, by the bodily or psychically
conditioned position it occupies and from which the
child receives either lasting or intensified feelings of
inferiority. The object of the conflict-attitude is the
conquest of power and importance, an ideal of superiority
constructed with an infant's incapacity and over-evaluation and the fulfilment of which presents compensations

and super-compensations of a most general kind, in the pursuit of which there always occurs a victory over the constraints of society and over the will of the environment.   As soon as this conflict has taken on more acute forms it evolves, from within itself, an antagonism against compulsions of all kinds, whether they be education, reality, common interest, external force, personal weakness, as well as all the compulsions presented by such factors as work, cleanliness, acceptance of nourishment, normal urination and defecation, sleep, treatment of disease, love, tenderness, friendship, loneliness and its opposite, sociability.   In toto we get the picture of a man who does not want to play the game, a dog in the manger.   Where antagonism is directed against the awakening of feelings of love and comradeship there arises a fear of love and marriage that can assume many and manifold degrees and forms. At this place let me call attention to a number of forms of compulsion hardly perceptible to the normal individual, which are nevertheless almost regularly prevented from developing by the appearance of a nervous or psychotic condition.   These compulsions are :—to recognize this compulsion, to be attentive, to subordinate oneself, to tell the truth, to study or to pass examinations, to be punctual, to entrust oneself to a person, a carriage, the railroad ; to confide the household, business, children, spouse, or oneself to other people ; to become a landlord or adopt a profession ; to marry, to acknowledge the correctness of the other man's view, to be grateful, to bring children into the world, to play a proper sexual rôle or recognize proper love-responsibilities ; to rise in the morning, to sleep at night, to recognize the equal rights and equality of others, the rights of women, to keep a measure in everything, be loyal, etc.   All these idiosyncrasies may be conscious or unconscious but they are never grasped by the patient in all their bearings.

This examination teaches us two things :

1. The concept of compulsion in the neurotic has been tremendously enlarged and embraces relationships, even if only from a logical point of view, that a normal individual does not include under the category of compulsion.

2. The antagonism is no final-phenomena but extends further. It has a continuation and is followed by a state of fermentation. It signifies at all times a conflict-attitude and shows us as though at an apparent resting point, the striving of the neurotic to triumph over others, the striving for a directed violent twisting of the logical inferences drawn from human communal life. "Non me rebus, sed mihi res subigere conor". In this passage taken from a letter of Horace to Maecenas, the former shows in what this infuriated lust for importance ends: in a headache and sleeplessness.

A patient, thirty-five years old, complained to me that he had for a number of years been suffering from sleeplessness, from brooding and masturbation-compulsions. The latter symptom was particularly significant, for the patient was married, the father of two children and on excellent marital relations with his wife. Among other torturing phenomona he spoke of a kind of "rubber-fetichism". From time to time, in any exciting situation, the word "rubber" forced itself to his lips.

The results of an extensive individual-psychological examination lead to the following facts: starting from a period in childhood characterized by marked depression, at a time when the patient used to wet his bed and was regarded as a stupid child because of his clumsiness, he had developed *along the guiding-line of ambition* to such an extent that the latter had grown into a *megalomania*. The pressure of his environment, which actually did exist in a very high degree, brought close to him the picture of a *definitely inimical external world* and invested him with a permanently pessimistic outlook upon life. In such a mood he felt all the demands of the external world as unbearable compulsions and retorted by wetting his bed and by clumsiness, until he met a teacher in whom, for the first time in his life, he came into contact with the counterpart of a good fellow-man. He then began to mitigate his defiance and rage at the demands of others and his conflict-attitude toward the community, to the extent of it becoming possible for him to stop wetting his bed, of developing into a "gifted" student and to work for the highest of ideals in life. His hostility against the compulsion of others he solved, in the manner of a poet and philosopher, by a flight into the transcendental. He developed an emotionally-steeped idea as if *he were the only living being* in existence, and that everything else, particularly human beings, were merely appearances. The relationship with the ideas of Schopenhauer, Fichte, Kant is not to be dismissed. The deeper purpose, however, lay in his robbing existence of value in order to obtain a feeling of security, and escape "the scorn and questionings of our times". All of this was to have been accomplished by *magic*, comparable to that which unreliant children use when they wish to deprive facts of their power. In this way the *rubber - erasure* became the symbol and sign of his power, because to the child, as the destroyer of the visible, the rubber appeared like a possibility fulfilled. The whole situation called for over-evaluation and generalization, and thus the word and concept "rubber" became the conquering watchword, whenever school, the parental household and later on man or woman, wife or child, presented any difficulties or threatened him with coercion.

So, in a well-nigh poetical manner, he arrived at the goal of the isolated hero, fulfilled his striving after power and renounced society. His steadily improving position in the world prevented him, however, from entirely pushing aside the actual and ever-present communal feelings. Little was consequently lost *of the love and the logic that binds us all together*, and so he was spared the fate of developing *a paranoic disease*. He went only as far as a compulsion-neurosis.

His love was not based upon pure communal feeling. In fact it came under the attraction of the main line of his striving after power. Since the concept and the feeling "power" were united with the magic word "rubber", he sought and found a catchword that would free him from his sexuality in the picture of a *rubber-girdle*. Not a woman but a rubber girdle, in other words, not a personal but an impersonal object influenced him. And thus while making his power-intoxication and his derogatory attitude toward women secure, he became a fetichist, for these traits are found regularly as the starting point of fetichism. Had the belief in his own virility been slighter we would have seen suggestions of homo-sexuality, paedophily, gerontophily, necrophily and similar traits appear.

His masturbation-compulsion had the same basic character. It likewise served to enable him to escape from the compulsion of love, from the "magic" of women.

The sleeplessness was directly caused by his brooding-compulsion, the latter struggling against the constraint of sleep. An unquenchable ambition compelled him to spend the night solving the problems of the day. Has he not like another Alexander accomplished so little as yet? This sleeplessness had however another side to it. It weakened his energy and his power of action; became the justification for his disease. What he had so far accomplished had been done so to speak with one hand, had been done despite his sleeplessness. What might he not have done had he been able to sleep! But he was not able to sleep and in this way, by means of this nocturnal brooding-compulsion, he obtained an alibi. Thus he rescued his uniqueness and his god-likeness. All blame for any deficiency could now no more be attributed to his character but to the puzzling and fatal circumstance of his not having been able to sleep. Thus his invalid state had become a disagreeable accident, and for its continuation not he but the insufficient knowledge of the physicians, was responsible. If he is not able to prove his greatness, it will be the concern of the physicians to do so. As can be seen it was of no small importance to him to remain an invalid and he was not going to make the task of the physicians easy.

It is interesting to see how he solves the problem of life and death in order to save his god-likeness. He still has the feeling that his mother, who has been dead for twelve years, is alive. But there is a marked uncertainty about this assumption, manifesting itself more strongly than that tender feeling which so frequently appears shortly after the death of a near relative. This doubt concerning his wild assumption does not at all emanate from cold logic. It is to be explained through the insight given by individual-psychology. If everything is but appearance then his mother has not died. If she is alive, however, then the idea of his being unique falls to the ground. He has no more solved this problem than philosophy has the idea of the universe as an appearance. He answers the compulsion and mischief of death with a doubt.

The interconnection of all the manifestations of his disease he regards as a justification for securing all his privileges as against his wife, his relatives and his inferiors. His high opinion of himself can never come to harm, for taking his sufferings into consideration, he is always greater than he appears to be and he can always evade difficult undertakings by pointing to his disease. But he can also act differently. Toward his superiors he can be the most conscientious, the most industrious and the most obedient official and enjoy their complete approbation although secretly always aspiring to surpass them.

This over-intense striving after the sensation of power had made him ill. His emotional and sensational life, his initiative and his capacity for work, even his power of reasoning, fell under the self-imposed compulsion of his lust for omnipotence, so that his feelings for humanity and with it love, friendship and adjustment to society, all disappeared. A cure could only have been attained by dismantling his whole prestige-mechanism and by inducing the development of a feeling for society.

IV

Individual-Psychological Treatment of Neuroses

(1913)

INTRODUCTION

To treat the extensive field of psycho-therapy concisely
at a time when the discussions concerning the value of
its principles are still so rife, is a fairly hazardous enterprise. Permit me consequently to refer to the basis for
my views given in the material containing my experiences, that has been at the disposal of the public since 1907.
In 1907 I proved in my book on Organ Inferiority
(Vienna) that the inherited constitutional anomalies are
not to be regarded as manifesting themselves merely
in degenerative processes, but as causing the appearance likewise of compensatory and hyper-compensatory
activities and significant correlation-phenomena to which
the reinforced psychic activity essentially contributed.
This compensatory psychic exertion in order to conquer
the psychic tensions, frequently strikes out along new
and different lines. To the observer this compensatory
activity appears to be of a well-tested nature, thus fulfilling its purpose of covering up some imagined deficiency in a most wonderful manner. The most widely
distributed method adopted by the *feeling of inferiority*,
appearing during childhood, to prevent its being unmasked, is the creation of a compensatory psychic
superstructure, *the neurotic modus vivendi*. This seeks
to regain, by means of fully tested preparations and
defences, a point of vantage and superiority in life.
Any departure from the normal can subsequently be
explained either by a greater ambition or by a more
marked degree of precaution. All the devices and
arrangements, including therein the neurotic character,
traits and symptoms, derive their value from previous
attempts, experiences, identifications and imitations that

are not entirely unknown even to a healthy individual. The language they speak, rightly understood, makes it evident that an individual is here struggling for recognition, actually attempting to force it ; that he is aspiring ceaselessly to a godlike domination over his environment from out the region of his insecurity and his sense of inferiority.

Placing on one side this,the root of neurotic behaviour, we find the latter to consist of a variegated assortment of incitements and potentialities for incitement, which do not represent *the cause*, but rather the consequences of the neurosis.   In a short treatise : " Aggressionsbetrieb im Leben u. in der Neurose " (*Heilen und Bilden*, 1914), I have tried to present this frequently intensified "affective activity" and to show how, in order either to achieve some purpose or escape some danger, it is often converted into an apparent "aggression-check".   What is customarily known as "disposition to neurosis" (*neurotic disposition*) is a real neurosis already, the more suitable neurotic symptoms appearing more definitely and as proofs of disease, only on those actual occasions when *an inward need demands the calling forth of strengthened devices*.   This demonstration of illness and the "arrangements" associated with it, are specifically needed for the following purposes :

1. To serve as excuses if life denies the longed-for triumphs.
2. So that all *decisions may be postponed.*
3. To permit those goals already attained to appear in an intenser light, since they have been gained *in spite of suffering.*   These and other devices clearly exhibit the striving of the neurotic *for the semblance of things.*

The inference to be drawn is in each case simple. The neurotic in order to ensure success for his actions, in all of which he has been guided by an imagined goal, keeps to lines of direction typical for him and which he actually follows literally and unwaveringly.   In this manner, by means of definite and adapted traits of character, tested affect-preparations, and a neurotic perspective of the past, present and future, the neurotic personality gains its fixed form.   The urge to ensure security for this superiority operates with such strength

c

that every psychic phenomenon, when analysed from the comparative psychological view, discloses superficially the similar characteristic, namely, to free itself from a feeling of weakness that it may reach the summit of its ambition ; to lift itself from "below" to "above" and by the use of devices not always easily intelligible, become completely supreme.   In order that by planning, thinking and a grasp of the world, he may be able to obtain a pedantic kind of order and *security*, the neurotic resorts to every rule and helping-formula he knows, the most impoitant of which correspond to the primitive antithetic scheme.   He consequently attaches importance only to affect-values that correspond to an upper and lower and attempts—as far as I can make out—to relate these to the contrast between "masculine" and "feminine" that appears so real to him.   Through falsification of conscious and unconscious judgments, there is thus given, as if by means of some psychic accumulator, an occasion for *affect-disturbances* and these latter are in turn adapted to the personal life-line of the patient.   Those traits of his psyche felt as "feminine", *e.g.* passive attitude, obedience, softness, cowardice, memory of defeat, ignorance, lack of capacity, tenderness, he attempts to push with an exaggerated orientation towards the "masculine," thus developing hatred, defiance, cruelty, egoism.   He seeks triumph in every human relation.   He may, however, on the contrary markedly emphasize his weakness and, in this way, force upon others the burden of serving him.   This procedure increases the patient's precautions and prevision enormously and leads to planned evasions of impending decisions.   Where the patient believes it incumbent upon him in life to bring evidence of "masculine excellences", for instance, in struggles of every nature, in professions, in love, or in those cases where he fears he may become "effeminate" through defeat, (and this applies also to the masculine sex), he will even, when far removed, try to approach the problem circuitously.   We shall then always succeed in finding a life-line, deviating from the direct path, which, on account of fear of mistakes and defeat, is searching for safe side-paths.   The falsification of his sexual rôle results, in consequence of which the neurotic seems to exhibit a tendency toward "psychical hermaphrodism", which he actually believes himself to possess. Viewed from this side the neurosis might easily be suspected of having a sexual causation. In reality, however, the same struggle takes place within the sexual domain that we have found within our entire psychic life ; the original inferiority-feeling forces itself forward along by-paths (in sexual life along the road of masturbation, homosexuality, fetichism, algolagny, over-evaluation of sexuality, etc.), so as not to lose its orientation toward the goal of superiority. The schematic formula, " I wish to be a complete man ", then serves as the abstract and concretistic goal of the neurotic. It is a compensating termination for the basic feeling of an inferiority interpreted as feminine. The scheme that has been apperceived in this manner and upon which the individual has proceeded, is antithetic throughout and it has, in conscious falsification, been interpreted as containing within itself *hostile elements*. We can consequently always recognize as the unconscious premises of the neurotic goal-striving, the following two facts :

1. *Human relations in all circumstances represent a struggle.*
2. *The feminine sex is inferior and by its reaction serves as the measure of masculine strength.*

These two unconscious presuppositions that both masculine and feminine patients reveal in equal degree, are at the bottom of the distortion and poisoning of all human relationships, of the appearance of affect-disturbances and strengthenings, and the occurrence of permanent dissatisfaction instead of frankness. Dissatisfaction generally becomes lightened after intensification of the symptoms and after a successful demonstration of the existence of a disease. *The symptom is a substitute, in a way, for the neurotic lust for superiority with its associated affect.* In the patient's emotional life it leads more certainly to a sham-victory over the environment than would be true in the case of a straight-forward battle, a definite trait of character, or resistance. *For me the understanding of the symptom-language has become the main condition for the success of the psycho-therapeutic cure.*

Since the purpose of the neurosis is to help an individual in the securing of the end-goal of superiority and since the feeling of inferiority apparently, excludes

the possibility of direct aggression, circuitous routes
which possess vaguely active, sometimes masochistic
and always self-torturing characteristics, are preferred.
Generally we encounter a mixture of psychic stirrings
and disease-symptoms making their appearance either
synchronously during the same period of illness, or
following one another.   When torn from their context
in the disease-mechanism, they at times give the impression of being contradictory or of indicating a split
in personality.   The context shows that the patient
can draw from two contradictory lines to reach his *ideal
situation of imagined superiority*,   just as he actually,
with the same object in view, will argue correctly or
incorrectly, and judge and feel quite independently of
his goal.   We must, on all occasions, expect the neurotic
to   possess   those   view-points,   sensations,   memories,
affects, character-traits and symptoms that are to be
presupposed in him by reason of his recognized life-line
and goal.

Thus the neurotic in order to conquer along the line
of obedience, submissiveness, "hysterical impression-
ability", in order to chain other people down through
his weakness, fear, passivity, need for tenderness—has
at his hand all kinds of reminders, of fear-inspiring
pictures of horror, affect-preparations and identifications
with properly adapted feelings and character-traits, in
the same way that a neurotic, subject to compulsions,
possesses definite principles, laws and prohibitions
supposed to apply to himself only, but which in reality
invest his sense of personality with a god-like power.
As a goal we always find the acquisition of some ideal
"income" for which the patient battles with the means
his immediate experiences have shown to be the most
suitable, just as tenaciously as a neurotic suffering from
compulsion of meeting with accident, struggles for his
material "income".   The same holds true in those
cases where active affects like rage, anger and jealousy
make the path to pre-eminence secure.   These latter are
frequently represented by attacks of pain, fainting-spells
or epileptic seizures. (Cf. "Trotz und Gehorsam" in
Heilen und Bilden.)   All neurotic symptoms have
as their object the task of ensuring the safety of the
patient's feeling of personality and the life-line with
which he has identified himself.   In order to prove his

ability to cope with life, all the "arrangements" and neurotic symptoms necessary for the patient come into existence, as an aid in necessity, as an unduly developed coefficient-of-security against the dangers he anticipates and toward whose prevention he has been unceasingly working when, under the influence of his inferiority feeling, he has been constructing his plans for the future.

The " Arrangement" of the Neurosis

The feeling of inferiority, afterwards purposely adhered to and emphasized, developing from the impressions of reality, incites the patient continuously in his childhood, to fix some goal for his striving, a goal extending beyond human limits, one which approaches a deification and which coerces an individual to march along lines rigidly determined. The neurotic system, *the life-plan of the nervous man*, lies between these two points—his feeling of inferiority and his striving for superiority. This compensatory psychical structure, this nervous "willing", utilizes all of one's own and foreign experience, purposefully distorting them, it is true, and falsifying their value at times, yet, on the other hand, employing their correct content whenever it suffices for the neurotic objective.

On closer inspection we find a perfectly explicable phenomenon, namely that all these lines of direction are provided, on numerous sides, with warning-signs and encouragement, with reminders and summons to action, so that it is really possible to speak of the existence of a widely ramifying safety-net. Everywhere we encounter the neurotic psychic life forming a super-structure built over a threatening infantile situation, a super-structure, changing in the course of years and adapting itself to reality more than would have been the case in the child's ordinary evolution. It is not to be wondered at then, if every psychic phenomenon of the neurotic is permeated by this rigid system and appears *like an analogy* in which the lines of direction always stand out in relief. Such phenomena are : the neurotic character, the nervous symptom, the de-meanour, every device used in life, the evasions and deviations that occur as soon as decisions are about to threaten the god-like state of the neurotic, and finally

his view-of-the-world, his attitude to men and women
and his dreams.   I presented my interpretation of the
last-named phenomenon in 1911.   Bringing my views
upon dreams into harmony with those on neuroses, I
found their *main function to consist of simplified early trials,
and of warnings and encouragements favourable to the life-
plan ; and to have as their object the solution of some future
problem.*   A more detailed exposition is to be found in
the chapter on " Dreams and Dream-interpretation ".

How does this striking similarity in psychic phenomena arise, where everything seems to be permeated
with and guided by the same tendency—a striving
upwards, a striving toward the masculine, toward the
feeling of god-likeness?   I pointed out these facts in my
neurological study, "Ueber Zahlenanalysen und Zahlen-
phobie" (*Neurolog.-psychiatr. Zeitschrift,* 1905), a work
that was regarded, when viewed from the position then
generally taken, as incomplete and along wrong lines.

The answer can be easily extracted from the above-
mentioned work.   The hypnotic nature of the goal of the
neurotic, forces his whole psychic life into an integrated
adaptation.   As soon as the patient's life-line has been
recognized, he will always be found at that particular
place where we should expect to find him according
to his presuppositions and previous history.   The strong
urge toward the integration of his personality, flows from
an inward necessity and has been created by his tendency
to safeguard himself.   The path is made secure and
unalterable by the proper schematic "arrangements"
of character-traits, affect-preparations and symptoms.
At this point let me append some remarks about "affect-
disturbances", and neurotic "sensibility" in order to
prove the existence of an unconscious "arrangement"
for the purpose of keeping them within the life-line, thus
employing them both as a *means to an end and as an
artifice of the neurosis.*

For example, a patient with agoraphobia, in order
by a complicated mechanism, to raise his prestige at
home and force his environment into his service and to
prevent himself likewise from losing, while on the street
or in open places, the "resonance" so fervently desired,
unites unconsciously and emotionally into a "junktim",
the thought of being alone, of strange people, of
purchases, search for the theatre, society, etc., and

the phantasy of an apoplectic stroke, a confinement on the street, disease infection through germs on the street.[1] The exaggerated size of the *safety-coefficient as contrasted with the thought potentialities* is clearly seen. In this way the discernible purpose can be followed to its final objective and the life-line recognized. Similarly the neurotic precaution of a patient subject to attacks of anxiety, who wishes furthermore to withdraw from making a decision, be it in an examination, a love-affair or an undertaking, will force him by thus establishing a proof of illness, to connect his situation with that of an execution, a prison, a shoreless sea, being buried alive and with death. In order to evade a decision about the success of a love-affair, the following connection of ideas may be resorted to as serving the desired purpose : a man, a murderer or a burglar, a woman, sphinx, demon or vampire. Every defeat is felt as all the more threatening because of being brought together with the thought of death or pregnancy, (encountered among neurotic men also). The transferred affect compels the patient to avoid a certain undertaking. Father and mother are at times invested by phantasy with the rôle of lover or spouse until the bond is firm enough to secure an evasion of the marriage problem. Religious and ethical feelings of guilt are, as is so frequently the case in compulsion-neurosis, constructed and utilized in order to attain a sensation of power, (*e.g.* "if I do not pray at night my mother will die"; the statement should be made positively in order to understand the fiction of god-likeness : "if I pray she will not die").

Together with the exaggerated personality-ideal and the "anxieties" of a neurotic type designed to secure it, we also find exaggerated "expectations" whose certainty of disappointment leads the patient to reinforced and definitely conditioned affects of mourning, hatred, dissatisfaction, jealousy, etc. In these cases the insistence upon principles, ideals, dreams, castles in the air, etc., plays a tremendous rôle and the neurotic can, by connecting these with some person or situation, deprive everything of its inherent value and so exhibit

---

[1] "Junktim": purposive connection of two thoughts and affect-complexes that have in reality little or nothing to do with one another, in order to strengthen the affect. The metaphor has a similar origin.

his superiority. The great importance of love in human life and the neurotic's search for superhuman influence and importance in love, bring about the frequent occurrence of an "arrangement" like that of disappointed expectation, so that the patient may in this manner evade the sexual problem. Masturbation-compulsion, impotence, perversions and fetichism are found to lie along some indirect route of such a main line.

As a third type of construction designed to prevent defeat or a marked inferiority feeling, I shall briefly mention the *anticipation* of sensations, feelings and apperceptions, that have the significance, in connection with threatening situations, of acting as preparations, warnings, and encouragements such as occur in dreams, hypochondriac and melancholic conditions, in illusions in particular, in psychosis, in neurasthenia and in hallucinations.[1] A good example is provided by the dream of children who wet their bed, picturing them-selves in the toilet so that they may be able to develop their generally revengeful and obstinate enuretic attitude, *uninfluenced by the intellect*. Similarly, images derived from tabes, paralysis, true epilepsy, paranoia, heart and lung affections etc. can be employed to produce fears or secure safety.

In order to present an intelligible, but admittedly schematic picture of the peculiar orientation of neurotics and psychotics, I suggest that we present the common attitude towards nervousness in a formula and then compare that formula with another representing the above views and corresponding better with reality. The first formula would appear as follows :

$$Individual + experience + environment + demands$$
$$of\ life = a\ neurosis.$$

In this formula the individual is regarded as weakened either by a feeling of inferiority, by heredity, by "sexual constitution", by emotionality or by his character. Furthermore his experiences, the environ-ment and the external demands weigh upon the patient so heavily that they induce him to "take refuge in sickness". This interpretation is manifestly wrong

---

[1] This view-point has since then, in consequence of the study of war-neuroses, been accepted by practically all writers.

and gains no support from the secondary hypothesis
that the deficiency in wish-fulfilments or the "libido"
that exists, in reality, is corrected by the neurosis.

A better formula would read as follows :—

Evaluation $(I + E + M) + Arrangement$ $(Experiences +$
Character + Emotionality + Symptoms) = Personality-ideal.

In other words the only *definite and fixed point conceived of is the personality-ideal.* In order to approximate
more nearly to his god-likeness, the neurotic makes a
tendentious evaluation of his individuality, his experiences and his environment. But since this does not by
any means suffice to bring him to his life-line or nearer
to his goal, he *provokes experiences* which his previously
determined favourable applications make easier—of
feeling set - back, deceived, suffering — all of which
give him the trusted and desired basis of aggression.
That he constructs so much from real experiences
and from possibilities and builds just the type of
character-traits and affect-preparations that fit into his
personality-ideal, follows from the above description
and has been discussed by me in detail. In a similar
fashion the patient identifies himself with his symptoms,
all his experiences taking the form that appears necessary
and useful for the heightening of his feeling of personality. Not the slightest trace of a predetermined
autochthonous teleology is to be found in this modus
vivendi, projected and tenaciously adhered to by means
of a self-suggested principal goal. The neurotic life-
plan is maintained and teleologically arranged only by
the urge toward superiority, by the careful evasion of
dangerous-looking decisions, by previously tested
wanderings along a few clearly determined lines of
direction and the enormously increased safety-net. In
consequence, the questions relating to the conservation
or loss of psychic energy lose all their meaning. The
patient will create just so much psychic energy as will
enable him to remain on his path of superiority and
express his masculine protest and god-likeness.

Psychic Treatment of Neuroses

The most important element in therapeutics is the
disclosure of the neurotic system or life-plan. In its

entirety this can only be conserved if the patient
succeeds in keeping it away from his own self-criticism.
The partially unconscious course of the neurosis, working
in opposition with reality, is explained first and foremost by the definite tendency of the patient to arrive at
his goal.[1]   Its opposition to reality, *i.e.* to the logical
demands of the community, is in this system connected
with the limited experiences and differences in the type
of the relations which were efficacious at the time of the
construction of the life-plan, *i.e.* in earliest childhood.
An insight into the meaning of this plan is best obtained
through artistic and intuitive self-identification with
the patient's personality.   A person will then realize
for himself how unconsciously comparisons are made
between himself and the patient, between different
attitudes of the latter or similar actions of other patients.
In order to bring order into the material apperceived,
into the patient's symptoms, experiences, manner of life
and development, I make use of two prejudices of my
own gained from experience.   The first deals with the
origin of the life-plan under aggravated conditions—(organ-
inferiorities, pressure in the family, a neurotic family-
tradition)—and centres my attention upon identical or
similar reaction-types in childhood.   The second lies in
the *assumption of the above empirically obtained and fictitious
identification* according to which I estimate my apperceptions.   Further on I shall explain this by an
example.

From my remarks it is apparent that I always expect
from my patient the same attitude that he has shown,
in conformity with his life-plan, toward the persons of
his early entourage, and at a still earlier period, toward
his own family.   At the time of his meeting with the
physician and frequently earlier, the same connection
of feelings is found as that which exists in persons of
greater ability.   That the transference of such feelings
or the opposition to them seems to begin later, must
be based on some mistake.   The physician probably
recognizes them in these cases later.   Often too late,
especially in those instances where the patient, in the

---

[1] Cf. "On the Rôle of the Unconscious" in this volume—'Genius' (*Geist*)
does not seem to protect an individual against a purposive concealment of
the facts.   And the god-likeness at times plays curious tricks upon the
practitioner too.

consciousness of his hidden superiority, brings his treatment to an end or where through an aggravation of the symptoms, an unbearable condition has been created. That the patient is under no circumstances to be offended I need not inform psychologically trained doctors. But this may occur without the knowledge of the physician and harmless remarks may be purposefully revaluated if the latter does not clearly understand the nature of the patient. It is therefore essential, particularly at the beginning, to proceed with caution and to fathom as quickly as possible the neurotic system of an individual. As a rule, with any experience, this is discovered on the first day.

Even more significant is the necessity of *obviating the possibility of positive aggressive preparation for an attack.* At this place I can only give a few hints, designed to prevent the physician *from falling into the position of being treated by the patient.* First of all, not even in the safest cases, should a *successful issue of the cure* be promised ; it should never be made more than a possibility. One of the most important devices in psycho-therapeutics is to *ascribe the work and the success of the cure to the patient,* who is to be employed as a fellow-worker and treated like a friend. The custom of having *payments* depend upon the success of the treatment creates enormous difficulties. It is best, at every point, to keep to the assumption that the patient *craving for superiority as we know him to be, is going to use every promise of the physician—that which he makes with respect to the duration of the cure as well*—to secure the discomfiture of the doctor. Consequently all the necessary questions—the visiting-time, a friendly and open welcome, the question of payments, free treatment, the physician's pledge to secrecy, etc. — should be regulated immediately and strictly adhered to. It is under all circumstances a tremendous advantage if the patient goes to the physician. *To prophesy, where it is certain, an aggravation of the disease as in cases* of fainting-spells, pains or agoraphobia, saves an enormous amount of work at the beginning, because the attacks, as a rule, do not then take place, a fact that corroborates our view about the marked negativism of neurotics. *To clearly show pleasure at a partial success or to boast about it would be a great mistake.* The situation would soon take a turn for the worse. It is therefore best to centre all interest upon the difficulties patiently, without annoyance, and in a calm scientific manner.

In complete agreement with the above is the basic principle never to allow the patient, except under great protestations and explanations, to force upon anyone a superior rôle such as that of teacher, father, saviour, etc.   Such attempts represent the beginning of a movement on the part of the patient to pull down, in a manner to which he has been previously accustomed, *all persons standing above him and by thus administering a defeat, to disavow the physician.*   To insist upon any superior rank or right is always disadvantageous with nervous patients. The best thing is to be open and to avoid, bearing in mind the danger of a mistake in technique, being dragged into any undertakings by him.   It would be even more dangerous to take him into your own service, put requests to him, expect anything from him, etc. To expect secrecy from a patient indicates a complete absence of an elementary knowledge of the psychic life of a neurotic.

While these and similar measures dictated by the same attitude bring about the best adapted relationship of equality, *the uncovering of the neurotic life-plan* proceeds apace in friendly and free conversation, it being always the *better tactics to let the patient take the initiative.* I found it the safest course to search for and merely unmask the neurotic line of operation as shown in expressions and in the train of thought, and at the same time unobtrusively educate the patient for the same kind of work.   The physician must be so convinced of the *uniqueness and exclusiveness of the neurotic direction-line,* that he is able to call up the true content (of the patient's mind), always telling him beforehand his disturbing "arrangements" and constructions, and trying to discover and explain until the patient, completely upset, gives them up in order to place new and better hidden ones in their place.   How often this will occur it is impossible to say beforehand.   Finally, however, the patient will give in, all the more easily, if his relation to the physician has not permitted the feeling of a (possible) defeat to develop.

Just as there are these "arrangements" lying along the path of the feeling of superiority, so there are also definite subjective sources of error utilized and conserved merely because they possibly deepen the feeling of inferiority and thus furnish irritations and stimulations for further constructions. *Such errors and their tendencies* must be brought within the vision of the patient.

The patient's primitive apperception-scheme which *definitely and distinctly evaluates all impressions* and then groups them in a purposeful manner (above-below, victor-vanquished, masculine - feminine, nothing - everything, etc.) is always to be indicated, unmasked and shown to be immature, untenable and with a purpose in view : namely, that of continued hostility. It is this scheme likewise that shows us, in the psychic life of the neurotics, traits similar to those found in the beginnings of culture, where necessity has forced people to such types of safety. It would savour of the fantastic to suspect in such analogies anything more than mimicry, possibly a repetition of phylogenesis. What impresses us in primitive man and in the genius, is the overbubbling power, the Titan-like defiance, the raising of one's self from nothing to the godhead, constructing out of nothing a world-dominating sanctuary. In the neurotic as in dreams, this can easily be seen to be a " bluff" even though it is the cause of great suffering. The fictitious triumph that the nervous patient gains by his manœuvres exists only in his imagination. We must show him the view-point of others, who generally feel their superiority demonstrated in a fashion similar to the love-relation of the neurotic or his perversions. At the same time there takes place, step by step, the *uncovering of his unattainable goal of superiority, the demonstration of the purposive veiling of the same*, of his all-dominating, direction-determining power and of the patient's lack of freedom and hostility toward mankind conditioned by the goal. In a similarly simple fashion we find, as soon as sufficient material is at hand, the proof that all neurotic character-traits, neurotic-affects and symptoms, serve as means partly to continue along the prescribed path, partly to make that path secure. It is important to understand the nature of the genesis of the affect and the symptom, which as we have shown above, owes its efficiency to a frequently meaningless "junktim" also operating according to plan. The patient often discloses the "junktim" quite innocently. At other times it has to be extracted from his analogizing explanations, his previous history, or his dreams.

The same tendency of the life-line is disclosed in the world-view and the life-view of the patient, as well as in his outlook upon and his grouping of experiences. Falsifications and conscious additions, purposive special applications markedly one-sided, unbounded fears and expectations clearly impossible of fulfilment, are encountered at every step and they always serve the patient's life-plan with its glorious last act. Many derailments and checks will have to be unearthed and this only succeeds after a careful, ever-increasing understanding of the unified tendency (of the life-plan) has been attained.

Since the physician obstructs the neurotic strivings of the patient he is regarded as an obstacle in the way, as an obstruction preventing the attainment of the superiority-ideal along the path of the neurosis. *For that reason every patient will attempt to disqualify the physician*, deprive him of his influence, conceal from him the true state of affairs and he will always find some new turn of affairs to hold against the practitioner. Particular attention is to be paid to these, for in a well-planned treatment they disclose most clearly the tendency of the sick person, by means of a neurosis, to maintain his superiority. And especially is it to be borne in mind that the further the improvement has progressed—(when there is a standstill there exists almost always a hearty friendship and peace except that the attacks continue)— the more energetic will be the patient's attempts, by means of unpunctuality, waste of time or non-attendance to jeopardize the success of the treatment. At times a marked hostility arises which like all the phenomena of resistance possessing the same tendency, is only to be neutralized if the patient's attention is drawn again and again to the realization that his behaviour is quite natural. *I always find the hostile relation of the patient's relatives to the physician of advantage and I sometimes have carefully attempted to stir it up*. Since generally, the tradition of the entire family of the sick person is neurotic, it is possible by uncovering and explaining it, to greatly benefit the patient. *The bringing about of a change in the nature of the patient can emanate from him alone*. I always found it most profitable ostentatiously to sit with my hands in my lap, fully convinced that the patient, no matter what I might be able to say on the point, as soon as he has recognized his life-line, can obtain nothing from me that he, as the sufferer, does not understand better.

Appendix

I shall in this Appendix give, in excerpts, some notes bearing on the above-described life-analogy of the neurotics, taken from the psychic life of a twenty-two year old patient who came under my care in connection with masturbation - compulsion, depression-manifestations, unwillingness to work and timid, embarrassed behaviour. Let me state that answering to this analogy, the more intensely the patient has undertaken the evaluation of his person, all the more will he be called upon to accomplish it by way of arrangements—(relating to experiences, character-traits, affects and symptoms)—whether his evaluation be conscious or under the pressure of defeats in life. *It is in this way that both the neurotic attacks as well as the choice of neuroses, that is to say, the chronic attacks, are to be explained; both must be able to stand the test of being utilizable for the life-plan.* From the differential diagnostic point of view, an insight into this connection is of the greatest importance. However, the practitioner needs an exact knowledge of organic nervous diseases and of pathology, because mixed forms are frequently found.

Let me now in order to make the matter clearer to my reader, assume, as is done in certain problems of mathematics that can only be solved by this artifice, that my task is provisionally solved and let me attempt, in so far as this is possible in a sketch, to prove the correctness of my solution by examining my data. Let us start with a provisional premise—that the patient is striving after a modus vivendi *to attain the goal of perfection, superiority and god-likeness.* In our unconstrained conversations the patient very quickly furnishes us with ample justifications for this assumption. The special kind of aristocracy of his family is described, its exclusiveness, its principle of "noblesse oblige" and how an older brother had brought down upon his head universal criticism for marrying below his rank.

This insistence upon the high position of the family is quite intelligible and is to be regarded as necessary because in this way *his own position also rises*. As a matter of fact, he attempted to dominate all the members of his family either by amiability or force. An external attitude exhibited the same urge upward: he was particularly fond of climbing on the roof of his family house, went to the further-most edge but would not permit any other member of his family to attempt to go so far. Only he!—He showed great excitement in childhood whenever he was punished, fought against every form of compulsion and never tolerated the slightest influence. He generally did *just the opposite* of what other people, particularly his mother, asked him to do. He would sing and hum to himself on the street, at public places in order to show his contempt for the world (i.e., *he is arranging* feelings of superiority). In his very first dreams he already found the warning not to allow himself to be cowed by me. He was very careful not to step on the shadow of a person, in order— (this is a frequent superstition)—not to absorb the latter's stupidity ; (positively interpreted : I am brighter than all of you !) Strange door-latches he would only touch with his elbows not with his hands. ("All people are dirty, that is, only I am clean". This is also the impelling-motive of washing-compulsion, of cleanliness-frenzy, fear of infection, fear of contact.) Occupational phantasies : to become an aeronaut, millionaire, to make all people happy. (He, in contrast to all others)—Flying-dreams.—What is to be inferred from this ensemble all points to a high self-evaluation.

Looking more closely at the matter, from these spasmodic exertions and peculiarities of the patient, we obtain the impression of great unhappiness and insecurity. He always came back to his weak constitution, described in detail his female build, emphasizing the fact that he had always been reproached for it and that he had been tortured in childhood with the doubt as to the possibility of his ever becoming a mature man. Statements to the effect that it would have been better had he been a girl, had made a deep impression upon him. That, at an early period, a neurotic system had been developed in which the necessary emotionality for enabling him to force his way through life was not absent,

is proved by the early appearance of traits of defiance, rage, desire for power and cruelty, all of which
tended towards the masculine side and were directed in
particular against his sister and mother. These traits
became clearly discernible when, for instance, at the
suggestion that he play a female rôle in some minor
theatrical performances, he flew into a rage. He pointed
heatedly and with purposive fears to the late appearance
of his body-hair and to a phimosis (organ-inferiority !).
The doubt concerning his ability to play a masculine
sex rôle was deeply rooted in him and urged him to
exaggerations in many directions of a type considered
masculine, to professions of narcissism and closed the
extension of his life-line in the direction of love and
marriage. Thus he developed to the point of masturbation and remained there. No matter how publicly and
definitely he may exhibit this attitude of superiority, as
soon as we examine the presuppositions of his actions,
we come into unmistakable contact with a deep-set and
easily deepened feeling of inferiority. In order to obtain
the feeling of security he was compelled to extend his
life-line in such fashion that he approached the whole
problem of hetero-sexuality in a circuitous way—and
thus got the *sexual-direction that fitted into his system*,
masturbation. He was compelled to stabilize this as a
compulsion, to fall back upon it as a security against
any threatened approach of a woman, to force it upon
himself by means of a headache in case of resistance,
and to ameliorate it by sleepiness. In order to intensify
his fear of women he collected all the instances in his
experience indicating the ruinous rôle they have played.
Instances to the contrary he disregarded. What possibility of love or marriage still remained, he excluded on
some such principle as, for example, only to marry
according to "Gotha"[1] or by positing an ideal that
appeared even to him unattainable.

Apart from masturbation in half-sleep he tried a
number of other devices of which the most disturbing
socially, was his tendency to change of profession and
his complete unwillingness to work. The meaning of
both was easily decipherable. His "*hesitating attitude*"
he conserved as useful, in order not to be compelled to
approach the marriage problem. His construction of

[1] The *Almanach de Gotha*, the equivalent of *Debrett*. [Tr.]

D

ethical and aesthetic schemes had protected him from prostitution and from " free-love ". These prejudices must not make us blind to the neurotic tendency inherent in them.

At the same time this "arrangement" of the "*hesitating attitude*" made it possible for him with the large number of fatal experiences inherently conditioned, (in consequence of delays, laziness, postponements etc.), to reinforce a second safety construction—that of an intense family feeling. This always brought him back again to his special relationship to his dogmatic, domineering mother. It was just the difficulties of his life that had forced the latter to turn all her attention to him and he could thus feel that there really was a female personage over whom he ruled despotically. He knew, in masterly fashion, how to attract her by describing his depressions, by self-drawn ornamental decoration of his letters which were supposed to represent revolvers. Hostile attacks as well as occasional indications of tenderness always rendered her tractable. Both were his weapons, his devices for dominating his mother, and since *in this case the sexual problem was excluded* there existed in this relationship an analogy to his lifeline, the attainment of domination. In order to be able to evade other women he developed a mother-fixation. In some cases a caricature of an incestuous relation might in this way arise, in others this might be reflected as an "incest-analogy" of a patient's life-line, a "bluff" of the nervous psyche that should not be allowed to deceive the physician.

The psycho-therapeutic treatment has for its object consequently, to show the patient how in his preparations while awake and occasionally in his dreams, he is always attempting in an habitual manner to fall into the ideal situation of his main path ; to show him that first, through negativism and later on of his own free will, he can change his life-plan and with it his system and so gain a contact with human society and its logical demands.

V

Contributions to the Theory of Hallucination

(1912)

THE facts connected with brain and nerve stimuli, the seat, according to most assumptions, of sensations, apperceptions, and occasionally of memories and reflex and motor impulses, do not carry us any further than the vibration and undulatory theory of nerve-substance and its chemical transformations. To look for more than plausible, or at best ultimately, undemonstrable connections is a logically incorrect inference, permissible only in folk-psychology. The building up of the psychical life out of mechanical, electrical, chemical or analogous stimuli is to such an extent incomprehensible that I prefer to fall back upon the hypothesis which assumes that in the nature and meaning of " life ", there must be included a soul-organ whose function is not that of subordination but co-ordination and which, starting from small beginnings, develops ultimately the final function of responding to these stimuli.

At whatever point we examine the workings of this psychic organ we find it engaged in reacting to inward and external impressions and always clearing the way for the actions and practices of the individual. However, it is not the will alone that is here to be considered but, likewise, the planned ordering of the stimuli, our understanding of them and their connection with the world, be it conscious or unconscious ; our anticipating and piloting conation in the direction characteristic for each individual. The character-path is always in motion and tends definitely in the direction of an amelioration, of the supplementing and heightening (of life), as if all the sensations connected with our personal situation conditioned a feeling of restlessness and insecurity at times light, at times intense. The always-wakeful needs and instincts check the sleep of the psychic organ.   In every one of the manifestations apprehended by us we may interpret the restlessness as past history, reaction to environment as the present and a fictitious goal of salvation as the future.   It is not to be assumed that in all these instances attention is operating with unbiassed readiness, dispassionately taking memories and uniting them with impressions that possess no specific tendencies in order to produce a final integration.   To an experimenter and observer not versed in the individual-psychological method, even the gross differences disappear and he will never become aware of decisive individual under-tones.   To such a person, for example, fear is fear.   But it is far more vital, if we are to obtain an understanding of mankind, to know whether the fear is of a kind impelling him to run away or to call in the aid of a second person.   If I were simply to examine an individual's capacity to remember, strength of memory, receptivity or quickness of response, I would not in the least know what objective he had. Consequently experimental psychology, by itself, is not able to teach us anything about a man's talents or values, because it can never tell us whether an individual is going to use his psychic capital for good or evil, quite apart from the fact that some people may be specially apt at a test and not successful in life.   The success of a test, too, is dependent upon the nature of the relation existing between the examiner and examined, between the examined and the field covered by the examination.

Every apperception and perception is concerned with complicated activities in which the particular psychic situation plays a great rôle and enormously influences attention.   Even simple perception is not merely an objective impression or experience ; it is a creative act consisting of anticipatory and subsidiary thoughts causing the whole of our personality to vibrate.   Yet perception and apperception are not fundamentally different acts.   They are related to each other in the same way as is the beginning and temporary ending of some incident.   Everything flows into apperception that we at any given moment need and that we expect will enable us to approach our individual goals.   The degree of pleasure and pain experienced is exactly sufficient for furthering the attainment of an anticipated

goal.   It may in fact be said to spur us toward it.
That apperception is in the nature of a creative act is
to be inferred from the fact that we are able to apperceive
objects and persons just as in memory, but from an
angle not permitted by the immediate perception, when,
for example, we see ourselves in a memory-picture.
This creative act of a capacity inherent in the psyche,
unfolding itself and at the same time possessing definite
contact with the exterior world, is also the explanation
of hallucination.   It is an identical psychic power that
permits, though in different degrees, the creative and
constructive activity found in perception, apperception,
memory and hallucination.

This quality which might roughly be called that
of the hallucinatory components of the psyche, is more
clearly apparent and more easily discerned in childhood
than afterwards.   We are compelled either to greatly
limit or even to completely exclude hallucination as
such because of its contradiction with rational thinking,
the fundamental function and condition of the life of
society.   The psychic power contained in hallucination
is confined within the frame of perception, apperception
and memory, all of which are very easily demonstrable
and possess attributes of value for society.   Only in
those cases where the ego has separated itself from the
community and approximates to a condition of isolation,
are the clamps removed; in dreams, for example, in which
the ego seeks to overwhelm its neighbour; in the terrible
uncertainty of a death in the desert, where the torturing
thought of slow destruction allows an hallucination to
develop like a consoling fata morgana, and finally, in
the neurosis and psychosis which portray, in reality, the
situation of an isolated man struggling for prestige.
With ecstatic fervour such individuals rush drunkenly
into the realm of the unsocial, the unreal, and construct new worlds in which hallucination gains a value
because rational thinking is not so important.   As a
rule enough community feeling still persists for the
hallucination to be felt as unreal.   This holds generally
both for the dream and the neurosis.

One of my patients who had lost his sight through
atrophy of the optic nerve, suffered continually from
hallucinations which, so he insisted, were exceedingly
painful.   The current assumption that the irritable

condition of the optic nerve associated with this disease, leads to excitations which are then reinterpreted and rationalized, shirks the problem involved.   Excitations within the sphere of vision we freely grant.   The peculiar reinterpretation into contents of definite type whose common element always appears in the form of suffering for the patient, forces us to the assumption of a tendency working uniformly, with the object of appropriating and using these excitations as data.   It is in this manner that we arrive at explanations of a psychological nature.   Up to the present, research has been concerning itself with the question of the nature of hallucinations, answering by a meaningless tautology that they are excitations in the sphere of vision.   We individual-psychologists start with the assumption that it is impossible to give a name to or recognize the nature of all the fundamental facts concerning life and nature, the objective fact of life itself, of organic assimilation, of electricity ; we look upon hallucination as an expression of the psyche as contrasted with the true and logically determined content of society prefigured in apperception and memory, the nature of which is to a certain extent also hidden from our view.   Our examination thus teaches us that the victim of an hallucination has taken himself out of the domain of the community feeling and by evading logic and gagging the feeling for truth, has been striving for a goal different from the usual one.

The objective in such a case cannot be extracted from the hallucination without some difficulty.   Like every psychic phenomenon torn from its context, it is multiple in meaning.[1]   The true meaning of hallucination, its significance, the where and the whyfor — these are the questions put by individual-psychology— can only be given after a knowledge of the complete individual and his personality has been attained.   We regard the hallucination as the expression of a personality when in a peculiar position.

In the case in question we know that sight has gone and the hallucinatory capacity intensified.   The patient complained ceaselessly about " perceptions " that did

[1] Some interpretive artists, like the psychologists of sex, stress very superficially the double meaning of the phenomenon and then speak of an inner-psychology.

not always appear agonizing to us, for example, when he saw colours or trees or the sun following him into the room. We must here call attention to the fact that this man had himself tormented people all his life and tyrannized over his whole family. The impression obtained from the history of his early life was that this man believed his greatness to consist in setting the tone and in compelling his entire family-circle to concern themselves continuously with him. Since his blindness, he could no longer achieve this in the course of his normal business-activity or in the superintendence of the household, but he could accomplish it by continuously referring to his agonizing hallucinations. He had merely changed his tactics. As his sleep was extremely fitful, the impulse to dominate worked at night also. Out of the excitations emanating from the sphere of vision he constructed a supplementary hallucination which gave him the opportunity of binding his wife to him absolutely. He saw (in his hallucination), gypsies rob and maltreat her. On such occasions, in an attack of cruelty and very likely also in revenge for the loss of his eye-sight he would repeatedly wake his wife in order to convince himself of the falseness of his hallucinations and, at the same time, to prevent his tormented spouse from being removed from his proximity.

Just as this patient, through intensive pre-occupation and the development of a hallucinatory capacity, again reasserted his lust for domination after all power had apparently been taken away from him, so my experience teaches me many individuals behave who are subject to hallucinations and whose illness has the same etiology. The following is a splendid case, of an instructive kind, obtained subsequently. A man of good family, of fair education but conceited, stingy and unwilling to meet life, had completely failed in his profession. Too weak to ward off, by himself, the threatening catastrophe or yet to endure it, he turned to drink. A number of attacks of delirium tremens accompanied by hallucinations brought him to the hospital and freed him from the necessity of accomplishing any task. Such a turning toward alcoholism is frequent and intelligible— exactly as indolence, crime, neurosis, psychosis and suicide, represent both the flight of puny, unstable and ambitious men from the anticipated defeat and their revolt against the demands of society. After leaving the hospital he was completely cured of alcoholism and became a total abstainer. His history, however, had become known and his family refused to concern themselves with him, so that there was nothing left for him to do but to make his living by means of poorly-paid navvy work. Shortly after, hallucinations set in and disturbed him in his work. He repeatedly saw a man whom he did not know and who made his work distasteful to him by making mocking grimaces. He did not believe in the reality of this figure. Incidentally, he knew the significance and nature of hallucinations from the period of his alcoholism. One day he threw a hammer at the figure in order to free himself from all doubt. The figure jumped aside nimbly and subsequently gave him a good thrashing.

This remarkable reaction naturally suggests the thought that our patient was occasionally capable of mistaking a real man for an hallucination, just as is described in a passage of Dostoevsky's "The Double".

This case teaches us another thing also. It is not always enough to make a person a total abstainer. He must be transformed into another man, for otherwise he will fall a victim to some other form of evasion, such as, in this instance, hallucination and its disturbing consequences appear to be. Just as in the first case, the position of the patient prevented his removal from the sphere of his family because his prestige-policy would suffer, so in the second the fear of admitting defeat in life, in other words the same prestige-policy, led to a declaration of illness and of taking refuge in a hospital. Only in such a manner can the above be understood, namely that hallucination, like alcoholism previously, was to furnish consolation and be the excuse for the disappearance of ambitious egotistic hopes. This man was only to be saved by freeing him from his isolation and restoring him to the community.

We see here likewise how alcoholism with its power of inducing hallucinations serves both as the material and as a suitable soil for the subsequent development of the latter. Had there not been this previous alcoholic stage some other preoccupation, some other neurosis, would surely have set in.

Our third case dates from a time subsequent to the war and is concerned with a man who after the normal inhuman and frightful war experiences, took ill with manifestations of fugue, great irritability, attacks of anxiety and hallucinations.   He was, at the time, under medical examination in connection with a request for an invalid grant to which he felt himself fully entitled on account of his greatly depreciated power of making a living.   He claimed that frequently, particularly when he was walking alone, he noticed a figure following him and causing him great fear.   All these phenomena taken together with a marked absent-mindedness, had made it impossible for him to accomplish as good work as formerly.

The complaint of reduced capacity for earning a living, of a loss of formerly possessed capabilities was found often after the war, in people who had taken part in it.   It cannot be denied that many people did actually lose a good deal of their working-capacity in consequence of so many years of disuse.   Nevertheless some of that lost capacity could have been regained.   We do not always, however, find preparations whose object is the recovery of lost capabilities.   In some cases it is noticeable, indeed, that hope has been abandoned to an extent quite contrary to common sense.   As soon as we know their previous history, these all turn out to be neurotic individuals of old standing who have always recoiled from decisions and who now, when confronted with new tests, fall back, as on previous occasions, upon a *neurotic stage-fright*.   Their "hesitating attitude" is still further intensified by the lure of a sick-grant, and by the fervent search for a privilege which will obviate both the necessity of further trials and the expenditure of effort.   They look upon this invalid-grant as a sign of tenderness and of petting, a confirmation of the justice of their cause and the injustice of the world. The monetary value seems only of apparent interest to them, merely an admission by society of the extent of their sufferings.   The neurotic manifestations must therefore rise to a point disclosing adequately the patient's inability to work.

Their earlier history removes such people from the suspicion of simulation.   Frequently this is the only evidence.   The patient, in the case before us, had always

been isolated.   He had had no friends, no love-affairs,
and had lived a retired life together with his mother, he
himself completely rupturing all relations with his only
brother.   It was the war that again brought him into
contact with a social group.   The social group itself
would never have succeeded in regaining him.

One day when a grenade burst near him, fear-mani-
festations set in and the above-mentioned hallucination
which is also to be interpreted as fear.   His illness
made it possible for him to again withdraw from a social
group unpleasant to him.   His attitude toward society
had become even more hostile.   The secret revolt had
of necessity to express itself in his profession, for that
in the fullest sense of the word, implied an affirmation
of willingness to co-operate with society.   Weaned even
more than formerly from the desire of co-operating, he
very likely did regard himself as suffering from reduced
capacity for work.   His absent-mindedness rather indicates his lack of absorption in his work.   Society,
whose enemy he had always been (he said to himself),
would now be made to pay for its last attack upon him.
It was to pay him in the form of a pension just as a
conqueror received tribute.   When he returned from
the front he deprived the normal processes of thought
of their validity and took refuge in a hallucination that
would save him.   This remained with him after the war
until he received his pension which, to him, was a
symbol of triumph.   In this, as in the former case, a
cure could only have been attained had a more adequate
adjustment to society been possible.   A disappearance
of the symptoms, such as at times occurs even without
treatment in conditions where a lesser degree of tension
prevails, would only have been an apparent success.

VI

The Study of Child Psychology and Neurosis

Lecture delivered before the International Congress of Medical Psychology and Psychotherapy, 1913

I

IF we were compelled to name a common element in the relations of the child and the neurotic to the environment, we should select lack of independence as that trait. Neither the child nor the neurotic has advanced to the point of being able to cope with the problems of life without the aid of others. The neurotic requires this aid to a far greater degree than the necessities of society exact. What in the case of the child the family naturally perform, that the family, physician and the rest of the environment together do for the neurotic. With the child it is helplessness and weakness, with the neurotic, "being sick" that is selected for the purpose of imposing increased tasks upon the previously mentioned persons, of burdening them with greater requirements or demanding sacrifices on their part for the sake of one's own personal advantage.

The similarity in the *increased demands* of child and neurotic would alone justify our comparison. More important are the results obtained by "comparative individual - psychology", which tells us that in the individuality of a man we must try to find, focussed in one single point, both the past, present, future and the goal. We must assume—our proofs will have to follow after increased study of the subject—the possibility of recognizing the traces of external influences from reactions in the various attitudes and modes of expression, in short from the modus vivendi of an individual.

Starting with this view-point, we insist that our task in individual-psychology is to interpret completed concepts like will, character, affect, temperament, and indeed

every psychic characteristic, in the light of the specific
means at their disposal corresponding to and bringing
to realization, a conceived life-plan.   If proof of illness
is necessary it will appear as the will of a patient to
undergo treatment.   In this way his life-plan, such, *e.g.*
as limiting the sphere of action to the house as in agoraphobia, is tremendously furthered.   The same patient
will probably later on show a desire to give up the
treatment if, in the prosecution of his plan, it seems
necessary for him to utilize some error in the cure.
That is simply equivalent to saying that if an individual
pursues a course with two contrary purposes, he may
still desire the same thing.   The two will-efforts may
also be distributed between two people:—thus if two
people do not do the same thing, it is still the same
(Freschl, Schulhof).   That in this case no knowledge
is to be obtained from an analysis of the phenomena,
can be safely claimed.   What interests us is the existence of the individually-conceived element, the personal
essence, as a preparation anterior to the actual event
and as a goal posterior to it, the event itself being
found at the point of intersection.   In both cases the
sum total of everything necessarily appertaining to the
event—the energy, temperament, love, hate, understanding, lack of understanding, pain and pleasure,
amelioration and lack of amelioration—will all be
present in exactly that degree that the patient regards
necessary for securing the desired outcome.   That the
conscious and unconscious nature of thinking, feeling,
and willing is conditioned by the *urge toward the formation of personality* can easily be proved.   It is in this
way that *repression makes its appearance* and it is to be
interpreted, not as the explanation of the individual ego,
but as the *means* and mechanism employed by it.

The same inter-connections hold, I have shown,[1] for
the determination of character and its rôle in the service
of the personality.   The gradations in the powers inherent in the constitution (of an individual), the child's
evaluation of them and the experiences obtained from the
environment, influence both the goal set and the life-
line.   *As soon as both are definitely fixed*, character and
instincts will be seen to fit into them exactly.   We must not,
of course, off-hand regard every departure or variation

[1] Adler, *The Neurotic Constitution* : London, Kegan Paul.

in the means adopted, as indicating a fundamental difference in the purpose of the psychic life. No matter how great the dissimilarity between a hammer and a pair of tongs we can put in a nail with either. In neurotically-disposed children of the same family we, at times, see one striving for domination in the family by defiance, the other by submissiveness. A five-year-old boy suffered from the habit of frequently throwing everything he could lay his hands on out of the window. After he had been thoroughly punished he took ill, possessed of a *fear* that he might again throw something out of the window. By the utilization of these symptoms he succeeded in chaining his parents to his side and of becoming their master. One of my patients, until the appearance of a brother, had been a frightfully spoiled child. His antagonism to his younger brother, for a time, took the path of defiance and laziness and so that he might regain the attention of his parents and chain them down, he developed an enuresis and refused all nourishment. He succeeded in this way in displacing the younger child. Having gained his object he became an exceedingly pleasant, industrious boy, but since to retain his favoured position permanently, he had to live under great tension, he developed a severe *compulsion-neurosis*. A markedly developed *fetichism* easily betrayed the main basis of his operations, which was unmasked as an arrangement *for depreciating woman through fear of her*. *The supremacy* this patient tried to obtain through violent aggressiveness, was obtained by his at one time favoured younger brother, more easily by a marked display of amiability. A slight tendency toward stuttering revealed in the latter, likewise, the lines of defiance, ambition and the feeling of fundamental insecurity.[1]

Thus the entire course of psychic life, that of neurotic will, feeling and thinking and the relation of neurosis to psychosis, exhibits itself in the form of a completed arrangement of long standing, as a method for the triumphant overpowering of life. Its beginnings invariably take us back to early childhood. It is during this period that, from hints thrown out by our constitution, and from the nature of the psychical framework of the environment, we should look for the first tentative

---

[1] Cf. Appelt, "Fortschritte der Stottererbehandlung"—in *Heilen und Bilden*.

attempts leading subsequently to the ever-impelling *goal of superiority*.

In order to understand in what the arrangement of the life-system consists, let us visualize the manner in which the child confronts life. Whatever be the epoch in which we care to place the first beginnings of consciousness, it must clearly be at a period in which the child has already collected some experiences. Now it is of the greatest significance to remember that this collection of experiences can only then succeed if the child already has some goal in its mind. Otherwise life would be a meaningless groping and every evaluation impossible ; it would be senseless for us to speak of necessary groupings, of the application of higher viewpoints, of interconnection or of utilization (of experiences). Every evaluation would be lost if, in a purely fictitious mass of matter, a fixed goal were absent. Consequently it ought to be clear *that nobody really permits experiences as such to form, without their possessing some purpose.* Indeed experiences are moulded by him. That simply means that he gives them a definite character, being guided by the way in which he thinks they are going to aid or hinder him in the attainment of his final goal. What is active within our experiences and continuously at work, is the life-plan with its goal. This it is that gives us the impression that former memories can encourage or frighten us, memories we can only understand and properly evaluate after we have recognized in them some guiding voice.

At whatever point in the life of the child, or during anamnesis, we undertake the examination of an experience or a memory, we find the manifestation as such telling us nothing. In itself it is multiple in meaning. Every interpretation must be read into it and demands proof. That is equivalent to saying that what interests us, *does not inhere in the phenomenon itself* but lies, one might say, in front of and behind it ; that we can only then understand a psychic manifestation if we have previously intuitively felt it to possess a life-line. A life-line, however, must have at least two points and our first task then becomes the union of these two points of psychic life. In that way we obtain an impression which is then either extended or limited by the addition of new elements. What occurs in this process is perhaps

best to be compared with a *portrait-painting* and its value
to be measured not by fixed rules but by what it actually
represents. Sometimes the attitude takes on a plastic
form, as in the case of one of my patients suffering
from attacks of hysteria accompanied by loss of consciousness, paralysis of the arm, and amaurosis. An
examination showed that *in order to keep a secure hold
upon her husband*, she had, in addition to successive
attacks every day, developed marked suspicions against
everybody, particularly against physicians. To demonstrate to her graphically her hostility to the world, I
told her that she was like a person who, *from some distance, stood* warding off people with outstretched hands.
Thereupon her husband, who was present throughout
the treatment, informed me that *is exactly what had
happened during her first attacks;* she had suddenly
stretched out her hands as though to ward off someone.
The patient's first attacks began at a time when she
suspected her husband of unfaithfulness. As was disclosed through anamnesis the patient was then behaving
as she had done in childhood when, on one occasion
being left alone for a short time, she had almost become
the victim of an attempted rape. Only when these
two widely separated manifestations are connected, do we
first get an impression and realize—and this is contained
in neither of the two phenomena—that *she is afraid of
being left alone!* As such a possibility she feels is now
to present itself again, she directs against it the whole
force of her valuable and useful accumulated experiences.
We now for the first time are in a position to realize
what we should have assumed at the beginning, that
the following conclusion *has been drawn by her from her
childhood experience:*—a girl should always have some
one near her. At that period her father could alone
serve that purpose. He served all the better because
all thought of sexual connection was, at that early stage,
excluded and because he represented a counter-balance
to her mother who was extremely partial to her older
sister.

The above considerations, which I and my co-workers
have frequently discussed, adequately demonstrate the
untenability of other interpretations, that of the French
school who aim to explain the illness as due to former
experiences and those of Freud and particularly Jung,

who emphasize the point mentioned above as though the patient were the victim of some form of earlier recollections. The later modifications of this theory are more in consonance with the actual conflict but still suffer from a defective understanding of the patient's life-line. For both the event and the actual conflict are held together by an activating life-line. The goal that continually holds the patient in its grip has led *at one point to the making of an experience and at another to the lifting of an event into the realm of an individual experience and conflict.*

For psychology, particularly for child psychology, it follows as a necessary corollary that we are always to draw interpretations and conclusions from the entire context and never from a single fact.

Pursuing our individual-psychological interpretation of the above case it is apparent that but slight insight into the disease was gained by knowing that the patient was afraid of being alone. A nervous condition like the latter has a multiple significance and a few facts tell us little. One fact must be connected with another. The early childhood memories of our patient are permeated with thoughts and feelings of rivalry against her sister. These memories rise to the surface more specifically in connection with the fact of her sister always accompanying (her parents), while *she had to remain home alone.* We here find in an infantile recollection given by the patient as her earliest, the same theme often recurring, and the likelihood of our assumption about the patient's life-line is increased. Can, however, another of the patient's symptoms, the sporadically occurring and 'splitting' headache be explained on this interpretation? And why does this pain always occur during the menstrual flow? In anamnesis the statements of the patient suggested that this symptom manifested itself shortly after a scene with her unjust mother. Her mother had seized her by the hair and the patient who was having her menses at the time, ran directly to the freezing river flowing past the estate, in the hope of either getting ill or dying. Such attacks of rage, designed to hurt another person and going so far as to endanger the patient's own life, she had frequently witnessed in the case of her older brother. But in imitating her brother's behaviour she had at the same time sinned, in a marked manner, against a rule demanding unconditioned obedience from a girl : she had been in ice-cold water in winter during her menses! Her rage had carried her beyond her feminine nature! Although she did not understand her procedure, and fell back on causes and activities lying on the surface, she was in reality making a résumé along the following lines : my brothers revolted and became the masters of the house ; my sister enjoys the favour and love of my mother ; I am a girl, the younger sister, in fact, and yet I am left alone ; sickness and death can alone prevent my humiliation! *The longing for equality* is so definitely expressed in this mood and its corollaries that it would have been superfluous for it to have become conscious. The result obtained by its expansion is in itself sufficient. Other reasons admittedly exist explaining why this situation should remain in the unconscious. There is really no need for the mechanism becoming conscious. A full consciousness of the process might indeed jeopardize the desired success. It would be impossible for the personality of this girl to remain intact, were she to behold with her own eyes what we know, that the main presupposition of her life, her life-plan, is based upon a deeply-rooted feeling of the *inferiority of woman!* In order to protect herself against such an admission she draws from all her experiences the moral that seems to attach to them, that *to maintain her importance she must not be left alone!* When, consequently, she fears the recognition of her importance and her influence and hold upon her husband slipping from her, *the offensive* and *defensive mechanism* developed all this time and to whose most important element we give the name neurosis, comes immediately into action to demonstrate first, the need of her power and finally to regain in appearance at least, her former dominance. *She must not be left alone.*

Having now forged forward to the central point of all our action, feeling and thinking, with the psychic physiognomy of the patient thus sharply outlined, as a natural corollary of this very distinctness of the psychic portrait, a large number of additional characteristics and individual peculiarities follow. The fear of being alone would necessarily have driven her to seize

E

upon the most obvious weapon—anxiety. The question has but to be put, to obtain its corroboration. For instance, an attack of fear regularly supervenes whenever she sits alone in the back of a carriage while her husband drives. This symptom-complex is the answer to the feeling of subordination, to the exclusion of her will, the *absence of the required "resonance"*. She regained her calm only when she also sat in front. The tectonic form of this attitude demands no further discussion. Indeed it becomes more clear when we discover that these fear-attacks occur at every turn in the road, at every encounter with other carriages. She would then immediately seize the reins held by her husband, although realizing that she was the unskilled one and he the practised driver. She was also seized with fear when the horses ran fast. Her husband would on such occasions in order to tease her, spur the horses on to even greater speed. Then her fear-weapon deserted her! It is interesting and important for our understanding of apparent cures to see what has happened : the attack of fear did not take place lest her husband continue to urge the horses on ![1]

A new and highly significant insight has thus been obtained without trouble. We find ourselves consequently in a stronger position when called upon to answer the following quite justified question :—why in her striving for equality with man did not the patient reach the point of herself seizing the reins? Her whole past answers this unhesitatingly :—she *has in fact no confidence of obtaining this equality with man* and falls back consequently upon the alternative of using man as a means, as a support, as a protector, *in order thus to establish her superiority over him.*

II

The study of the psyche must like the study of pedagogy be prepared to rely more than it has hitherto done upon the results of neurology and psychiatry. There is no need of my dwelling upon this point before so well-qualified an audience. Similarly psycho-therapy

[1] In the treatment of war - neuroses the strong - current specialists, hypnotists, and charlatans were led astray by such apparent successes; with them of course both patients and science.

induces us to attempt the investigation of the psychic life of children. If our assumption, as I have tried to show again to-day, be correct, that life's experiences, the teachings of the past, the expectations of the future, are all *grouped* around the fictive life-plan formed in childhood, that what is required is but a slight falsification of accounts, a little *autism*, (*this being probably its purpose*), to restore the old lines and give either open or disguised expression to our intensified aggressiveness against the demands of society, then there remains nothing for us to do, if we desire to eradicate the consequences of the life we have been living in our phantasy, but to resort to a thoroughgoing *revision of this infantile system*. The *synthetic view this necessitates*, I have, I believe, placed in the proper light by insisting that *symptoms, traits of character, affects, evaluation of the patient's personality and his sexual relations must all be given the same position as the neurosis and psychosis viewed as complete units.* They are all means, contrivances, sleight-of-hand performances subserving the tendency which impels what is below to force itself above. In a patient's experience of the vicissitudes of life, as well as in the manner in which the practitioner is moved by the contemplation of the psychic physiognomy, the impression of *increased tension* is always present, taking the form of a kind of *maliciousness* that has sprung up between the patient and the world and suggesting the means to be employed if he hopes to successfully overwhelm it. We are really describing infantile circumstances and the child's psyche, in demonstrating *how fear has become a weapon in the service of self-love;* how an individual personal compulsion has been posited *in order to cancel the alien compulsion of society*, the latter represented by what we have spoken of as the *hesitating attitude* when a decision is to be formed ; when activity is *limited to a small circle, when there is an unwillingness to play the game*, and a desire to *remain alone* or finally, when *ideas of greatness* are found. It would be utterly wrong to interpret all these manifestations, without exception, as infantile traits. What we actually perceive is that an individual who feels weak, be he child, mature person or savage, is forced to take recourse to the same methods. Their discovery and training takes us back to the *childhood of an individual.* There we

know it is not direct assault or action that promises
best success but obedience, submission and the various
forms of childish defiance such as refusal to sleep or
eat, indolence, uncleanliness and the manifold forms of
definitely demonstrable weakness.   In certain respects
our civilization resembles childhood :—it gives the weak
special privileges.   But if life is the continuous struggle
the neurotically disposed child by his demeanour seems
to think it is—this being his main presupposition—then
it inevitably follows that every defeat, every fear of
an impending decision must entail a nervous attack,
serve as a weapon, as a sign of revolt of a man who
feels his inferiority.   The *hostile attitude of the neurotic*
which from childhood gives him a definite orientation,
is reflected in hyper-sensitiveness, intolerance to every
form of compulsion including that of civilization itself
and in the insistent striving singly to defy the whole
world.   It is this same attitude that repeatedly spurs
him on to transcend the limits of his power, resembling
in this respect a child who experiments until burnt by
the fire or becomes bruised by knocking itself against
the table.   The re-inforced attitude of hostility, of
competing and comparing, planning and day-dreaming,
the artificial training of technical tricks of the organs
and finally the obtrusive, defiant and sadistic stirrings,
the belief in magic, the idea of god-likeness, the admirable *evasions taking the form of perversions* originating
in fear of one's partner, all these are regularly found
in children who have grown up either under an unbearable feeling of pressure, under conditions making for
softness and effeminacy or with retarded development
of body or mind.   An exceptionally large *coefficient of
safety* makes possible a progress upward and protects
the individual from defeat.   Yet at the same time, as
if by *some miracle, all kind of obstacles*[1] *force their way
between the patient and the fulfilment of his task.*   Among
those playing a decisive part and assuming the rôle of
an excuse is illness.   Unimportant details, over-evaluated
as in the compulsion-neurosis, are carried along without
serving any purpose until the proper time for action
has been wasted.

    It cannot be denied that this heightened incitement

[1] Cf. the chapter on "The Problem of Distance, a fundamental Element
in Neurosis and Psychosis ", in this volume.

toward certain success does occasionally lead to excellent results. But what we nerve-specialists behold is generally a sad *ut aliquid fieri videatur*, in which the natural meaning of organs must be falsified so that the brakes can be applied to their functions. The weak man is likely in his fanaticism to pervert every function. To evade a demand of reality, to give the semblance of suffering a frightful martyrdom, thought stops and brooding is substituted. *An artificially constructed system interferes with the night's rest, preparing, in this way, for tiredness in the day-time and consequent inability to work.* The sense-organs, mobility, the vegetative apparatus lose their functions by means of the operation of ideas with a definite bias and the purposive directing of the attention into other channels. The ability to identify one's self with harrowing sensations gives rise to pain ; fixation upon nauseating memories to nausea and vomiting. Through a long prepared tendency whose object is the careful evasion of a sex partner, strengthened by ideals, arguments and lofty demands of like import, the capacity for love, sufficiently narrowed in scope to begin with, is then entirely destroyed.

In many cases the specific individuality of the patient demands so peculiar and circumscribed an attitude toward the problem of love and marriage, that both the type and the time of the illness can almost be said to be determined beforehand. To what an extent such a life-plan goes back to childhood may be gathered from such instances as the following :—

I. A woman about thirty-four years old who a few years before had become ill with agoraphobia, was at the time of treatment still suffering from fear of railroads. It was enough for her to be in the neighbourhood of a railroad station to be seized with a violent attack of trembling, forcing her to turn back. These and similar occurrences suggest the idea of an *obstacle* as though she were confined within the limits of some *magic circle*. Her earliest recollection was a scene between herself and a younger sister in which she tried to usurp the latter's place. The multiple meaning of this occurrence is clear. If we were to draw a line from this early incident to the railroad-phobia, the last of her manifestations, and compare the two as though implying that she was trying to compete with the railroad as she had with her sister, then we would immediately realize that the patient was avoiding those places where her desire for domination found no encouragement. She remembered many such instances in connection with her demeanour toward her older brothers who always forced her to obey. We may consequently expect that this patient will in life try to dominate women and withdraw from the authority of the man, be he driver or the locomotive engineer and will eradicate love and marriage from her programme of life. During girlhood she was accustomed for long periods of time to walk through her estate whip in hand and strike the male servants. We must expect occurrences that clearly imply attempts to treat man as a subordinate. Practically in all her dreams men appear in the form of animals and are either conquered or put to flight. Only once in her life and then only for a short time, did she come into close contact with a man. He turned out, as might have been expected, to be a weakling, was homo-sexual and used his impotence as an excuse to break his engagement. Her railroad-phobia was the equivalent of her fear of love and marriage. She dared not trust herself to the authority of a stranger.

II. The mechanism of the "masculine protest" can, of course, be studied in childhood also. It manifests itself with especial clearness among girls. The direction taken by the expansion-tendency is found in many variations, and we soon discover to what a white heat the actual expectations and tensions of the child in relation to its environment are aroused. In no case have I ever found this *masculine delirium* to be absent.

From this *feeling of curtailment* there develops regularly the fanaticism of weakness, thus opening a door to the understanding of all the child's forms of hyper-irritability, negativism and neurotic artifices. An otherwise healthy girl of three years showed the following manifestations:—continuous trials of strength with the mother, frightful sensitiveness to every form of compulsion and relegation, stubbornness and defiance. Refusal to take food, constipation and other revolts against the ordinary household arrangements took place continually. Negativism developed to a degree that it became almost unbearable. Thus one day, when her mother suggested to her gently that she should take her afternoon tea the following monologue occurred: "If she says milk then I'll drink coffee and if she says coffee then I'll drink milk!" Her longing to be like a man was frequently indicated. One day she stood in front of a mirror and asked her mother: "Did you always want to be a man also?" As the impossibility of any change in sex became clear to her, she suggested to her mother that she would like to have another sister but under no conditions a brother; that when she was grown-up however, she would only have boys. Later on, she still betrayed an unquestionably high estimation of the male.

III. Because of its exceptional clarity let me give the following details from the life of another healthy girl three years old: Her favourite occupation consisted in dressing herself in the clothes of an older brother, never in that of her sister, at least not at the beginning. One day, when on a walk with her father, she stopped in front of a boys' clothing-shop and tried to persuade him to buy her some boy's clothes. When he pointed out to her that a boy did not wear girl's clothes, she pointed to a little cloak that might, at a pinch, be made suitable for a girl and asked that she at least be allowed that. In this instance we have what is a not infrequent change in the form assumed by the main path (of character), one at the same time dependent upon the masculine terminal goal and one which insists that even the *semblance* of being a man *suffices*.

In these cases, which I consider typical, and in both of which we observe a fairly general type of development, it is essential to ask the following question. What method has pedagogy heretofore offered for reconciling one half of mankind with an unalterable condition which it dislikes? For one thing is clear — that if such a reconciliation is not successful, we shall at all times have before us the condition which I have just discussed in detail; a permanent feeling of inferiority will continually give occasion for dissatisfaction and lead to various attempts and contrivances for proving one's own superiority *in the face of all* obstacles. In this fashion arise those weapons in part connected with reality, in part of an imaginary kind, that form the external picture of the neurosis. That this condition has advantages, that it enables a person to live in a more intensive and subtle manner, is not to be pleaded when our task is that of pondering over some means to be adopted for cancelling the far greater disadvantages. This mood with its feeling of inferiority at one pole, and its longing for quasi-masculine recognition at the other, is still further intensified when the girl is relegated to the background by the boy, when she sees her possibilities of development curtailed, and when the female molimina, menses, child-bearing and climacteric, with their new disadvantages, appear. *It is well-known that these periods are decisive in neurotic revolts and we may consequently predict these revolts beforehand.* Although one of the roots of neurotic troubles has thus been laid bare, we must unfortunately admit that neither in our pedagogic nor in our therapeutic equipment, has any method been found of preventing the consequences of this natural situation and that imposed by society. From our point of view we may provisionally draw the following conclusion :— the necessity of impressing upon the child early, both prophylactically and therapeutically, the unchangeableness of the organic sexual character; that the disadvantages are *not* to be regarded as *unconquerable* but to be looked upon as difficulties inherent in life which others know both to appreciate and, if need be, to battle against. With that I think the uncertainty and resignation present to-day in woman's work will disappear and with it, that exaggerated desire for recognition that so frequently makes her appear inferior.[1]

IV. This is the case of a ten-year-old boy. I give it to show how, after poison has once entered social relationships, in this instance the masculine protest of the female sex, it can also pass over to the other sex, to the boy and there induce the same manifestations. It is to be assumed from the very beginning considering the well-known nature of man, that the boy not only feels himself honoured by the high estimation sometimes openly expressed, at other times, indicated by social conditions, but that he also feels more duties

---

[1] Cf. Schulhof, *Individualpsychologie und Frauenbewegung* (Reinhardt, Munich, 1914).

imposed upon him.   Consequently, in his case, the tension in his relation to the world is also increased.   This tension, in so far as it has given rise to actual achievements, has produced our culture the latter being, to a large extent, based upon it.   Any normal pressure that bars the road of cultural aggressiveness, suffices for bringing to the front powerful hostile attitudes, maliciousness, lust for power, phantasies.   The boy frequently is afraid of not fulfilling his duties properly, of not being able to obtain that degree of recognition he feels necessary for masculine perfection.   We therefore find very early, in cases of organ-inferiority, among depressed and petted children, the beginning of plan-weaving, and a haste and greed in the pursuit of superiority *whatever* the difficulties.   *This often leads consequently to a utilization of their weakness, a general hesitating attitude, a leaning toward doubt and vacillation, an ever recurring order to retreat; or again it may lead to an open or concealed revolt and a definite unwillingness to play the game.   Here we have come to the basis of the neurosis and should stop to contemplate the damage inflicted.*

The next case concerns a very near-sighted boy who, in spite of all his efforts, was not able to cope with a two-year-old sister.   His aggressiveness showed itself in numerous quarrels.   Over his mother he likewise had no influence.   The father, who in importance and influence dominated the others, kept strict discipline and frequently swore at what he termed "woman-rule".   The boy in every way resembled the father, as I shall prove later on.   In his somewhat hard-pressed situation it was not quite so easy to bring positive proof of his former equality with his father.   On account of his short-sightedness he generally had bad luck in his boyish exploits.   On one occasion when he wanted to make use of his father's type-writer, his father rather abruptly called a halt to this scientific pretension.[1]   The latter, a passionate hunter, occasionally took the boy with him, and this finally seems to have become the particular masculine attitude proving to the boy his equality with his father and his superiority over "the females".   Whenever he was not taken along the boy took ill with enuresis, his father always becoming fear-

---

[1] This appears to us, contrary to the opinion of others, not as an experience but as indicating the relation between father and son.

fully agitated in consequence.   Later a night-attack
occurred whenever the father exercised his authority over
the boy.   These inter-connections were brought to light
after several conversations with the boy and it was
furthermore discovered that *enuresis had been made
possible by bringing together the necessary elements in
dream-hallucinations.*   The suffering quite clearly represented a violent revolt directed against the father.
The boy would generally dream, either before or after
his night attack, that his father (who had not taken
him on the hunt), had died.   When asked about his
plans for the future he answered that he wanted to
become an engineer like his father and have a housekeeper.   I asked him whether, like his father, he did
not wish to marry.   He dismissed this suggestion with
the remark that women were of no value and were only
interested in finery.   The prepared attitude that this
boy was going to take, his arrangement of life, is thus
clearly discernible.

V. Similar and yet entirely different, were the manifestations of the masculine protest encountered in a boy
of eight years suffering from status lymphaticus and
who was somewhat retarded in his intellectual and
bodily growth.   He came under my care on account
of masturbation - compulsion.   His mother devoted
herself almost entirely to the younger sisters and brothers
and left him in the care of servants.   His father was a
man of quick temper always giving orders.   The boy's
inferiority feeling showed itself in a timid retiring nature
and in a grateful attitude to all who paid any attention
to him.   The most far-reaching compensation he found
in an untiring interest in juggler's tricks to which his
attention had been directed in connection with fairy
tales and cinema performances.   Far more than other
children, did he succumb to their influence and he was
always prepared to find a magic wand that would take
him to fairy-land.   He deceived himself to such an
extent, with a partial realization of this idea, that he
always allowed others to do everything for him, this
being in reality a distorted picture of what he saw in his
father who was likewise compelling everyone to serve
him.   Along this path he could proceed only if he remained *clumsy* and *incapable*.   Therefore he remained so.

The masturbation was discovered after some time by the mother who, thereupon, again turned her attention to the boy. He gained, in this way, an influence over her and his importance considerably increased. In order not to lose it again he would have to continue masturbation. *So he continued it.*

His goal, that of being the equal of his father, showed itself incidentally in a desire, partaking of the nature of a compulsion, which led him to wear the stiff hat of grown-up people—just like little children who desire to be grown-up—and also of holding cigarette-butts in his mouth.

Permit me to briefly extend the knowledge of the neurotic manœuvres developed in childhood to the history of mankind. The belief in personal and alien magic properties was far more definitely met with formerly than to-day, but it is to-day likewise the almost general pre-supposition of human behaviour and of deficient belief in one's self, *i.e.* of the feeling of inferiority. The masculine neurotic's fear of his wife and his maliciousness, find their analogies in witch-mania and witch-burning; the female patient's fear of the man and his masculine protest, in fear of the devil and of hell, in attempts to practise witch-craft. By humiliating woman her present ingenuousness in love suffers and our education, in the main, aims at creating a mutual attraction instead of evaluation. In endeavouring to forcibly impose man's authority we are far less likely to further a psychic hygiene than to encourage illusory thinking.

Concluding Remarks

I. The organic and psychic mechanism which confronts us at every point as the "incitement to the positing of a goal", exists preformed in our conception of "life". Life insists that we act. Through action we establish the *final character of psychic life.*

II. The *uninterrupted attraction* that striving after a goal gives us, is conditioned in man by his feeling of curtailment. What we call instinct is in fact the path (of life) and can be shown to be oriented toward some goal. The conative faculty, in spite of apparent contradictions, is ready to forge forward toward this *integrated* goal.

III. Just as an *organ inadequately* prepared for the work it is called upon to do, creates an unbearable situation, and becomes the cause of innumerable attempts at *compensation* until finally it feels itself strong enough to meet the demands of the environment, so the psyche of the child, in its doubt, turns to the store-house containing the accessories to the powers that are to serve as the superstructure of its feeling of uncertainty.

IV. The foremost task in the study of the psychic life is to reckon with the tentative attempts and exertions of strength, growing out of the constitutionally given *powers* and the initial and subsequently well-tested efforts for utilizing the environment.

V. Each psychic phenomenon must therefore be interpreted as *a partial manifestation of an integrated life-plan*. All explanatory attempts that refuse to follow this course and, instead, attempt to penetrate into the child's psychic life, to analyse the manifestation itself and not its synthesis, must be regarded as unsuccessful. For the "facts" of the child's psyche are not to be taken as *finished products* but rather as preparatory movements in the direction of a goal.

VI. According to this view nothing consequently takes place without *subserving some tendency*. We shall therefore attempt at this point to call attention to the following guiding principles which we consider the most important.

Realities.—(*a*) The development of a capability for attaining superiority.

(*b*) Coping with the environment.

(*c*) The feeling that the world is hostile.

(*d*) The amassing of knowledge and piling up of achievements.

(*e*) Use made of love and obedience, hatred and defiance, of community feeling and the lust for power.

Imaginary.—(*f*) Development of the As-If (phantasy, symbolic successes).

(*g*) Use made of weakness.

(*h*) Procrastination in making decisions. Search for protection.

VII. The unquestioned presupposition for these lines of direction is to be found in one factor — *a high-set goal* of omnipotence and god-likeness, that must remain in the unconscious in order to be efficacious. Depending upon the experiences and constitution of the individual this goal may, in a marked degree, take a concrete shape and in this form rise into consciousness as psychosis. The unconscious nature of the power-goal is conditioned by its unbridgeable contradiction with the real demands of the community feeling.

VIII. The most common form in which it appears, although when necessary other apparently contradictory ones are to be found, is the scheme "man . . . woman" and hints at the sum total of all the powers the child wishes to possess. The contrast contained therein is, as a rule, the feminine element interpreted as hostile and to be conquered.

IX. All these phenomena are very prominent in a neurotic individual because the patient has to a certain extent, through his attitude of hostility, withdrawn himself from a thorough revision of his false infantile judgments. His ingrained solipsistic standpoint is of great help to him in this connection.

X. We ought not to be surprised, therefore, if every neurotic behaves as if he were always called upon to furnish evidence for his own superiority in general and for that over his wife specifically.

VII

The Psychic Treatment of Trigeminal Neuralgia

(1911)

THE *individual-psychological* method perhaps more than any other possesses characteristics of a definite kind and it is essential thus to limit its field carefully. That it is only of value in diseases of psychical origin is to be understood from the beginning. The possible psychic utilization of the material at hand ought, at the same time, not to be complicated by any intellectual derangements such as imbecility, mental deficiency or deliria. How and to what an extent, psychosis is amenable to treatment must remain an open question; but it certainly yields to analysis, shows the same main principles as neurosis, and may become of tremendous service in the study of *abnormal psychical* attitudes. That cases of psychoses complicated by intellectual degeneration, and which had made no progress, can upon more intensive application of the method of individual-psychology, both improve and be cured, I can demonstrate from my own experience.

If the field included in the individual-psychological method is thus to be fully utilized, it is of primary importance to know whether there is any possibility of recognizing a psychogenic disease.

The scientific conviction of the psychogenic origin of the typical psycho-neuroses, neurasthenia, hysteria and compulsion-neuroses, is so firmly established that criticisms are only hesitatingly advanced. The most important is that which stresses the *constitutional factor* and groups all manifestations as inherited degeneration, including therein both functional, organic and psychic phenomena, *but not taking into consideration the transition from organ inferiority to the development of a neurotic psyche.* *That this transition* does not always take place and lead, like other transitions, *to genius, crime, suicide, psychosis,* I demonstrated long ago.[1] In that and other

[1] Adler, *Studie über die Minderwertigkeit der Organe* (1917).

works I came to the conclusion that inherited inferiorities of gland or organ, if they make themselves felt psychically, were inducive to a neurotic disposition, *i.e.* if *they caused a child with some inherited stigma to feel a sense of inferiority in relation to his environment.*[1] The decisive factor in such a case would be *the situation* in which *the child* finds itself and its personal appraisement of this *position* with its naturally infantile errors. Upon more careful investigation, the neuroses show themselves to be not so much disposition as *position - diseases*. In this way external signs of degeneration, if they have led to any disfigurement or ugliness, or if they represent externally visible indications of a more deeply rooted organ-inferiority and unite with them, may, apart from their objective symptoms, evoke *a feeling of inferiority and uncertainty in the child's psyche.* For instance, deformed ears with inherited auditory anomalies, colour-blindness, astigmatism or other refraction anomalies accompanied by squinting, etc. In a similar way will organ inferiorities operate, particularly if it is not life that is threatened but the possibility of psychic disturbances developing. Rachitis may interfere with the development of stature and thus become the cause of marked shortness and plumpness of figure ; rachitic deformities — flat-feet, bow-legs, knock-knees, scoliosis etc., may diminish both the child's mobility and self-esteem. *Insufficiency* of the *suprarenal glands*, the *thyroid gland*, the *thymus*, the *hypophysis*, of the *internal genital glands*, particularly inherited types of unimportant character whose symptoms generally call forth censure more than active intervention, become of momentous significance not only for organic but, above all, for psychic development, by either evoking or suppressing a feeling of humiliation and inferiority. Similarly, *exsudatic diathesis, status lymphatico-thymicus* and *asthenic habitus, hydrocephaly* and slight forms of *imbecility*, all exert a ruinous influence upon both feelings. *Inherited inferiority of the urinary and digestive apparatus* creates both objective symptoms[2] as well as subjective feelings

---

[1] *Adler*, " Ueber neurotische Disposition "—in *Heilen und Bilden* (1914).
[2] *Adler*, " Zur Etiologie, Diagnostik, und Therapie der Nephrolithiasis " (*Wiener Klin. Wochenschr.*, XX, no. 42).
Adler, " Myelodysplasie oder Organminderwertigkeit" (*Wiener Med. Wochenschr.* 1909, no. 45). Among other things this paper treats of the superiority

of inferiority that frequently, due to infantile mistakes, find an outlet in some circuitous fashion ;—in enuresis and incontinentia alvi.   The demands made by the body, the fear of punishment and pain, also lead to exaggerated precautions in eating,drinking and sleeping.[1]

Considerations and demonstrations of this kind relating to the subjective and objective radiations of organ inferiority, seem to me to be of great significance for *they throw light upon the development of neurotic symptoms, particularly upon the development of neurotic character-traits, by the utilization of inherited organ inferiorities*.   At the same time they show the secondary nature of constitutional organ-inferiority and the primary nature of psychogenic factors in the etiology of neurosis.   The actual basis for what might be characterized as the rather tense relation between the organic and psychic, is easily recognized.   It has its roots in *the relative organ inferiority of the child*, even of the healthy child, as compared with the adult.   Among the latter it gives rise, likewise, to a feeling of inferiority and uncertainty, one however that is bearable.   In cases of absolute, permanent and poignantly felt organ-inferiority, those unsupportable feelings of inferiority arise that I have found among all neurotics.   It is a trait *of our civilization that the child is at all times desirous of playing the rôle of the grown-up*, that he dreams and weaves phantasies about just those successes that, from their very nature, present difficulties to him.   A short-sighted individual wishes to see everything, one possessed of auditory anomalies to hear everything ; one afflicted with speech-defects or stuttering, will desire to speak incessantly, one with inherited mucous growths, septum deviations or with adenoid enlargements preventing sniffing, will want to smell continually.[2]

of my view over the subsequent one of A. Fuchs.   Cf. also Zappert, *Enuresis und Myelodysplasie*, published 13 years later :   *Wien. Klin.*, *Wochenschr.* 1920, no. 22.

[1] Jean Paul's *Schmelzle* excellently describes the fear of night, indicates the "safety devices" to be discussed later, and allows us to infer clearly the inferiority of the urinary and digestive apparatus.

[2] In all these cases of organ-inferiority due to a "*qualified inferiority feeling*", altered or refined functionings, valuable enhancements of the impressions of the sense organs, such as increased sensibility, increased sensations of tickling to be detected within the periphery of feeling, are to be interpreted as a changed method of functioning of the organ of inferiority.   The foot is an atrophied hand yet its achievements when adjusted to the ground are quite evident.—Tickling sensations in the nose, in the throat and the air passages, constrictions of these passages, induce.

Slow-moving, plump individuals throughout their lives possess the ambition of occupying the first place just as do second-born or last-born children. A child not particularly nimble - footed will be continually afraid of being late and can be easily urged on by all sorts of reasons to make haste or to run, so that throughout his life he appears to be under the compulsion of indulging in a competitive race. The desire to fly is most likely to occur in children who have already experienced difficulty in jumping. This antithesis between organically conditioned limitations and wish, phantasy and dream, in other words the psychic compensation-strivings, is of so thorough-going a type that *a fundamental psychological law might be deduced from it of the following nature : an indirect reversal of organ-inferiority into psychic compensatory and hyper-compensatory strivings through the subjective sensation of inferiority.*

The external demeanour and the inward psychological behaviour of a neurotically disposed child generally shows, therefore, the indications of this indirect line of evolution at a very early period of childhood. His behaviour, however great the differences in individual cases be, can best be interpreted to imply that he desires to be *"on the crest* of the wave" in all life's relations. *Ambition, conceit,* desire to know everything, to discuss everything, to be distinguished for bodily strength, beauty, distinction in dress, to be the chief member of the family, of the school, to have all attention focused upon him either *by good or bad actions,* all these things characterize the early phases of abnormal development. The feeling of inferiority and insecurity forces its way through easily, expressing itself in *fear* and *timidity,* both to be regarded as neurotic character traits. In this fixation (of neurotic traits), the child is guided by a tendency closely related to ambition, which, put in words, would be :—*I must not be left alone ; someone*

---

ment of flow of secretion by intensified nasal inspiration (desire to smell), these all play a leading rôle in *nervous asthma, spells of sneezing* and probably in *hay-fever.* A delightful description of nervous nasal conditions of irritation and the feeling of inferiority connected with it is to be found in Vischer's *Auch Einer.* The inflation and artificial intensification of this " defect ", to secure one's self against marriage and against entering into social and love relations, are so correctly depicted that we are justified in assuming that the gifted philosopher had derived his facts from actual observation.

(*father or mother*) *must help me ;* people must be friendly
to me ; treat me tenderly ; (here we are to add : for I
am weak, inferior).   All these inward conversations
become the guiding principles of psychic stirrings.   A
permanently irritable *hyper-sensitiveness, mistrust,* and
querulousness, prevent *humiliation* or *slights* from finding
room to develop.   The case may be reversed, and the
child may develop remarkable keenness, *anticipate its
feelings, grope about for all possibilities leading to humiliation,* so that he can *secure himself against* it either by
active intervention in the form of definite precautions,
presence or agility of mind, or by obtaining the pity
and the sympathy which his exaggerated description of
suffering has awakened in the breast of some stronger
individual.   The child may likewise call to his aid real
or simulated illnesses, fainting-spells and death desires,
extending to the point of impulses toward suicide with
the ever-present purpose of either evoking pity or taking
revenge for some humiliation.[1]

The feelings of hate and revenge that burst forth, the
wild anger and *the sadistic desires, the craving to indulge
in forbidden acts, the continual disturbance of educational
plans by indolence, laziness and defiance*—all these are
indications of a neurotically-disposed child's revolt
against imaginary or real oppression.   Such children
make much ado about eating, washing, dressing,
cleaning of teeth, going to sleep and learning ; resent
every reminder to attend to defaecation and urination.
Or they "arrange" accidents, vomiting, for instance,
if forced to eat or urged to go to school ; soil themselves
(by defaecation or urination), develop enuresis so that
people are always around them, see that they are not
left alone or allowed to sleep alone ; interrupt their
sleep to obtain expressions of love, or to be taken into
their parent's bed, in short, do everything to get recognition, resorting either *to defiance or falling back upon the
sense of pity their environment extends to them.*

These facts, as a rule, stand out clearly and are quite
consistent with one another whether they are obtained
from life, from a neurotically disposed child's traits of
character, from the anamnesis of a neurotic or by the clear-
ing-up the dynamics of his symptoms.   Occasionally

---

[1] See Adler—" Ueber den Selbstmord insbesondere im kindlichen Alter "
—in *Heilen und Bilden.*

we have to deal with imagined "child-paragons" who exhibit an astounding obedience.   Every now and then, however, they too betray themselves by some unintelligible outburst of anger; or we may be led on the right track by their hyper-sensitiveness, continuous condition of feeling hurt, copious tears; their various causeless pains and aches (headache, stomach-ache, pain in the legs, migraine, exaggerated complaints of cold and heat, tiredness).   It is thus easy for us to understand how this *obedience, modesty, ever-ready willingness to submit* are but means adopted for the purpose of obtaining recognition and reward, of drawing out expressions of love, just as holds true for the neurotic in the "*dynamics of masochism*" as I have been able to show.[1]

We must now mention a number of manifestations found in the neurotically-disposed child and closely connected with what has previously been described.   They all disclose the desire to annoy parents by obstinate adherence to unnecessary or disturbing activities designed to draw attention to themselves even though this attention take the form of anger.   In such tendencies are to be included some of a playful nature like pretending *to be deaf, blind, lame, dumb, clumsy, forgetful or crazy, stuttering, making grimaces, stumbling, soiling one's self*.   Normal children likewise possess such inclinations, but it requires the diseased ambition, the defiance and urge towards obtaining recognition possessed by the neurotically-disposed person, to enable anyone to adhere for any length of time to such make-believe games and fooleries or actually utilize them.   Such children may either with malicious intent or in order to torment others—but frequently, I will admit, to escape from tyrannical oppression—adhere to and practise, for a long time, disease-symptoms or bad habits either personally experienced or observed, such as biting nails, picking the nose, thumb-sucking, playing with genitals (with the anus, etc.).   Even timidity and fear can be stabilized for these purposes and employed with a definite object, such as not being left alone, of being served by others.   In all these instances the assumption of some corresponding organ inferiority plays a rôle (vide my book on Organ Inferiority).

From these peculiarities of the neurotically disposed child, transitions lead to the symptoms of hysteria, com-

[1] "Psychische Hermaphroditismus" in *Heilen und Bilden*.

pulsion - neurosis, accident - neurosis, accident-hysteria, neurasthenia, convulsive tic, fear-neurosis and to those *apparently* mono-symptomatic functional neuroses (stuttering, constipation, psychic impotence, etc.), all of which, on the basis of my experiences, I regard as *integrated psycho-neuroses*. Those manifestations accepted during childhood, without full realization (of their nature), *on the basis of some reflected attitude* and whose purpose is to reach the line of least resistance for *the well-equipped aggressive instinct*, are all provided with typical superstructures and elaborately endowed with the neurotic's symptoms. To what an extent increased suggestibility (Charcot, Struempell), hypnotic condition (Breuer), the hallucinatory character of the neurotic psyche (Adler), *i.e.* identification, come into question, I shall not discuss here. It is certain, however, that every hallucinatory attack, as well as the permanent neurotic character, develop uniformly under the influence of an infantile attitude, an attitude that has taken on abnormal forms owing to childish wish-phantasies, errors and false evaluations.

The wish-phantasies of the child possess by no means merely a platonic value. They represent the expression of a psychic stimulus which completely dictates the child's attitude and so necessarily his acts. This impulse is differentiated into grades of intensity and grows enormously in the case of neurotically disposed children, compensating in this way for their increased feeling of inferiority. Investigation will at first bring to the surface, recollections of events ("infantile experience, dreams") toward which the child has assumed a definite attitude. I have already pointed out, in discussing the "aggressive instinct" (l.c.), that the "importance of the infantile experience lies in the fact that it must be interpreted to mean *that the power-instinct and its limitations—(both as wish and as wish suppression)—there find expression;* and that furthermore the contact with the external world, whether it be in the form of non-pleasurable experiences or be due to the expansion of the desire for culturally denied goods, unquestionably occurs *where organ inferiority exists and so compels a transformation of the instinct.*" The perceptible extension of instincts in neurotically disposed children, springs indirectly from the feeling of inferiority, taking the form of a tendency to overcome weaknesses and the longing for triumph and is clearly visible in dreams and wish-phantasies, the hero rôle, the whole attitude being but an attempt at compensation.

In this more deeply hidden neurotic layer, analysis also discloses *sexual wishes and stirrings that, in rare instances, are of an incestuous nature.* We also find attempts at and actual sexual activities, directed toward complete strangers. *These facts, quite unknown in child psychology before the phantastic analyses of Freud, naturally do away definitely with the previous assumption of the child's innocence and purity, yet we will learn to understand them better if we remember the frequently limitless expansion instinct can acquire and the compensatory balance possessed by the neurotically disposed child in the shape of its feeling of inferiority.* In other directions beside that of sex does this uprooting of instinct activities make itself felt. *We meet with intensified instincts of gorging, of seeing everything, of filth, of domination, of sadistic and criminal tendencies, defiance, rage, assiduous reading and extraordinary attempts to achieve distinction for one's self in some way or other.* All these tendencies become really clear only if we are successful in bringing to the surface, the early awakened desire for domination and its various manifestations.

The meaning of this desire for power is : *I want to be a man.* It permeates both boys and girls to such a frightful degree that we are *from the very first, forced to assume that this attitude came to the front to counter-balance the non-pleasurable sensation of not being masculine. The neurotic psyche is, as a matter of fact, under the coercion of a (psychic) mechanism, the psychic hermaphrodism and subsequent masculine protest previously described.*[1] The fixation of the inferiority feeling in neurotically disposed children leads to the compensatory stimulation of instinct activity and constitutes the beginning of that peculiar development of the psyche which terminates in the exaggerated masculine protest. These psychic processes become the cause of the neurotic's abnormal attitude toward the world and impress upon him, to a very marked degree, traits of the kind already mentioned, and which *can be deduced neither from the sexual nor ego instincts.* They, on the contrary, take in him the form of the *ideas of greatness,* frequently actually modifying and obstructing the sexual

[1] Adler, " Psychische Hermaphroditismus " in *Heilen und Bilden.*

instinct and, at times, even opposing that of preservation itself.

Accompanying the contact of the exaggerated instinct-expansion with the culturally denied gratification of instincts, are other traits, feelings of *guilt, cowardice, irresolution, hesitation, the fear of a fiasco, of punishment.* I have described them in detail in my work on *The Neurotic Constitution.* Quite often *masochistic stirrings, exaggerated willingness to obey, to submit, self-punishment,* are discovered and we may infer the nature of the psychic mechanism as well as the earlier history (of the case) from these character-traits. The strongest hindrance to the extension of instinct is encountered when on the border line of the community feeling. This event is in the nature of a reminder and thereafter takes over the task of weighting down the organic instincts with all sorts of obstructions. *The neurotic feels himself a criminal, becomes extremely conscientious and just, yet all the time his attitude is determined by the fiction that he is really wicked, dominated by uncontrollable sex desire, given over to unlimited self-indulgence, capable of any crime or license.* He is in duty bound, consequently, to take specific precautions. Through his one-sided striving for personal power he becomes in fact an enemy of society.

The arrangement of this fiction though clearly overdone, serves *the main object of the neurotic, which is to guard himself against defeat.*[1] The tendencies for security, help to build up a third group of character-traits that are all adjusted to the leading principle which is "precaution". Distrust, doubt are the most prominent of these precautions. *Just as frequently, however, we find exaggerated tendencies toward cleanliness and order, economy and continual examination of people and things, and it is in* consequence of this, that the neurotic never finishes anything.

All these traits interfere with the spirit of initiative, with the development of social responsibilities and are closely connected with the indecision due to a sense of guilt. Everything is previously considered, *all consequences taken into consideration,* the neurotic being in a

---

[1] In this respect the neurotic resembles that character in the Nestroy play who says: "If I once begin!"—"But I never begin!" He is afraid of his own urge toward activity. Cf. also *The Neurotic Constitution.*

continual state of extreme expectation of possible contingencies and his rest disturbed by assumptions and anticipations about the future. A magnificent defence-mechanism pervades all his thinking and acting and *shows itself unfailingly in his phantasies and dreams.* Frequently it is forced to fortify itself *either by some reminder, or by the unconscious arrangement of defeats, forgetfulness, tiredness, laziness and painful sensations of all kinds. A tremendous rôle in this defensive mechanism is played by neurotic fears, expressed in the most varied forms—phobia, anxiety dream, hysteria and neurasthenia and obtruding itself in the form of an obstruction directly or indirectly ("as an example"), in front of the attempted aggression.* The training of all these tendencies making for safety leads at times to a perceptible intensification of the intuitive faculty and intuitive penetration. If not that, it at the very least brings about the semblance of such an intensification. It is upon this that is based the claim of some neurotics to *telepathic faculties, knowledge of certain kinds of predestination, and their possession of the power of suggestion.* These traits then unite with those of the first group, those that had their origin in ideas of greatness. *We must, at the same time, regard the distinctiveness assumed by the ideas of greatness as compensatory and as a defence against the feeling of inferiority.* I am also acquainted with other safety devices among which might be mentioned the following :—*masturbation, serving the purpose of protection against sexual intercourse and its consequences, psychic impotence, ejaculatio praecox, sexual anasthesia and vaginism.* These are always to be found among individuals who are not capable either of devotion to others or the community. In a similar manner infantile errors, functional diseases and pains are given an evaluation and become fixed if they prove to be adapted to strengthening the neurotic in his doubts or keep him away from participation in life. Not infrequently the ball is started rolling *by the question of marriage or the adoption of some profession.* On such occasions, the tendency to seek safety expresses itself in a diseased fashion, the warning-signs often being placed so far apart, that all meaning and connection seem to be absent. The neurotic, however, always acts logically. He begins by avoiding society, imposes all sorts of restraints upon himself, interferes with his studies and his work (by headache for instance); paints the future in the most sombre colours and begins to hoard. At all times he is warned by a hidden voice whispering: " How can a man possessed of such faults and deficiencies as you, with such poor prospects dare make up his mind to such a momentous act!" *What, for lack of a better name, we call neurasthenia, is full of such arrangements and tendencies all aiming at security.* They are absent from no neurosis and show us a sick individual, as it were, on his line of retreat.

A fourth *group* of tell-tale indications of a neurotic attitude consists in the way in which actions, phantasies, dreams, subsidiary details clothed in the language of sex, show the desire to be a man as in group I. In my works on *The Neurotic Constitution* and *Psychic Hermaphrodism* I discussed these facts in detail. *The neurotic is destined to outgrow his actual situation of uncertainty in his search for security.* Uncertainty however is, upon analysis, still shown to exist in the neurotically disposed child's judgments as to his real sex rôle. Many of my male patients had during childhood and often until puberty, feminine features or secondary feminine marks to which afterwards they attributed their feeling of inferiority ; or they had anomalies of the external sexual organs, cryptorchism, adhesions, hypoplasia and other growth-anomalies upon which they felt they could fall back whenever an excuse was required. Photographs and pictures taken of children at a very early age have taught me that the wearing of a girl's dress for a lengthy period of years, laces, necklaces, curls, and long hair evoke this same feeling of insecurity and doubt in a boy. The same in an intensified degree holds true for the threats such as circumcision, and castration, or the falling off or rotting of the penis, with which parents menace their children who are detected practising masturbation. The child's strongest tendency is and always remains the same : to grow up to be a man, a longing which may be symbolized by the male sex organs of the adult. The same longing is manifest in girls where the feeling of inferiority engendered by their situation as compared with boys leads regularly to a compensatory masculine attitude. Thus by degrees the whole world of ideas of the neurotically disposed child, all the relations of society, fall into two groups, masculine and feminine. The wish to play the masculine rôle, the hero's rôle, is present at all times even if, as in the case of girls, it takes the queerest forms. Every form of activity and aggression, of power, riches, triumph, sadism, disobedience, crime are falsely evaluated as masculine just as in the grown-up's world of ideas. As feminine are reckoned suffering, waiting, enduring, weakness and *all masochistic tendencies. These latter when they forge forward in the neurosis, are never to be regarded as end-goals, but as always having as their object—since they are in reality pseudo-masochistic traits—the clearing of the path for masculine triumphs, i.e. for that desire for recognition so prominent in the first group.* The other traits of this (fourth) group belong to the masculine protest—the forcible exaggerations of the sexual feeling and desire, exhibitionist and sadistic stirrings, early sexual maturity and compulsion onanism, nymphomania, spirit of adventure, strong sexual craving, narcism and coquetry. Feminine phantasies (pregnancy and childbirth phantasies, masochistic stirrings and feelings of inferiority), appearing at the same time, serve as reminders that the masculine protest is to be strengthened or security to be obtained against its consequences and frequently takes the shape of the requital commandment : "What you do not wish others to do to you, do not you do to others"![1]—The concept of compulsion is enormously extended, even the merest suspicion of it being energetically resisted by a continuous struggle, so that normal relations like that of love, marriage and every other adjustment are felt as unmanly, *i.e.* as feminine and consequently rejected.

[1] In the case of a man suffering from *asthma nervosum* and who now, after treatment, has for a long time been free from attacks, definite pregnancy phantasies made their appearance as soon as the patient wanted to embark on any undertaking. These pregnancy phantasies accompanied by feelings of oppression in the breast, ended in ideas of greatness :—he became a millionaire, benefactor, saviour of the country, etc. *Accompanying this feeling was the quick breathing that occurs in a race.* The dynamic importance of the pregnancy phantasy is to be sought in its reference to the endurance and suffering of the woman, which is both a self-criticism and at the same time an added irritation : "You are only a woman ! It serves you right if you suffer"! Thereupon follows the masculine protest.—A reinforced scaffolding is here utilizing the pregnancy phantasies and the asthma *in the manner of an anticipatory repentance.* Now he was permitted to be a man and oppose his environment inimically. "I may take greater liberties than others because I am ill". For this illness he thus brings a true proof, an alibi.

Thus in the neurotic, we have *an extremely large number of interconnected character-traits*, which aid or obstruct one another according to a definite plan and which *permit an inference as to the nature of the abnormal attitude. All, in the last analysis, are to be traced back to the exaggerations and false evaluations of masculine and feminine features.* If any criticism is to be passed on the above presentation it is perhaps this, that the arrangement is too schematic, cannot possibly exhaust the exuberant interrelations of single traits but at best give only one part, that however the most significant to be gleaned from the study of the neurotic's character. *Nevertheless I am convinced that, given these facts, it would be legitimate to infer the existence of a psychogenic disease.* Often we are able to prove it. If now I turn to the problem under discussion, *whether trigeminal neuralgia is a disease of psychogenic origin,* I can on the basis of information obtained from diseases similar in nature, answer in the affirmative. The psychical structure of trigeminal neuralgia, its psychical dynamics, are so identical in the three cases examined by me and exhibit so clearly traits of a psychogenic nature, that all criticism is completely disarmed. Of great importance too for our problem is the fact that not merely does trigeminal neuralgia follow the above described main outlines of the neurosis, *but that every single attack represents a transference of some psychical happening.* We can now attempt to explain the relations of the neurotic psyche and the neurotic character to this disease and to individual attacks.

My patient O. St. was a state employé twenty-six years old. He came to me with the information that an operation had been advised for the trigeminal neuralgia from which he was suffering. His illness had already lasted a year and a half. It had seized him one night and affected the right side of his face and had, since then, recurred repeatedly every day in the form of acute attacks. During the last year he had been compelled to take morphine injections every three or four days because of particularly severe pains. This had always relieved him. He had tried a number of treatments which consisted either of medicines containing aconite or of being subjected to electrical and thermal treatments, all without success. He had also been given two alcohol injections which had only served to intensify the pain. A lengthy stay in the south had brought some relief although there too he had had daily attacks. He was now quite dispirited and in order not to ruin his career had resolved to submit to an operation. It was only because his very conscientious surgeon would not promise certain relief from the operation that he had decided to ask my advice.

I had at about this time collected an enormous mass of data concerning the psychic origin of neuralgic attacks and of trigeminal neuralgia and had also been able to make use of older observations. The uniform conclusion to which I had come from analysis and the comparison of individual attacks might be formulated in this way : *trigeminal neuralgia and its individual attacks regularly appear when an affect of rage has been linked with the feeling of humiliation.*[1] Having arrived at this result it was then possible to understand the abnormal attitude of patients afflicted with trigeminal neuralgia and *to recognize the dependent disease manifestations as the equivalents of affect processes.*[2] This was corroborated by a fact obtained within a short time. *The patient was expecting degradation, was, so to say, lying in wait for it, and this concept of humiliation had thus been tremendously enlarged. Now in general in neuroses, in some less in others more, a patient actually looks for and arranges such depreciations in order to draw from them the inference that he must protect himself, that he is not properly appreciated, that he has always been followed by bad luck, etc. Such an attitude characterizes neurosis in general* and not trigeminal neuralgia alone. When analysed and referred back *to some pathological situation of childhood, the psychic habitus of the neurotically disposed child is always clearly visible. It is a feeling of inferiority compensated by the masculine protest.* Coming back to our case, analysis disclosed the following :—

I. *Cryptorchism.*—His own discovery of it. The feeling of inferiority and uncertainty as to whether with this defect he could develop into a mature man. Added to

[1] Cf. the formulation in " Aggressionstrieb " in *Heilen und Bilden.* The formulation could also be :—it takes place in situations in which others have had an affect of rage.
[2] There is no need of wasting a word about the superficiality of those critics of my position who accuse me of being " intellectualistic ".

this are recollections from his 6-8 year concerning sexual attacks upon girls with the purpose of obtaining some light upon sexual differences, and the emotionally tinged recollections of children's games in which he had been the hero, or at least a general or the father of the family, which has the same purport.

II. Apparent or real preference shown to his brother five years younger, who was allowed to sleep in the parents' bedroom. Subsequent to this came recollections of his attempts to get into his parents' bedroom. There were a number of means at his disposal in childhood. First was fear, fear of being alone (pavor nocturnus), which he occasionally succeeded in expressing to such a degree that his mother took him into her bed. Then came *auditory hallucinations* also capable of evoking fear (fear as a means of safety), or noises attributed to burglars which always came from the direction of the parents' bedroom, so that he had to go there to look: at this point he could introduce the game of playing the father, a clear masculine protest against the uncertainty of his sexual rôle. The meaning of this infantile behaviour, which represents the most frequent type of escape from a pathological childhood situation, is now definitely indicated:—"I feel insecure, I am not successful; I am not given sufficient recognition (witness the preference shown to my brother); I must be helped; I wish to be the father; I wish to be a man". As a contrast to this, as we shall see, false evaluation, we should imagine the following: "I do not wish to become a woman"!—The thought, "I wish to become a man", is only made tenable and only becomes bearable when joined to the contrasting thought:—"I might also become a woman" or "I do not wish to become a woman".[1] A third way of circumventing the preference shown the brother, of playing the rôle of the father in order to obtain equality and to learn how adequately to fulfil his sex rôle, secure his manhood, was given by illness, particularly by illness attended with pains. Analysis brought to light, as is so frequently the case, recollections of actual, and of exaggerated pains and simulations of such. We are interested here in their nature. They

---

[1] Among the newer psychologists Julius Pikler, starting from entirely different premises, has come to similar conclusions with regard to " *contrast-thinking* ". Cf. also *The Neurotic Constitution.*

were almost always toothaches. Now for the first time in the analysis do we obtain a feeling of having come to a somewhat deeper understanding *of the reason the choice of the neurosis to be adopted in this particular case, fell upon trigeminal neuralgia.* The patient was a strong healthy boy who probably knew no other pains but toothache. We are thus forced to the assumption that at some point in his life there must have been a phase in which he equated the following conditions :—*pain—feeling of inferiority*—increased recognition by the environment.

We have so laid bare the dynamics of his pathological childhood situation. The possibility of his being forced to play an inferior, painful and feminine rôle has led indirectly to exaggerations of his masculine protest. As such are to be reckoned *defiance* and *obstinacy*, of a type which his mother still recollects with shuddering. Of the many activities that allow the child an opportunity to exhibit defiance, I have already mentioned *eating, washing, teeth cleaning and going to sleep.* It is therefore exceedingly significant that all patients I can think of suffering from trigeminal neuralgia—and this is in agreement with the descriptions of others—have had most of their attacks while eating, washing, teeth cleaning or going to sleep. Attacks also occur when in contact with anything cold. My patient shortly after the first appearance of the disease had retired to the country where his mother lived, thus gratifying an old infantile longing. The mother, carrying to excess her solicitude and love for the sick son, supervised his diet carefully and always provided him with warm water for washing. When he was compelled during his treatment to eat in Vienna he had severe pains ; when he ate at home none occurred. When he had progressed far enough to go to his office he had to live in Vienna, and on the very first day on which he washed himself with cold water in the new residence, he was seized with another attack.

Another group of attacks was connected with *his desire for recognition in society.* In this way seizures could occur either in connection with real, supposed or feared humiliations. He wanted to play the most important rôle at all times, was put out if occasionally he was not included in the conversation or if he could not hear the conversations of others. The scheme of the infantile pathological situation is easily recognizable here:—father, mother and younger brother with himself as the inferior person. The symptoms of fear of society, of agoraphobia found in other neurotics, whose *safety devices against defeat take the form of fear*, or occasionally *vomiting, migraine, etc.* and where *fear of humiliation guides the patient*, is in our case represented by an attack. I know of other instances of trigeminal neuralgia in which *the patient withdrew from all participation in society giving his suffering as an excuse*. In still other examples symptoms such as migraine, nausea, general and apparently rheumatic pains,[1] ischias, blushing and flow of blood to the face, preceded the trigeminal neuralgia.[2]

Sexual considerations played an important part in this triangular situation (parents, brother, ego), and lay at the root of the attacks. His sexual life was both normal and satisfactory. One marked trait was present however that is typical for a large group of neurotics, namely that love became strong *only when a rival made his appearance*, *i.e.* when love came to be connected with the masculine characteristic of robbing and fighting. This trait ran through his entire erotic life. It brought back to him vividly the triangular situation of his pathological childhood, thus showing to what an extent his erotic life had been poisoned by his prestige-seeking policy. While living in the south he met a girl whom he began to court until he found out that her dowry was very small. This sufficed to make him desist; but his love was again inflamed when another applicant for her hand appeared. This increase in love was paralleled by an increase in the severity of the pains that set in; *when, for instance, he saw the two alone and the girl smiled at the latter*, etc. During his treatment we could refer a few of his attacks to this affair; he had pains when the girl told him in a letter that she had had a good time in the company of the other man. A number of attacks were associated with the period

---

[1] Cf. Henschen's theory of the rheumatic origin of trigeminal neuralgia.

[2] The examples of trigeminal neuralgia in ageing people, particularly among women, are especially complicated, most specifically on account of real and imagined humiliations caused by age. That our society treats the ageing woman so inhumanly, constitutes one of the saddest chapters in our civilization. Among my patients, attacks were due to the following:—lack of interest, fear of ridicule, fear of preference shown to other people, the mirror, choice of clothes (she might be laughed at) and expenditures of money which might interfere with her standing and make her poor.

during which his letters were taken away by us.   On this occasion he began to *wonder why the girl had not written for so long a time ; she was very likely having a good time with others*, etc.   Day-dreams and phantasies also appeared.   He would let the girl marry and then incite her to break her marriage vow.   This trait, we will admit, *had become greatly intensified* shortly before his illness *by an unusual circumstance.*   While he was on a short journey a colleague of his had seduced his mistress.   He planned all kinds of revenge.   Into this markedly emotional period of his life fell another event. He had reason to believe that the wife of one of his superiors was making advances to him.   Apparently the husband also noticed it and began to annoy him in the office.   In order not to spoil his career he submitted, though with continual secret revolts.   *The night before the superior's return from his vacation he had the first attack of his trigeminal neuralgia* and one of such severity, that he raved and yelled and could only be calmed by a morphine injection.   He did not go to the office the next day and took out a sick leave in order to undergo treatment.   To all physicians, including myself, he reiterated the wish of returning to his bureau as soon as possible and everything that could be done to facilitate this was promised him.[1]   The alcohol injection was to have restored him to health immediately.   We saw above the effect it had.   But we now know why it so intensified the pain, *for his real unconscious striving had as its object the desire to remain incapacitated for work, and not to return to his office.*   One thought alone he could not suppress, the thought of emerging out of the situation as a man, as victor ; expressed in terms of the infantile pathological situation : *"I want my mother !"* When with her his condition improved a little, but not before he had demonstrated by means of successive and rapidly following attacks, particularly during meals, the extremely dangerous nature of his disease and the possibility of death through starvation thus through fear and fright making his mother even more amenable to his desires.

An analysis of one of his dreams during treatment exhibits the most important conditions for his uncon-

[1] Notice here *the agreement with the dynamics of accident neurosis and hysteria* which likewise appear only in neurotically disposed people.

sciously false attitude and his neurosis. He dreamt as
follows :—

*"I found myself naked in the room of my sweetheart.
She bit my thigh. I cried out and awoke with a severe
attack of my neuralgia".*

The events responsible for this dream occurred the
evening before and were as follows :—the patient had
received a picture post-card from Graz and among those
who had signed it was the name of his brother and the
girl in the dream. Nothing seemed to have any taste
during supper and he had a slight attack. In explanation
of the dream, he added that the girl had been his mistress
for a time but that he had very soon become tired of her
and given her up. A short time before his dream his
brother had become acquainted with her. He had
warned his brother but, as the card indicated, without
any effect. This upset him all the more because he
possessed as a rule great influence with this brother and
had so to speak taken his father's place since his death.

"Naked". He had an aversion to undressing in
the presence of girls. This is clearly connected with
his cryptorchism.

"She bit me in the thigh". In explanation he said
that the girl had all sorts of perverse tendencies and had
once bitten him. The somewhat leading question as to
whether he had ever heard of anyone being bitten in
the thigh, he answered with a reference to the stork
fable.[1]

"I cried out". This he always did in severe attacks.
Then his mother would always come out of the neigh-
bouring room to soothe him and, if necessary, eventually
give him an injection of morphine.

The interpretation of the dream is so apparent that
there is no need of any further detailed discussion. The
patient answered a feeling of humiliation by a train of
thought leading to an attack but yet permitting the
attainment of his symbolical goal, that of dominating

---

[1] This reference will give the experienced psychologist no difficulties.
We are dealing with a patient *whose illness is of a kind to make him fear pain.*
Further inquiries indicated his early knowledge of the pain experienced by
women in child-birth. This pain had been made plausible to him in childhood by the statement that the stork had bitten his mother in the leg. "She
bit me in the thigh" has the following meaning here :—*she has degraded me to
the position of a woman* and by her relation with my brother, humiliated and
emasculated me. We must bear in mind his cryptorchism.

his mother. In other words *he transformed himself into a dominating man.* His emasculating stigma — cryptorchism—would then fall from him and he would be able to exhibit himself naked. He was now a man, need not bow to anyone, was freed from all service even if it lead through the circuitous path of pain. *He safeguards this feeling of masculine superiority — as in his infantile pathogenic situation—by means of pains and isolation.*[1]

The transition in a dream from a feeling of submissive femininity to one of masculine protest is not always found as clearly as in this case. *Particular appearances* at times often mislead even us *into assuming primary homo-sexual tendencies. The masculine rôle played by the neurotics of both sexes in life and in the dream, is explained by the masculine protest. If a rival of the same sex was involved then the victory was often symbolized by the sexual act in which the neurotic, either in a dream or in phantasy, played some kind of a masculine rôle.* The problem of the active homo-sexual individual is, according to my experience, to be interpreted in the same way. There, however, the sexual instinct is placed directly and not merely symbolically, in the service of the lust for power, of the masculine protest. The homo-sexual individual passes from a phase of uncertainty of his sexual rôle to that of sexual inversion. The passive homo-sexual arranges his transference to the feminine, for the purpose of making himself quite definitely felt afterwards; of getting recognition by jealousies, conquests or exactions; above all, however, he makes this transference in order not to disclose his erroneously assumed lack of masculinity in normal love.[2] On the other hand the fundamental problem, the starting point of the psychic hermaphrodism with its subsequent masculine protest is, for the above reason, rendered less

[1] I.e. with apparently "feminine" weapons. I have already pointed out this mechanism, one that can easily mislead us to the conception that the neurosis is entirely a "feminine offering". An examination of *neurotic dynamics* would prevent this error from arising. *"Feminine" final goals just as "masochistic" ones are quite untenable assumptions, are only excuses;* they are "feminine" methods for the "masculine" protest.

[2] Just as the previously mentioned masochist who, by erotic submission, *i.e.* from his point of view, striving for recognition, attempts to awaken the sexual desire of a woman. From this point a number of perversions branch off that have as their object, through over-estimation of the person courted, *to awaken a woman's love and thus conquer her.*

"Put to flight he believes himself hunting". Cf. Adler, *Problem der Homosexualität* (Munich, 1918).

G

visible both in the neurosis and the dream, so that we are in consequence generally compelled to work with fragments belonging to the psychic mechanism and whose complements we have first to find.

The treatment of our patient took place under propitious circumstances. Previous treatments had been unsuccessful. However, much time was necessarily consumed and the patient's career suffered more and more. Fortunately favourable prospects presented themselves of his being transferred to another office where his feeling of being subjected to the tyranny of his hated superior would certainly be lessened. The treatment closed with a provisional success and that has now lasted a number of months. He now works in a new bureau and lives apart from his mother. His friends and acquaintances frequently express their astonishment at his having changed from a violent, restless and quick-tempered man, into a quiet and adaptable one and that he no longer feels his connection with his office to be in the nature of a compulsion. For us this has the specific significance *that his former false attitude has been corrected*, a correction that should not merely prevent attacks but also other forms of neurosis.

My two other cases refer to patients who had passed their climacteric. They developed severe symptoms of the illness when placed in a situation they regarded lowering. They had however been neurotically disposed from childhood. As in our first case, analysis showed, in both instances, organ inferiority, a feeling of inferiority and the masculine protest. Their whole life had been spent under the dominating thought:—I wish to be a man. It was easy to refer this attitude back to the feeling during childhood of uncertainty as to their sex rôle. On the whole the interconnections were more complicated, and the causes for attacks more frequent, than in the case of the man, because we were here dealing with women of more advanced age. The prospect of realizing any of their masculine protests was exceedingly poor and the adjustment to their lot at the same time difficult. Yet in spite of all the obstacles, the treatment brought about a marked reduction in the number of attacks and in their severity, inspired the patient with a greater enjoyment of life and I expect ultimately to succeed completely in both cases.

These are the data that I can bring forward at present, to prove my contention concerning the psychogenic origin of trigeminal neuralgia and I suggest an examination of every case from this characterological point of view. I will not deny that occasionally a case occurs whose etiology is to be sought in pathological and anatomical lesions. Its course would however have to be different from the examples with which we are acquainted and it should not be possible to connect an attack with a psychical happening. The absence of the above-mentioned character-traits ought to put us on the right track quickly.

Another theory that might be regarded as a rival of the psychogenic theory of the neurosis, namely *the toxic basis of neuroses*, I shall dismiss with the same remark :— the possibility of resolving the symptoms into psychic states disproves it entirely. Whatever toxins are found in the neuroses and psychoses become effective only through the intensification of the feeling of inferiority dating from childhood and the subsequent stirring up of the masculine protest. In other words the toxins can only call forth a neurosis in individuals so disposed, by evoking the feeling of humiliation, *in the same fashion as an accident does when it becomes the cause of an accident-neurosis.*[1]

The organic complement (of the disease) is probably to be sought in the direction of a tonus of the nervus symphaticus and an intensified irritability of the nerves of the blood-vessels such as exists in certain psychic irritations. The pain would become analogous to that which is experienced in attacks of compulsion-blushing, migraine, chronic headache, hysterical and epileptic unconsciousness in connection with pathological after-effects, all of which begin with acute vascular changes. An important rôle is played by its identification with an attack that is to secure safety. The starting point, however, always remains the neurotic disturbance of the psychic equilibrium.

[1] Awakening of a feeling of illness and the disclosure of inadequacy.

VIII

The Problem of Distance

(A basic feature of neurosis and psychosis)

THE practical importance of *Individual-psychology* is to be sought in the degree of certainty with which an individual's life-plan and life-lines can be determined from his attitude toward life, *toward society, toward the normal and necessary problems of communal life*, his plans of obtaining prestige and the nature of his group consciousness. Assuming the acceptance of many of my conclusions [1] let me direct your attention to the fundamental and at the same time, the determining factor in the psychic life of both healthy and nervous people—"*the feeling of inferiority*". Similar in nature must be reckoned the "*urge toward the positing of a goal*, toward the heightening of ego consciousness", a "*compensatory*" *function* as well as the "life-plan" obtruding itself upon the individual for the attainment of his goal through the employment of various "aggressions" and "deviations", along the line of the "masculine protest" or the "fear of taking a decision". I shall further assume a knowledge of the neurotic and psychotic psychic life, the fixation upon a "guiding fiction" in contrast to its absence in the healthy man, who regards his ideal "guiding principle" as giving only an "approximate orientation" and to be used as a means only. Finally, I assume the acceptance of the fact that, regarded as a whole, neurosis and psychosis are to be interpreted as a "*safety mechanism*" of the ego consciousness.

The manner in which the uninterrupted strivings of mankind "upward", have conditioned a cultural progress, perfecting at the same time, both a method and technique of life in which all possible eventualities and organic realities become of some utility even if not

[1] Cf. for instance—Adler, *The Neurotic Constitution*, and Adler-Furtmueller, in *Heilen und Bilden* (1914).

put to their proper use, must by this time, have assumed sufficient definiteness to place in a proper light the importance of the *dénouement* in psychic life as contrasted with causal attempts at explanation. The concrete evidence for the untenability of the so-called sexual-psychology—in which *the sexual attitude of the neurotic* is quietly seized upon by many people as a factor to be thought of *as an "analogy"* of the life-plan, is clearly presented and the untenability of this view is to be regarded as one of the fundamental principles of individual psychology.

In our investigations, we found the tendency to seek the "attainment of pleasure" to be a *variable* and in no way determining factor, adjusting itself completely to the orientation of the life-plans. *Traits of character and affects*, contrary to the almost generally accepted belief, were there shown to be well-tested and, in consequence, tenaciously fixed preparations for the attainment of a *fictive goal of superiority*. The theory of the "inherited sexual components, perversions and criminal tendencies", naturally becomes untenable as soon as this fact is disclosed. We are then justified in defining the general subject of psycho-neurosis to include the study of all those individuals who had possessed from childhood—be it in consequence of organ inferiority, an erroneous system of education or a bad family tradition—*a feeling of weakness*, a pessimistic perspective, and all those familiar and similar contrivances, prejudices, tricks and states of exaltation that develop in connection with the construction of an imaginary and subjective feeling of predominance. Every trait, every facial expression is so definitely connected with the promised goal of peace and triumph that we can justifiably claim that *all neurotic manifestations show a belief in an all-powerful ambition linked with deficient strength of personality, to be a necessary presupposition of their condition. Only when so viewed are they intelligible.*

Exactly similar psychic over-exertions as our school has demonstrated hold true for *phantasies, dreams and hallucinations*. The driving power is always something *in the nature of a preparation, a groping;* in the nature of an "if it were" tendency toward expansion, of a striving for power over others, of search for an outlet, of security against danger. Here we always have to remember that the second purpose lies nearer at hand, that the consequences of an act do not flow from the taking of a decision and that frequently, the social after-effects of the proof of really being ill or its imagined belief, suffice to satisfy the urge toward recognition. To what an extent, however, *all experience* is to the neurotic, merely the material *and means* for obtaining, through the employment of his life-perspective, renewed stimulations along the path of his neurotic leanings, that is proven by his utilization, at one and the same time, of apparently contradictory attitudes[1]—in "double vie", dissociation, polarity, ambivalence. To which we should add, the falsification of the facts of the external world, that may go so far as complete exclusion, the wilful and purposeful shaping of an emotional life and sensations with the externally directed reactions derived from them, and the planned interplay of memory and amnesia, of conscious and unconscious stirrings, of knowledge and of ignorance.

Once having reached this point and made certain that every psychic expression of the neurotic possesses within itself two presuppositions—the feeling of inadequacy, *inferiority* on the one hand, and the compelling, hypnotizing striving toward *the goal of godlikeness*, on the other—then the "multiple meaning" of the symptom which Kraft-Ebing had already pointed out, need no more deceive us. In the development of the psychology of the neurosis this multiple meaning represented no small obstacle. To this is largely due the fact that phantastic systems and narrow restrictions were permitted to dominate neurology, the first method leading to insoluble contradictions and the second to sterility (in results). The individual-psychological school is committed, on principle, to investigate the "scheme" of a psychic disease consisting in adhering to the route repeatedly taken by the patient. Our work has demonstrated the great importance to be ascribed to the actual material, and even more, to the patient's evaluation of it. A proper understanding of the individual and an individualistic discussion was, for that reason, a necessary preliminary. The perfecting of the life-plan, on the other hand, the

[1] We wonder whether it really is so difficult to understand the "semblance" in the so-called introversion and its opposite, to conceive both as means to an end?

rigid insistence upon complete superiority, bring to light its contradiction with the demands of reality— *i.e. with society ;* shake the patient free from his helpless behaviour and experiences and compel him to oppose the normal decisions inherent in social life with *a revolt in the form of an illness.* A clear-cut psychological-social element thus enters the neurosis. The neurotic's life-plan is always operating with his own individualistic interpretation of society, the family, the relations of the sexes, and discloses in its perspective the uncritical assumption of his own inadequacy in life and of the hostile attitude of his fellowmen. The recurrence of generalized human traits, although without inward adjustment and in an intensified degree, should impress us again with the fact that both neurosis and psychosis are not far removed from the essence of psychic life, that they are indeed but *variants* of it. He who questions this must be prepared then to deny, now and for all time, the possibility of any understanding of psychological phenomena, for the methods of normal psychical life alone are at our disposal for investigation.

Adhering to the conception of a determining neurotic line, rooted in a feeling of inferiority that has as its goal an "upward movement" as posited by our school, we obtain a ceaseless "here and there", a "half and half", as a sort of neurotic hybrid ; the attitude found in a *state of exaltation deprived of all force,* in which traits either of fainting or exaltation generally come to the front. As in the case of neurotic doubt, compulsion-neurosis or phobia, the terminal effect is either a "nothing" or almost a "nothing". At best it represents the pre-parations connected with an apparently difficult situation and a certification of illness, an arrangement to which—in more favourable instances—the actions of the patient seem bound. We shall see why later on.

This peculiar occurrence, demonstrable in all neuroses and psychoses, in melancholia, paranoia, and dementia praecox, has been described by me in detail under the term *"hesitating attitude"*. Favourable circumstances enable me to deepen this conception.

If we follow the patient's life-line in the direction indicated by us and try to understand how in his own individual manner—(that means simply by his manipulation of individually-gained experiences and personal perspective)—he is intensifying his feeling of inferiority *and yet freeing himself from responsibility* by attributing this inferiority to heredity, the fault of his parents or to other factors ; and if finally, we recognize both by his demeanour and his manœuvres, his insistence upon impeccability, then it must be all the more astonishing to notice how, *at a given place in his aggressiveness*, his behaviour deviates from the direction expected. To enable the reader to get a better idea of this I shall subdivide it into four modes, each one challenging attention by the fact that the patient attempts unerringly to interpose a "*distance*" between himself and the anticipated act or decision at that particular point.   As a rule the whole disturbance appears as a sort of stage-fright confronting us in the form of a symptom or neurotic disease.   Coincident with this purposeful "distance", frequently *expressing itself in some bodily sign*, the patient is giving shape, in varying degrees of intensity, to his separation from the world and reality.   Every neurologist will be able to dovetail this disease-habitus with his own experiences, especially if he take into consideration the manifold gradations.

I. *Retrogressive   movement.* — Suicide,   attempted suicide ; severe attacks of agoraphobia with great "distance"; fainting, psycho-epileptic attacks; compulsion - blushing and severe compulsion neurosis; asthma nervosum; migraine and severe hysterical pains ; hysterical paralyses; aboulia ; mutism ; severe anxiety attacks of all kinds ; refusal to take food ; amnesia ; hallucination ; alcoholism, morphinism etc. ; vagabond habits and tendency toward crime.   Anxiety and falling dreams as well as criminal ones are frequent and indicate what exaggerated precautions are at work —the fear of what might conceivably *happen !*   The concept of external compulsion is tremendously extended and every communal as well as humanitarian demand, rejected with exaggerated sensitiveness.   In severe cases, which must be included here, every useful activity is interdicted.   The sickness-certification naturally has its positive side in the assertion of one's own will-power and triumphs negatively likewise over the normal communal demands.   This holds true for the other three categories too.

II. *Cessation.*—The impression obtained is that of *some magic circle* drawn around the sick person preventing him from coming into closer contact with the facts of life, of confronting truth face to face, of permitting either an examination of his worth or a decision. *The direct cause* (for the neurosis) is furnished by professional tasks, examinations, society, love or marriage relations, as soon as they take the form of problems bearing on life. Anxiety, weakness of memory, pain, insomnia with subsequent incapacity for work, compulsion-phenomena, impotence, ejaculatio praecox, masturbation and completely disqualifying perversions, asthma, hysterical psychosis etc.—these are all safety arrangements to prevent any regional over-stepping. The same applies to the less violent attacks of the first category. Dreams of being confined, of impossibility of attainment as well as examination dreams, occur frequently and outline concretely the patient's life-line, how he breaks off at a definite point and then constructs his "distance". Niebuhr in his *History of Rome*, III, 248, says : " National like personal vanity is ashamed of non-success for it is a greater confession of limitation in powers than the most shameful disgrace, which carries in its train, slothful and cowardly cessation of all energy : the former utterly destroys all court-like pretensions while the latter permits them to survive ".

III. *Hesitation and mental or actual (oscillations)* " *to and fro*", make the "distance" secure and terminate with an appeal to the above mentioned diseases, to the doubt that is often combined with them or to a "too late" (fatal delay). We find definite exertions *to kill time.* This is an inexhaustible field for compulsion-neuroses. Generally the following mechanism is discernible :—a difficulty is called into life, *sanctified* and then an attempt made to master it. Washing-compulsion, pathological pedantry, fear of contact (found likewise as a spatial expression of arrangements of distance), tardiness, retracing one's steps, destruction of work begun (Penelope), always leaving something untouched—all these traits are frequently encountered. Just as often do we find work or decisions postponed because of "irresistible" compulsion toward unimportant activities, pleasures, until action is too late ;

or a difficulty, generally self-constructed (*e.g.* stage-fright), makes its appearance just a moment before a decision is to be taken.   This behaviour is clearly related to the former category but with the difference that in the above instances, the act of decision is pre-vented.   A frequent type of dream consists in any kind of a "to and fro" movement or in tardiness employed as provisional attempts at a life-plan.   The superiority and safety strivings of the patient betray themselves in a fiction, frequently mentioned, never unmentioned and never understood.   The patient "says it but does not know it"!   It begins with an "if" clause:—"if I didn't have (this disease), I would be the first".   That as long as he maintains his life-line, he never frees him-self from this life-falsehood is intelligible enough.   As a rule, the if-clause contains some unfulfillable condition or the patient's arrangement, and any change of it lies entirely in his own hands.

IV. *Construction of obstacles and their mastery as an indication of "distance".*—Here we encounter less severe cases always operative in life and occasionally taking on brilliant aspects.   At times they arise spontaneously or (secondarily) out of the more severe cases, by the aid of some medical treatment.   At times both physician and patient are under the credulous belief that a "remnant" is nothing but the old "distance".   But the patient is then utilizing it differently, with a stronger social mean-ing.   As formerly he constructed "distance" in order to break off, so now he creates it in order to triumph. The "meaning", the goal of this attitude is now easily guessed :—The patient is now protected both against his own judgment and, in the main, against others' evaluation of his self-complacency and prestige.   If the decision goes against him, then he can fall back upon his difficulties and upon his (self-constructed) sickness-certificate, if he emerges as victor then his thoughts will read " What might he not have accomplished had he been well, he who has accomplished so much though ill, with one hand it might be said !"   The arrange-ments of this category are :—slight conditions of anxiety and compulsions ; fatigue (neurasthenia) ; insomnia ; constipation ; stomach and intestinal disabilities con-suming both strength and time and demanding a pedantic and time-killing regime; headaches; poor memory; irritability; moodiness; pedantic insistence upon a submissive environment and uninterrupted preparations of hostility against the latter; masturbation and pollution with superstitious conclusions etc.—throughout, the patient is testing himself to determine whether he really is efficient, and arrives consciously, or without admitting it to himself unconsciously, at the conclusion of pathological inadequacy. Frequently this conclusion, unexpressed but easily recognizable, inheres in the very neurotic arrangement under the protection of the patient's life-plan. Once the "distance" has been effectively constructed, the patient can permit himself to appeal either to some "other will-power" or battle against his own attitude. His line is then composed of the following factors:—unconscious arrangement of "distance"—a more or less unfruitful attack against it. We must clearly recognize that the battle of the patient against his symptom, and his complaints, his desperation and possible sense of guilt in the stage of the developed neurosis, *are primarily designed to accentuate the importance of the symptom in the eyes of the patient and his environment.*

In conclusion, let me point out in these neurotic methods of life that *all responsibility* in connection with success appears to be *cancelled.* To what far higher degree this factor is concerned in psychoses I shall attempt to present later on. So the life of the neurotic, as is consistent with his atrophied community sense, is spent predominantly within the circle of his immediate family. If the patient frequents wider circles he always exhibits a tendency for and a retrogressive gravitation toward his immediate family.

It is but in agreement with the views of the individual-psychological school that the analogy of neurosis with the behaviour of healthy persons, should obtrude itself markedly. The psychic demeanour of either type is to be understood, in the last analysis, as a prepared answer to the questions suggested by society. We consequently regularly find the following constituent, immanent presuppositions and safety devices: a life-plan whose goal is unification, operating with a special purposeful self-evaluation; a goal of superiority and psychic manipulation which — in an inte-

grated connection—has developed out of an infantile
perspective.

Quite as convincing is the similarity of our types
with the creations of mythology and poetry.   This is
not surprising.   They are all creations of the human
psyche born of the same types of ideas and method of
thought.   They have naturally influenced each other.
In the life-line of these artistic figures the indication of
"distance" is again perceptible, most clearly in the
figure of the tragic hero where it begins as "peripetia,"
and is then linked with the "hesitating attitude".   This
"technique" has palpably been taken from life, and
the idea of "tragic guilt" points as an "illuminating
intuition" at the same time to activity and passivity,
to "arrangement" and the vanquishing of the life-plan.
Not merely fate, but predominantly, some prepared
experience is portrayed in the person of the hero, whose
sense of responsibility is only *apparently extinguished*, in
reality persisting, *for he has overheard the ever-insistent
question about his adjustment to the demands of society*, so
that as hero he may emerge victorious over the rest of
the world.[1]

Thus he who seeks new, strange paths for society is
threatened with an intensified danger of losing touch
with reality.   The interplay of vanity and insecurity,
common to all these types, brings to the front the
peripetia and within its individual "distance" constrains
it to decisive action.

---

[1] The "chorus", on the other hand, represents the voice of the community which in the later phase of dramatic evolution, is transferred to
the hero.

IX

The Masculine Attitude in Female Neurotics

IN a series of works on the mechanism of neurosis, I described the uniform result (at which I arrived), and which I regard as the main motive force in neurotic disease :—*the masculine protest against feminine or apparently feminine stirrings and sensations.* The starting-point of the neurotic constitution is rooted in an *infantile situation of pathologenic origin,* in which the most minute expression of this play of powers becomes visible : on the one hand uncertainty as to future sex-rôle, on the other, intensified tendencies to playing the masculine (domineering, active, cruel) rôle with the use of all available means.

Quite apart from the certainty with which the rather general aversion of the neurotic for his feminine line and the strengthening of his masculine line, can be shown to exist in his acts, wishes, dreams, it is not in the least astonishing that the period of sex discovery should take place under intense excitement for the child. Many patients speak of special doubts that persisted up to the later years of childhood — others carry such definite characteristics of exaggerated masculine protest along with them throughout life—so that their adjustment to the communal level, be it profession, family, love or marriage, went to pieces in consequence of it. All, however, and this testimony strikes us more forcibly in the case of female neurotics, definitely insist that they had, at all times, *longed to be complete individuals* and that they had given expression to this wish in various ways. I regard it, on the basis of my results, as fully proven that what in these remarks of our neurotics is but weakly forced into consciousness—the far larger portion of its power dwelling in the unconscious—is the compelling force that gives rise to the neurotic's symptoms, actions and dreams. Let me present the following fragments taken from various analyses of mine and which enable us to survey as from a vantage-point the adjustment of female neurotics.

First case.—A tendency by means of cleverness, courage and deceit to make good the fact of not being a man.

A female patient twenty-four years old, suffering from headaches, insomnia and from excessively severe out-bursts of rage predominantly directed against her mother, recounted the following experiences. — Re-turning home one evening she was the witness of a scene in which a man reprimanded a prostitute for having spoken to him. Other men in his company were gently attempting to pacify him. The patient, at the same time, was seized with an irresistible desire of herself interposing and explaining to the excited man the unreasonableness of his behaviour. Analysis dis-closed that she wished to act like a man, to transcend her feminine rôle which counselled reserve, and to behave just as the men were doing, but better informed.

On the same day it so happened that she was an auditor at an examination. The examiner, an educated witty man who was indulging in his "masculine protest", poked great fun at the candidates and rather frequently dropped remarks about "geese". The patient rose angrily, left the examination hall and was wrapped for the rest of the day, in thoughts of how she might have made a fool of the professor at the examination. That night she did not sleep except toward morning, and then she had the following dream :—

"I was completely wrapped in a veil. An old man approached me and pointed out querulously that the veil was quite useless because people could see right through it".

The old man bore the features of a well-known German pathologist and as the patient emphasized, is a *permanent dream accompaniment* of hers. Then came to her mind incidentally, a number of individuals, a strict but witty examiner. Extraordinary cleverness emerges as the common element of all these people. The expression "people can, after all, look through the veil" was taken from the treatment.

"Completely wrapped in a veil".—She is thinking of the apparent contrast, of the Venus of Milo. On the previous day she had spoken of it and praised it as a work of art. Other thoughts were connected with the covering attitude exemplified in the Venus of Medici and the absence of limbs in the Venus of Milo, as might easily have been anticipated. A third chain of thought questioned the validity of the remarks of the old man (in the dream). Would it not be possible, say with numerous shawls, as in the case of dancers, to cover nakedness?

I need not explain that the tendency of the dreamer was in the direction of concealing her sex identity. The position of the hand in the Venus of Medici, the absence of limbs in the Venus of Milo, all give clear expression to the wish disclosed some time ago not to be a woman and to be a man.

The two experiences of the day, the insomnia, the desire to behave like a man in the scene, to get the better of the strict professor and dupe me by means of protecting veils, represent one part of that continuum of which the neurosis of the girl forms the content. There is a slight doubt thrown out in the dream as to whether this transformation will be successful. This doubt, brought into relation with the infantile pathological situation, must correspond to some primitive uncertainty, an uncertainty bearing on the question of the future sex rôle. Later on the neurotic character-traits unite with this phase, which then consists of apparently masculine features and defensive tendencies, the last mentioned constructed to ward off the danger of leaning toward the feminine, of being pushed " below ".

Second case:—Brought up by a neurotic mother. Fear of child-bearing the cause of the errors of education.

A woman thirty-eight years old, under treatment for frequent attacks of anxiety, occasional attacks of heart palpitations, painful pressure on the breast and "appendicitis pains", *stood in a peculiar relation to her only child*, a girl of ten. She kept her under continued surveillance, was always dissatisfied with her progress and unceasingly found fault with the somewhat mentally retarded but good-natured child. Excitement occurred daily and frequently a whipping would be the termination of an unimportant controversy between mother and child, the father being called in to arbitrate. The child had consequently fallen into an unconscious attitude of defiance and created all sorts of obstruction, as is generally the case — at eating, dressing, going to bed, washing, learning.[1]

Her first attacks appeared when she was nineteen, shortly after her secret engagement to her present husband. Her engagement lasted eight years, was strongly opposed by her family and brought in its train many frustrated excitements. Shortly after the marriage, the attacks disappeared only to reappear after the birth of the child. During this period her husband had resorted to coitus interruptus. After a physician had called his attention to the possible danger of this habit and referred his wife's attacks to this fact, he took refuge in other protections against conception. The result was marvellous and attacks ceased for a while. Suddenly they set in again without the sexual habits having been changed and for three years now they have defied all treatment. Sexual relations are entirely satisfactory.

If there were such a thing as pure neurosis, an anxiety-neurosis, she undoubtedly might have—until three years ago—been said to possess it. Analysis disclosed her physical content and her hysterical build. Masculine protest traits stand out very clearly :— defiance, hyper - sensitiveness, domineering - desires,

---

[1] Friedjung has described the fate of the only child in an interesting series of statistics, and primarily holds psychic factors responsible : — petting, anxiety, etc. The case above, as well as other similar cases, both corroborate and further extends his view-point It uncovers what is perhaps the fundamental cause for the restless, fault-finding, bringing-up—*the mother's fear of another confinement.* The exaggerated solicitude, by day and by night, was to serve as a proof " that it is difficult enough to endure the trials of one child ". To this must be added the fact that the soil of the neurotic development of both mother and daughter was prepared by the existence of a number of organ inferiorities. Both had been quite weak since early childhood. The mother's menses did not begin before her eighteenth year and the birth of the child was rendered exceedingly difficult by parturition weakness and subsequent (weakness of the genital system). Shortly after the birth of the child a prolonged bronchial catarrh set in (weakness of the respiratory system). Her brother was suffering from laryngeal growth and her father had died of pneumonia. The daughter had had nephritis and uræmia following scarlet fever (kidney inferiority), and later on chorea (brain inferiority) and appeared intellectually retarded. The house-physician warned her against becoming pregnant again.

Thus do the neuroses of female patients reflect, in every individual case, the convulsion that is shaking our civilization to its foundations—the woman's horror of the feminine, her infantile fear of the coming parturition. Moll has recently corroborated the above-mentioned facts.

vanity. Her feeling of inferiority was kept intact *by the fiction of unusually strong erotic strivings.* These "libidinous" desires had existed since her eighth year, had at all times kept alive a fear of falling or giving birth to a child, and had inspired the patient with a fear of the feminine rôle. After becoming acquainted with her husband, and during the long period of their betrothal, she created for herself a dependable safety-device by utilizing this fear and unconsciously (by hallucination), "arranging" it. To this safety-device she added pains in the breast and stomach, in order to make all illegal (sexual) relations impossible. In her unconscious phantasy she beheld herself in the rôle of a passionate and yet weak-willed girl, a depraved being blindly following the lead of sex. Against this fiction of a libidinous female she protected herself by her fear and her neuroses. This struggle against her feminine nature was staged in her unconscious, but it had deposited from childhood something in the nature of a precipitate in her conscious self, consisting *in the definitely conscious desire to be a man.* Whenever, therefore, the situation became tense—be it that the apparently harmless coitus interruptus conjured up the picture of her pregnancy, or that the unfavourable economic situation in which she had been living during the last three years, *made her attach greater importance to the possible danger*—her reaction took the form of attacks directed against her femininity and her husband. Nocturnal seizures disturbed him in his well-merited repose : these were designed to bring concretely before his eyes how disagreeable it would be to be awakened at night by a child's crying. She was always able likewise to withdraw from her husband, or by an attack of breathlessness warn him of the threatening possibility of tuberculosis following pregnancy. She was thus able also to avoid society and chain her husband down to the house whenever it suited her ; and so she forced her somewhat bluff husband to subordinate himself to her in many ways.

The most important result of this analysis I would like to point out, is the manner in which her *fault-finding, tormenting method of education served her unconscious purpose.* She wished to prove by her haste, her continual restlessness and pre-occupation, that even one child was giving her too much trouble. Her circle of acquaintances had obtained the correct impression when they insisted "God be thanked that you have only one child". She followed the child mercilessly, corrected it, passed from one excitable state to another, carefully prevented the child from having intercourse with other children and thus aided a behaviour that had its origin in an unconscious attitude, to take the form of *a logical representation*, which said :—"my girl shall not become like her mother, she must not become sexually premature ! "

Other mothers with similar attitudes, act differently but the tendency is the same: *day and night they are bound to the child.* They pet it uninterruptedly, always busy themselves with it and, not infrequently, disturb its night's rest by unnecessary precautions. They keep untiring watch over its taking of nourishment, stool-functions, weight, measure, take temperature, etc. If the child takes ill, then the ruinous effect of the mother begins in earnest. "Sense becomes nonsense, kindness, misery". This continues until the child gradually begins to feel sensible of its powers and holds the mother in check ; until it begins to suspect in the most minute relations of the nursery, an attempt at domination and consequently rears itself up against her in permanent acts of defiance.

The dreams of this patient always represented a section taken from the ensemble of her psychic reactions and showed in clear outline the neurotic dynamics, the psychic hermaphrodism with its subsequent masculine protest. The symbolism of "above and below" is of frequent recurrence. One of her dreams was as follows :—

"I am fleeing from two leopards and climb on a chest. I awake in fear".

The analysis disclosed a train of thoughts referring to a second child from which she was taking refuge "above", to the masculine. Identical with the latter is her neurotic main symptom, fear, which is her most important safety-device against the feminine lot of child-bearing. At the same time in the upward oriented striving in the dream, there is brought to light an initiated attempt to dominate her parents, who she imagines, are an impending danger.

III. *Attempt at reversal as the masculine protest.*

1. That this desire toward "reversal", to reverse everything, is connected with the patient's thought of

behaving like a man, I can demonstrate from the analysis of the dishonest dream of one of my female patients (cf. *Zentralbl. f. Psych.* 1910 Heft 3) where I also give the analysis of the symptoms. As I am about to show the presence of this "reversal" in a dream analysis, I also feel it my duty to return briefly to a theme sketched, in its theoretical bearings, in the introduction to this book. *Sleep, in our interpretation of the psyche as a safety-mechanism, is a condition or brain-function in which the rectifying capabilities* of the psychic organism have in part ceased their work. From this view, "deep sleep" indicates the degree of this cessation. Biologically considered this arrangement may be regarded as designed, by periods of rest, to protect the most recent and most delicately organized of the specific brain functions to which we must assuredly reckon those dealing with rectification. The corrective, however, is produced by the concentrated and assiduous activity of our sense organs and in these we must include the motor mechanism. As this sensory apparatus whose function is to assure the safety of our being, beyond the range of the body must, in part, be excluded during sleep, the adjustment to the external world, in the widest sense of the term, is lost and with it the normal possibility of a corrective. Fiction, whose content can be shown to consist of a primitive, analogical and pictorial safety-device against the feeling of inferiority, develops in wild abundance. In this fiction the reaction is to a *real feeling of inferiority* as if there existed some danger of again being forced "below". Since this anticipatory sensitiveness is regarded as feminine, as a purposely exaggerated safety-tendency, the still wakeful psyche reacts to it with the masculine protest. From it arise, couched in the jargon of the infantile psyche, representations of an abstract, condensed, reversed symbolical and sexual nature, whose imaginary elaboration springs likewise from an originally intensified safety-tendency. The symbolical, *i.e.* fictive representation of the dream, certain dream complexes which are to be broken up into their constituent dynamic contents, seems to have vaguely been in Bleuler's mind when he speaks of the symbolic meaning of sexual occurrences. To Freud and his school they possess real, purely sexual significance, sexual representation, perverse (sexual) thought-connections, incest-complexes. The difference between Freud's and my dream and neurosis analysis lies, viewed from this angle, in the fact that Freud takes as real experiences, the consciously exaggerated fiction of the patient, passes over the purpose and incites the patient to give up this "phantasy that has become an element of consciousness". My view penetrates more deeply into the problem, attempts to break up the patient's fiction by showing it to be a creation of his own making, and to follow it back to its origin in feelings of inferiority and masculine protest. The corrective powers of the patient, constrained within the bounds of his affective attitude, are freed and utilized for the production and blending of masculine protest and reality. The essence of psychosis and neurosis lies in the fusion of the corrective faculties, a condition wherein the patient's fiction obtrudes itself definitely in the shape of the masculine protest. The selection of the neurosis is, however, conditioned by the infantile structure of this fiction and takes on the form best fitted to advance the recognition sought from the environment, something in the nature of a discharge along the line of least resistance.

The reversing type of procedure of many neurotics must consequently unite itself with a fiction of a primal nature which has as its object palpably the reversal of the relation felt, from the point of view of the masculine protest, as inferior and inherent. The tendency to reverse everything will thereupon influence decisively the nature of the neurosis. Our patient distinguished herself by the fact that she attempted to reverse morality, law, order, in and out of the house. And the starting-point for her protesting procedure was based on a false under-evaluation of her feminine rôle, whose dangers she felt in far too extravagant a manner. To free herself from it, she tried to track down her femininity in the hope of being able to translate it into the masculine, but got no further than two incidents in her attempts at explanation. She had come into the world from the wrong end as her mother had told her in early childhood in commenting upon her attempts to paddle in the water, and following upon a brother. So she desired to reverse everything, her birth and her late arrival. All her behaviour was to that end. She attempted to play the rôle of the superior with me at first, too, instructed me and broke in on the conversation. One day she sat in my chair. The following dream occurred in a later phase of the treatment.

"I am watching a game of rings with carousel. Afterwards I climb up. The director began a quick turn and I fell on another person, etc. I was on top. Then the director of the game said: 'Now we shall turn in the reverse direction'. Then suddenly we found ourselves in our old places".

The remarks of my well-trained patient disclosed the following:—"Ring-game might possibly mean 'life'. I possibly had heard the jocular utterance that life was a ring-game. That I should leap upon a person is a conception known from earlier explanations, meaning I am a man, am above, and is connected with sexual intercourse. Incidentally, in Vienna people say, 'I sleep on him', meaning I would like to possess him. The spatial conception of this scene is to be interpreted temporally:—I leap upon many. You must evidently be the director for you frequently tell me that I am reversing things, that I would like to have things otherwise. If you had anything to say about it I would be in my proper place, *i.e.* a woman".

The dream analysis has thus progressed to the point I postulated, so that we are in a position to predict that the dreamer will answer her realization of the feminine rôle with a masculine protest. From her view-point that means, to reverse her organically-conditioned nature, to change it into its opposite. How strong this protest is, can be seen from the frequent attempt of repeating this leaping upon a person, a trait which we must regard as characteristic of the psychology of the Don Juan and Messalina types, and of erotomania. In the Messalina type the restless conquest represents a vestige of the tendency of reverting to the masculine ; in the Don Juan type it is to be interpreted as an intensified masculine protest, *i.e.* as a compensation for a feeling of inferiority. A further indication of this strong longing for *"reversal"* is exemplified by that of the thought-connection in the dream picture. Here analysis discloses an "ascent" to masculinity ; the actual words, an ascent to her proper place, that of the female. Freud in his "Dream Analysis" has stressed the fact that dreams are to be read inverted but without being able to explain this remarkable phenomenon. Our assumption permits us to say it is a tendency of the dream-fiction to reverse the external structure of the dream.

I might add to the previous account, the fact that the patient frequently complained in the morning of headaches, as on this occasion after the dream, which she attributed to the peculiar position in which she found herself upon waking. Sometimes her head hung downward over the edge of the bed, at other times her position was entirely reversed and her head was at the foot of the bed. Both positions can be explained as attempts at reversal. I have a dream of hers in which all people are represented as standing on their heads. In this connection, another detail is to be emphasized ; one that her parents in particular regarded as pathological, namely, a dance-mania, that often seized her and compelled her to whirl around wildly. Analysis revealed " synchronous " phantasies due to a tendency commonly found, in which a man successfully courted her. The motive of the reversal occurs here too, but toned down by the erect attitude, appearing thus to obviate what the patient most fears, the superiority of man. In dancing according to her artificial evaluation equality reigns. Her emotionally-tinged impression was, "there I also can play the man".

The patient suffered chronically from incontinence of urine and of stool, because her mother had in early childhood already, assured her that this trouble might make marriage impossible.

Where did this feeling of inferiority reside which the patient answered by a tendency toward reversal?

The day before her dream, she had reprimanded a friend because the latter had visited a young man at his residence. Her friend retaliated by asking her whether in her life she had never committed some piece of stupidity. Subsequently the patient called to mind the fact that a number of years back, when there was no question of medical treatment, she had come to me to ask a personal favour without her mother being aware of it. Because of the nature of our relations there could have been no suggestion of the patient conceiving any tenderness for me. Nevertheless her resistance to the treatment caused her to take refuge in a fiction, as though like her friend, "she had leaped upon a man". She adhered all the more tenaciously because she could make a categorical imperative of it, never to visit a man, also being able in this way to make use of the feeling against me, since I was, in her opinion, threatening to vanquish her and appeared to be gaining influence over her. The dream represents a defiant "no" and neuro-psychologically, has the same value as her urine and stool incontinence. It reiterates the same thing: "I shall not let myself be persuaded by a man : I want to be a man ! "

During the treatment, after marked betterment in the patient's condition had already set in, it so happened that she saw a cousin living with them, attack the servant. She was so shocked that she spent the whole day weeping. She came weeping to her treatment terminating her tale finally by telling me indignantly, "*Now I am going to marry the first one that turns up* so that I can get away from this house !" It was easy enough to suspect that this idea, considering the previous history of the girl and her insistent wish to be a man, would be bound to culminate in a sort of reaction and I expected a turn for the worse to set in. Given the psychical constitution of this girl, the reaction ought to take that form which would give rise to severe scruples in her mind—her idea of marrying the first man who appeared—and make her realize the danger of her procedure. As a matter of fact I was able to observe the reaction the next day. She was more unruly than usual, unexpectedly came to the office on time, although somewhat defiantly calling especial attention to her punctuality. Then she told the following dream :—

"I seemed to see a number of marriage candidates placed in a row. You were at the end of the line. I passed all of them and selected you as my husband. My cousin, astonished at my behaviour, asked me why I selected a man with whose faults I was acquainted? I answered him, 'For that very reason !' Then I said to you that I would like to stand on top of one of the men who had a pointed head. You, however, said that I had better not do that".

"A series of marriage candidates"—Yesterday, she said she wished to marry the very first man she met.

In her dream, where she selects the last one in the line, this is *reversed*. Thereupon, a sentence from *Herbart's* Pedagogics comes to her mind :—if a series of ideas successively enter consciousness then the last one always cancels the one preceding. Comparing this remark of hers with the corresponding "sketch" of the man ("a series of marriage candidates"—), we infer that *she desires none of them*, a desire which might have been anticipated at the start. Dream-analysis disclosed further—"either no one or someone whom I know very well". That was myself. In continuation of my devaluation she adds—"because I know *his faults*". "My cousin is going to be astonished just as I was"— reversed—"at his behaviour". The man with the pointed head is one of her former admirers and she had been frequently teased on his account. He has been introduced into the dream in order to demonstrate to what an extent she would like to be superior to man ; how she would like to stand on his head in order to be "above". This "*wanting to be above*", one of the significant expressions for the masculine protest, is but another way of expressing the "reversal", co-operates in this dream with the "reversed" and appears logically in the humiliation of myself, "whose faults she already knows". I actually told her "she had better give up", *i.e.* give up the over-developed masculine protest.—She contented herself by subjecting me to a harmless depreciation.

Her hostile attitude toward men was still more intensified by the action of her cousin. This time, however, she contented herself by indulging in an exaggerated expression of her masculine protest consisting in locking the door of her bedroom *as though her cousin* wanted to attack her ; protecting herself now in this way and not as she had formerly protected herself against marriage, by soiling the bed.

This reverting to infantile situations is in the nature of intense abstraction. Neurotics are men who instead of actively breaking new paths like the artist, genius and criminal, hark back to the memories of childhood whenever they rebel and attempt to secure themselves against present and future dangers. Of as great importance is, likewise, the fact that their infantile analogical apperception is not corrected for society—but for that of gaining personal security at any price. We thus receive an impression of infantilism which is to be understood not as a psychic hindrance but as representing, after the infantile analogy, the manner in which the patient is trying to find his bearings in the world.

Quite frequently the tendency for "reversal" is encountered in the form of a *superstition* whose aim is to act as if really seeking the contrary of the gratification so ardently desired. The impression conveyed, is that of an attempt on the part of the patient to play a trick on God or fate, an attempt indicating the intense degree of uncertainty existing, and the extent to which the patient is aiming, by some device, to approach an individual, both hostile and stronger. Accompanying it, another trait is frequently found whose object is to have the person's personal situation create a bad impression in order to prevent other people's envy and hatred. The fear of the "*evil eye*" and "sacrifice" in folk mythology, the latter performed to prevent the dissatisfaction of more powerful beings, belong here. We have but to call to mind the "Ring of Polycrates".

2. E. W. twenty-four years old, youngest daughter of a tobacconist, suffering for five years from compulsion manifestations. Until about a year ago she had a noticeable speech defect. She would halt in her talk, search in vain for the proper words, and be possessed at the same time by the feeling that everyone was watching her while she spoke. In consequence she avoided society—as far as she could—became greatly depressed and was not even able to enjoy certain instruction that she had looked forward to with great pleasure and which was to further her education. Her mother, a nervous and eternally nagging woman, whose most marked characteristic was avarice, attempted at times by severity, at times by consulting nerve specialists, to wean her away from her depressing thoughts and cure her of her speech impediment. As this did not succeed, she sent her daughter to relatives in Vienna and upon her return the speech defect had actually disappeared entirely. During her visits to me, *i.e.* a year later, she showed no trace of it. Other symptoms however set in. The girl was, at definitely recurring times, seized with the thought immediately after exchanging a few words with anyone, that that person found her company both un-

pleasant and irksome. And this compulsion-idea with which she occupied herself even when she was at home alone, would in every case throw her back into a *mood of depression*, so that, as formerly, she avoided all society.[1]

I always find it a justifiable proceeding to utilize the first information given by the patient and to sketch out an approximate picture of the purpose she wishes her disease to serve her. This picture is to be drawn, as though it were a fiction, an "As-If", knowing that further analysis will bring out a number of additional features. In this connection you must permit me to fall back upon some personal experiences and both ask and answer the following question:—what picture should or could, the sick person have presented in normal health? Thus the necessary measure of comparison would be gained both for determining the extent of the deviation from the normal and the extent of the harm inflicted upon the social organism. The comparison shows that the normal picture, *for some reason or other*, *frightens the patient* and that he plans to evade it. In the above-mentioned instance, it is easy enough to see that it is the normal relation to a man, against which the girl is seeking to protect herself. It would be quite erroneous to imagine that this temporary supposition solves the riddle, although my psychological preparatory studies justify me in taking the main-motif of the evasion —a fear of the man, of defeat—as a tentative mode of explanation. Any expectation of a cure must however be linked up with the disclosure of the specific errors in the development and these must be unlocked by our pedagogical approach. This begins with the patient's relation to the physician, a relation that should reflect every phase of the sick person's social adjustment. This we must presuppose, for otherwise the stringing together of the patient's statements by the physician would become defective and the latter might very easily overlook important attitudes of the patient directed against himself.

The very first bits of information obtained from my patient corroborated and added to these suspicions. She claimed to have been a healthy child full of life and

[1] The paranoid trait — the guilt of the other one — appeared more definitely.

always *superior* to her playmates. From her numerous and diverse memories she brought to the surface the following:—

When she was eight years old, her sister married and her brother-in-law who laid great stress upon social standing and outward appearance, forbade her to have social intercourse with poor and badly brought-up children. As a matter of fact a number of people were continually *interfering* with her. She called to mind a school teacher who had treated her unjustly and she had often been *terribly humiliated* by him.

When she was eighteen, a young student who was a good deal sought after by all her female friends, entered her circle of acquaintances. She alone *was unpleasantly affected by his consciousness of success* and frequently took a determined stand against him. Her relation to him became less pleasant, in consequence, for he *annoyed* and *humiliated* her in every way and she more and more withdrew from the circle. One day he sent her, through a malicious girl, a message to the effect that he had now seen through her and that she was merely playing a game with him, her nature being in reality quite different. This superficial and unimportant remark threw her into a condition of marked indecision.[1] She dwelt continually upon this message and developed an extraordinary degree of absent-mindedness in her intercourse with people. In the midst of a conversation the student and his remark would always reappear and prevent her from being at her ease in society. She became excited, *weighed every word* and paused frequently in her conversation. Gradually she preferred being alone, which meant remaining in the company of her quarrelsome mother where, of course, she also found no rest. She was often under the care of physicians but showed no improvement. It is of great importance to keep the mother's attitude in view. She insisted doggedly that her daughter was suffering from "mere fancies", that she could easily change if she wanted to, a criticism that always irritated

---

[1] On account of the tense relation existing between herself and this man this experience was very much welcomed. She accordingly kept it fresh in her memory because she could utilize it to safeguard her "distance" from love. She needed this "*distance*" in order to evade being dominated or defeated. To her "sacrifice, service" or a gift to others on her part (*i.e.* any expression of social feeling), seemed a humiliation.

the latter who parried by claiming that her mother did not understand what was taking place within her.

Thus four years elapsed and the parents finally came to the decision of sending the girl, who went less and less into society, to relations in Vienna. She stayed there a few weeks and returned home apparently well, *i.e.* without any speech impediment. She had, however, become far more reserved and taciturn.

Shortly after her return the above-mentioned compulsion-idea developed, due to an excited scene with the student who again through a friend sought to humiliate her.

She gave me some further reminiscences. The student had, on one occasion, in revenge against a girl, concocted a successful plot for having this girl slighted at a dance by all the young boys and she had left the hall weeping. He had made a remark about another girl to the effect that she would stand on her head if he asked her to. To my question as to whether she found the student unsympathetic she answered unhesitatingly "Yes".

At our next meeting she told me a dream which, to show the connection of these impressions, I shall quote together with the interpretation. The dream was as follows :—

"*I was walking in front of a working-man accompanied by a young, blonde girl.*" *She continued hesitatingly, and insisting that she did not know how she had come to such thoughts, that the father had made a criminal attack upon the girl. I shouted out to him : "leave the girl alone"* !

After some friendly insistence, the patient consented to make the following statement. A year before, during her visit in Vienna, she noticed at a performance in a theatre, a man fondle his little daughter sensually. But this man was not a working-man. About the same time a cousin who was on an excursion with her tried to put his hand under her skirt. She pushed him aside and yelled : "Leave me alone" !

She herself in childhood had been the blonde girl. Shortly before she had read in the paper of a working-man who had attacked his own child.

The starting-point of this dream lay in thoughts connected with the illness and death of her father. Stimulated by a question that had come up during treatment, she asked her mother what this illness had been and she discovered that her father had died of consumption of the spinal marrow. When I asked her whether she had any clear notion as to the origin of this disease she told me she had heard that it was the result of "high living". I informed her that this was wrong but that until very recently, this origin of the disease had always been taken for granted. She told me further that her father had led an inactive life and much to her mother's annoyance, had spent the whole day either in a bar-room or coffee house. She was six when he died. A sister had committed suicide three years before *because her betrothed had deserted her.*

When I asked her why in the dream she had preceded the working-man, she suddenly said, "because all these events lie behind me". She was not able to explain the working-man. All she knew was that he was poorly dressed, tall and haggard in appearance. I reminded her—*having myself arrived at a definite conclusion*—of her desire to be ahead of men, to be superior to them ; and of the order her brother-in-law had given her (in youth) not to associate with poorly dressed or poor children. Her dream was merely carrying out this interdiction but with a different purpose, the interdiction in this case being to associate with men. To that my patient made no answer. When I asked her whether her father was tall and haggard, a question suggested by the connection of the conversation with her father and the clearly-expressed incest-problem that seemed present, she answered affirmatively.

The analysis of the dream as such, contained a definite warning against men, and this came out more clearly when brought into relation with the inferred psychic situation of the patient. Our working hypothesis, that the girl's illness was to serve the purpose of protecting her against men, received corroboration. The dream as well as the disease consequently represented *a precautionary device* and proved conclusively the nature of the illness to have been of psychic origin. Let me now, on the basis of my data, explain in greater detail this *essential point of both neurosis and dream-life.* To my mind it represents *an attempt at an anticipatory mental preparation designed to secure personal superiority.*

Normal human thought and its *pre-psychical* (unconscious) acts are under the pressure of the safety tendencies. Steinthal has, in an analogous manner, represented *the psyche as an organic constructive-force* fulfilling in a high degree the demands of expediency.   Avenarius and others have pointed out the empirical purposiveness of human thought.   Recently Vaihinger[1] expressed the same belief.   I became acquainted with his ideas long after I had arrived at the hypothesis of safety-tendencies and arrangements.   In his work there will also be found a rich storehouse of data taken from other authors, who had expressed similar views.   Claparède attempted quite frequently to explain neurotic symptoms as atavistic traits, an attempt that like Lombroso's, must be rejected, *for along the lines of least resistance,* the possibilities inherent in the whole of past existence may at any time reassert themselves without exhibiting any connection with previously existing protective measures.   *But the concept of purpose includes within itself the teleological problem,* although predicating nothing as to the type and inward nature of the adjustment.   My interpretation of this "purpose" insists quite dogmatically, *that the dominating tendency of the psyche lies in the nature of the precautions which, in the form of a compensatory super-structure, lift itself above the organically conditioned feeling of insecurity.*   The gnawing sense of insecurity and inferiority in children, either with inferior organs or with more marked feeling of inferiority in relation to their environment, compels them to a more intensive elaboration, a more intensive forcing of their safety-tendencies, processes which when pushed beyond the bounds of the individual's neurotic constitution, lead to psychosis and suicide.   Let us remember that the patient's sister, *when her love was spurned,* committed suicide while in a condition of intensified inferiority feeling, a psychical development that I regard as basic for the understanding of the suicide-complex.   *In the tremendous, all-enveloping dynamics of life, the masculine protest plays the part of fortifying the ego-line, "as-if" to be masculine were synonymous with certainty and completeness.*

Examining the data the patient has up to the present given us, we see it consisting of two types first, reminiscences in which a man gains or tries to gain

---

[1] *The Philosophy of 'As If'*: English translation (London: Kegan Paul & Co., in this Library).

the upper hand and second, dreams corroborating the last-mentioned interpretation by the fact that, in a sort of a sketch, she represents all men *including her father*—and in this instance that is the meaning of the incest-complex—as immoral and uncontrolled, and represents herself as trying to guard herself against their unbridled instincts just as deer protect themselves against a hunter.

This attitude toward possibilities of escape, and of falling back upon a line of retreat and preparation for defence, must have begun somewhere. We should, consequently, expect to be told of attacks of all conceivable kinds and of an attitude arising out of the girl's feeling of insecurity, an attitude disclosing the patient's type of reaction and indicating that it did not develop out of the unconscious fixation of some simple event, but in its final form, was the product of the girl's feeling of insecurity and her reactions to the demands of the external world. The results obtained from a careful interrogation of her earliest memories strengthen our expectation. The patient called to mind games she had played with other children when she was four or five years old. At first, she remembered "father and mother" games in which she generally took the rôle of mother. Her second recollection was that of playing "doctor", a game found everywhere. The first game is made up of the child's longing to become the equal of the grown-up. Erotic (additions) are quite frequent and these lead to the "doctor" game, which is almost completely erotic in character, and in which body exposure and touching of the genitals generally occur. My definite statement to this effect led to the patient's admission that they had also done the same. In connection with this statement she told me that when she was five years old she had been *locked into a room by the twelve-year-old brother of a girl friend* and been taught masturbatory practices which she continued until she was sixteen years old.

The patient then discussed the fight she had undertaken against masturbation. The basic motive of this struggle lay in her fear that, by continuing the practice, she might become highly sexed and thus *fall a victim to the first man who appeared.* Here we again approach our former belief that the patient was suffering from *a fear of men and that to make herself all the more secure, she had over-emphasized her own sexuality* which apparently was quite normal, but which it is impossible in the present "arranged" condition to correctly estimate. It can, however, be claimed with certainty that she is exaggerating her sexuality. We must be careful, consequently, not to adopt her estimate as ours.

These beginnings of an analysis already indicate that *in order to secure her own safety*, the patient depreciated man. "All men are bad—wish to oppress, besoil and dominate women!"

We should expect to discover a number of typical and atypical attempts having as their object the playing the superior rôle and, at all costs, nullifying the assumed privileges of man actually existing in our civilization; in short by developing certain traits or by occasional minor attacks, to find attempts to destroy man's prerogatives. *All the weapons employed in women's fight for emancipation should become visible in her behaviour. Only they will however appear distorted and changed into infantile, ridiculous and useless forms.* This individual struggle, in a way a private enterprise against masculine prerogatives, shows in its aspect as the analogue, precursor and often accompaniment of the great social struggle for women's emancipation, that it has arisen out of the woman's desire of *equality with man.* It has taken the line of evolution from inferiority feeling to compensation (cf. Dönniges' Memoirs).

The following traits of character will appear less definitely :—defiance particularly of man, (in this case of the student); fear of being alone; timidity frequently indicated by arrogance; dislike of company; open or concealed hostility toward marriage; deprecatory attitude toward men accompanied, however, not infrequently by strong desire to please and make conquests; embarrassment, etc.—Our patient's neurotic symptoms take the place of traits of character. Her stuttering is the substitute for embarrassment. Her desire to please and compulsion-ideas such as the hostility of the surroundings, lead to the same goal, and arise out of the realization of her own hostility toward her environment. An ever-ready feeling of distrust completes her safety-preparations. Morality, ethics, religion, superstition, may all be called in as aids. Frequently all sorts of inconveniences and contradictions occur ; desires that all might be changed arise, or an exceedingly active delight in opposition develops, making social intercourse with the patient more difficult. The physician like a good teacher will have to concern himself with all these traits not because the patient *brings them to his notice but because they are present* and actually constitute all the patient's tendencies and powers. Their concealment is due to the fact that the patient's attitude causes him to show his brusque side and aggressive attitude toward everyone.

Accompanying the above traits are at times found, attempts at raids (of a masculine type), and of attacks upon man which the physician can often detect. They can all be translated :—"No I shall not subordinate myself ; I shall not be a woman. They will not succeed with me. They are going to be put in the wrong !" Attempts are made to invert the rôles, to give orders in the treatment, to put oneself (literally and figuratively), in the physician's place, to be superior to him. For example, one day this patient came to me with the statement that the treatment had made her even more excitable. On another occasion she told me that on the preceding day she had for the first time, attended a course in stenography and had become more excited "than she had ever been before !" When I pointed out to her that this was directed against me, she gave up her resistance on this particular point, not because it had disappeared but because she realized that I did not take these attacks seriously and that, at the same time, I was not attempting to humiliate her.

The suggestions given above enable the physician to predict that a patient, in such a mood, will assume an attitude in which she desires to *invert everything*. "As if" in this manner the appearance of femininity could be avoided ! One of my patients, in such a mood, dreamt that all girls stood on their heads. Analysis disclosed a desire to be a man and to be able to stand on one's head as boys often do, an action forbidden to girls on ethical grounds. This emphasis upon the difference (in sex) is adhered to consistently, is employed in "examples" and becomes almost symbolical. A patient will often refuse to visit the physician and, on the contrary, ask that he visit her in her home. Most frequently the tendency toward inversion is expressed in the dream by a woman being substituted for a man, the depreciation of the masculine taking place at the same time.   This is more cautiously suggested by the hermaphrodite symbol or castration-concept as Freud, myself and others have often proved. According to Freud and others, the least important aspect of this idea is the shock experienced by the threat of castration.   I, on the contrary, have come to the conclusion, that in the castration phantasies, traces of the uncertainty of the sex-rôle are indicated and that they serve to give expression to the possibility of a transformation of a man into a woman.   One of the dreams of the patient illustrates the train of thought so well that it might be taken as a model case.

"I was being treated by a nose specialist.   The physician was away at an operation.   His female assistant cut out one of my bones ".

Upon analysis we found, as though it were a matter of no importance, the fact that some years before, the patient had been treated for adenoids.   She was particularly attracted to the physician and this sufficed to make her precipitately retreat.   The linking up of this recollection with a lecture indicated a definite connection with me.   I too had succeeded, by getting around her assumed prejudices against men and in gaining her good will and consequently her safety-tendencies manifested themselves in a dream to warn her against the future.   The dangers against which she wished to protect herself *beforehand* in the dream are her "marked sexuality" and the "brutal lust of man".   As a matter of fact the assistant was not a physician and had never performed an operation.   It is her dreams that have created female surgeons.   Taken in its proper context we are really dealing with a transformation of a man into a woman and of a still further depreciation of a physician into a female assistant.   This centres our interest upon the problem of transformation.   The bone that has been cut out is to be interpreted as the male genital.   As the patient admitted this, we may assume that, she had when a child believed she had been changed into a woman by castration, an assumption she denied.   Many examples have taught me, however, that such and analogous sexual theories can persist in a *pre-psychic* form, *i.e.* that all the conditions for the development exist and yet that these tentative beginnings never mature into a conscious judgment. In many other instances such a conscious fiction can be actually proved. Its frequency, as well as the circumstance that patients with predisposition for the fiction, behave as if the phantasy were conscious, warrants the following important conclusion : — *The motive power of the psyche is not desire for knowledge, but the feeling of specific inferiority and uncertainty which is sketched, at first, pre-psychically and then develops in consciousness into a judgment or a phantasy whenever necessary.* If, however, as it appears to be, the feeling of inferiority is based on sensations evaluated as feminine, then we must look upon the guiding fiction, upon the "tendency" of the neurotic, as a compensation taking the form of the masculine protest.

Our knowledge of the above - mentioned dream extends far enough for us to realize that the dreamer is complaining of her lost womanhood (the loss of the bone), and, at the same time, protesting against the fact that men are superior to her. Her masculine protest is part of her ideal of personal equality : — *the physician is to be transformed into a woman.* Anyone not addicted to merely literal interpretation of words, will realize that there is no difference between this desire of hers and her other wish—that of becoming a man. For is it not the cancelling of her sense of inferiority, the goal of her longing? This purpose is to be gained as much by raising her importance as by lowering that of man, who at present enjoys a higher evaluation. We are still not clear about the sentence—" The physician was away at an operation ". All the patient can tell us in its elucidation is that she never heard of the nose specialist making visits of that nature. In consonance with the tendency of her dream, the explanation seems to be that the man is to be done away with and replaced by a woman physician. In other words we might say, " All men can go to the devil ! "

The following surmise might also be quite justifiable. The above traits of thought seem to point rather definitely to the possibility of an *arrangement for homosexuality.* The dream-sketch, as well as the psychic situation of the patient, show clearly her desire to make a woman out of a man. Additional support for her tendency to withdraw further from any relation with men is furnished by recollections and impressions of a masturbatory nature going back to the erotic games with other girls.

Finally, let me say that the patient remembers the fact that her birth was not welcomed by either her mother or elder sister. The latter, in particular, always treated her harshly and a bad relationship had always existed between them. From the above-described line of retreat from any relationship with men, we must then draw the conclusion that she resisted *the idea of being in subordination to any woman too*. Throughout life her striving had been to be superior to girls and women and she strenuously fought all influence emanating from her mother. There is no indication of any primary, active or inherited homo-sexuality, in the strict sense of the term, no more than there is in other instances. Yet it is clearly to be seen how experiences and her tendencies force her into an "as if" homo-sexual attitude and in addition, determine the nature of this attitude although not expressing themselves decisively.

Her behaviour in many respects will be regarded "reversed" and in part as "perverse", because under the domination of her fiction of man-equality she tries to reverse, change and distort most if not all things. This desire which under certain conditions may develop into a mania,[1] remains in the unconscious and can only be cured if the patient is given the opportunity of understanding it and of deepening her powers of interpretation. This possibility depends upon the pedagogical tact of the physician.

Occasionally a patient allows us to realize that we are on the right track by other means than those mentioned. It may occur to her to indicate that she is not averse to developing a love-affair (with the physician), but everything pertaining to sex is to be excluded. So in this form too does the masculine protest assert itself.

The patient subsequently stated, with great hesitation, that the nose-specialist to whom she had been so strongly attracted, had kissed her a number of times and she had made but weak attempts to repulse him. When finally she found the courage to tell him, on one occasion when he wished to force a kiss from her, that she considered

---

[1] The relationship of this case with paranoidal dementia is not to be dismissed off-hand.

his attitude horrible and that she would not come again, her complaints disappeared, and she felt very well for about three months. Then came her contact with the student and shortly after his rather stupid remark that she was really other than she appeared, there arose compulsion-ideas to the effect that she could not mix in society because of the poor impression she made.

That she permitted the physician so easily to kiss her, appears on first thoughts rather strange and to contradict apparently the assumption of a masculine protest. Experience teaches us, however, that the awakened masculine adventure-spirit, not infrequently makes use of feminine weapons and that to be kissed and the awakening of love can be felt as a gratification of power. The very moment, however, that the man tried clearly to demonstrate his superiority and use force then she had to prove to him that she was his superior. This is so typical a case in its psychological make-up that it ought to be quite generally intelligible. Everyone knows that the individual who has not yet admitted his love, can thus intensify the love of the one who has confessed to it, just as that which appears unattainable is greatly desired and the more openly expressed love is generally rebuffed. Neurotic girls must therefore always fail in their attempts at establishing relations with men because they are immediately struck by the feeling of subordination and possessiveness in the love relation and it becomes unbearable. The improvement in the condition of the patient is easily enough intelligible, for she has triumphed both over the physician and those sexual desires regarded as feminine and of inferior value.

When, however, she saw herself defeated in her struggle with the student and when he even succeeded in capturing her friend, *then she gave to his words an old meaning*, her fear of people detecting the feminine sensuality as represented by her onanistic practices. The student's words were quite general—*one could see that she was different from what she appeared to be.* And so his words were given the meaning that everyone could recognize her sensuality and take the same liberties as the physician. She herself was too weak to protect herself against a man.

This postscript given very unwillingly had been

preceded by complaints lasting an hour about her condition and doubts as to the possibility of a cure. It was easy to see that this behaviour of hers was directed against me. It was as easy to see that she defended herself against me by falling back upon the fact that I had taken advantage of her " weakness " to force from her numerous admissions. In order therefore to remain in a strong position as regards me, she had to show that her condition had become worse, which at that particular stage of the cure was equivalent to saying—"He must not gain any power or influence over me ".

Let us point out briefly how the fear of men also has a tendency to " reverse itself ", in such a train of thought as, for instance,—"the man should get frightened ". This mode of thinking is identical for the neurotic feeling of the patient, with an emotional wave proceeding from " below to above ". This tendency toward reversing, expressing itself occasionally in turning " the bottom to the top ", and in turning tables, seats and boxes around, is found not only in neurosis, but also in psychosis. Its psychological equivalent is the well-known negative-istic attitude that can always be replaced mentally by a " reversal ". Let me point out the fact that in the case of our patient, other trains of thought also made their appearance with which we are quite familiar from the study of psychosis ; such, for instance, that people can look through her, that everyone experiences a disagreeable feeling in her presence, that she can be easily influenced. In contrast however, to psychotic individuals, we must insist that such a person always knows how to bring her infantile fiction into such harmony with reality that the impression of her suffering from a psychosis is absent. The lack of psychosis is consequently not due to any inherent trait of the fiction, which here only serves to make the patient even more careful, but to the weakness of the correlation between the lines of conduct to be corrected and the necessity of adhering to a logical procedure. Our patient may, in order to obtain security for her assumed feminine weakness, strengthen as much as she wishes the fiction that she is to behave like a man, she will always find another kind of safety-device given by the correlation of her rectifying mechanism with reality so that she will consequently behave " sensibly ". Here we approximate to Bleuler's views, that a "loosening of associations " is characteristic of schizophrenia. Our stand-point however, presupposes the relative inferiority of the rectifying mechanism whose compensatory capacity no longer suffices when the mechanism proceeds to undertake heavier tasks.

A number of years ago I made observations on a patient who had dementia praecox in its declining stage. One day he pointed to a pack of hounds and said with a significant gesture, that these were all well-known, beautiful women and gave me the name of every one of them. He was under the influence of the fear of woman and safe-guarded himself in belittling the sex by transforming all women into dogs, *i.e.* in " reversing " things. His rectifying apparatus was not strong enough to harmonize his facts with reality, to turn the whole thing into a joke, or to be able to regard his statement as an insult. The compensation of the rectifying apparatus was still functioning in connection with the depreciatory tendency of the safe-guarding mechanism.

A dream of our patient which she had the day after giving me the information about the behaviour of the specialist, shows the same psychic dynamics. Her dream was as follows.—

" I went to buy a hat. As I was returning home I saw, in the distance, a dog of whom I was very much afraid. I wanted the dog however to be afraid of me. I came nearer and he jumped upon me. I pacified him and stroked him on the back. Then I got home and lay down on the sofa. Just then two cousins came on a visit and mother brought them in, looked for me and said : ' There she is '. I felt embarrassed at being surprised in this attitude ".

Analysis disclosed angry thoughts connected with the information she had given me. She has to be on her " guard ". The strengthening of her safety-tendency demanded this. She had shown her weakness and had been defeated and I—the dog—had sprung upon her. She apparently thinks of her defeat in terms of sex symbolism, not however to be taken at full value. The actual symbolical expression used for " defeat " and for the feeling of femininity, and which clearly makes the antithesis too strong, she secures by establishing a reminder. Its origin is to be found in the warning safe-guarding tendency. Thus she lowers me to the position of a dog and in her supplementary statement clearly indicates in what way she is planning to "reverse" the admitted fact of my superiority. "I wanted him to be afraid of me!" During the first days of the treatment she felt fatigued (upon her return home) and used to rest upon the sofa. These symptoms were palpably "arranged" in order to prove—as she herself at times stated — that her conversations with me did not calm but on the contrary tired her. But what is more important, is that she had lain in the same way on the sofa after her nose operation in the office of the specialist who had then kissed her, a secret that I had "wrung" from her. Both cousins were at that time married. She had associated with them when they were single. Then they had often come for there were many house-parties. They always came in the company of either their mother or aunt. *They would have considered it immodest to have gone anywhere alone. She, however, had gone alone both to me for treatment* and formerly to the nose specialist where she had had the above-mentioned experience. In the dream she goes out alone to buy a hat. The last purchase of a hat had occurred in the company of her quarrelsome mother and perturbed her a good deal, for her mother was continually complaining about money-expenditures. The pacification of the dog refers to the way in which, on one occasion, she had consoled a rejected suitor. Thus it would happen to me.

The problem contained in this dream thus reads, "Shall I go alone or with mother? The latter alternative is unpleasant because my mother always tries to down me. I want to be the dominant one and I shall therefore go alone. As I am afraid of men I shall consequently try to change the rôle. Once I caused a man who wished to become intimate with me deep anguish, repulsing him because I was afraid of further advances on his part. I have often the same fear whenever I speak to a man. Only when I meet a man for the first time am I able to make him feel my superiority. The oftener I go to the doctor the weaker I become. But quite apart from that, it is not becoming for me to visit him alone". Her propriety-tendencies which she occasionally brought into play against me, arose out of the above consideration and had, of course, been "arranged". As a matter of fact, she absented herself from the treatment two days later without any reason.

In short her feeling of weakness arose out of her fear of man and the only possible corrective lay in behaving as though she were a man. To take this thorny path, brought her into numerous contradictions all of which could be traced back to the non-rational nature of her fiction. The world regarded her as a woman and she herself was open to feminine impulses which she markedly restrained, although by no means suppressed. This restraining of her feminine impulses led to a "reversal", to what might be called an acid reaction, which transformed into a safety-tendency reads :—" I do not want to be a woman ; I want to be a man ! "— She took this attitude toward everyone, toward her girl friends and toward her physician. In the latter case however her safe-guarding fiction would have then to break down and be brought into harmony with reality.

The continuation of the treatment is the most difficult pedagogical task of the nerve-specialist, for he must bring the patient into a mood where he will take kindly to being led. On one occasion the above patient appeared in my office markedly depressed and when I asked her what she wanted to say to-day, made no answer. Finally when I pointed out to her that her bad humour was necessarily part of the hostile attitude toward me, she exclaimed, "Why do you say that?"— This was not the first time I had heard these words from her. She had repeatedly used them when she introduced herself and her mother to me the first time and had used them whenever her mother, in narrating the story of her illness, added critical remarks of her own to the effect that her daughter was taking no trouble to be different. I must consequently assume that the patient had succeeded in foisting upon me the rôle of her mother, *i.e.* in regarding me as in the afore-mentioned dream of the doctor, as not being a man. This is her final purpose. As soon as she had depreci-ated me she proceeded to an attack. Other indications of hostility that came to light on the same day consisted in disguised reproaches against me in connection with the aggravation of her condition, of so subjective a tone that the idea that she would like to try her fortunes elsewhere was clearly discerned. She actually gave expression to the hostile thoughts directed against me and indicated that she intended to give up the treatment, at least for a short time. That this was all directed against me, is easily seen even though the patient denied having been conscious of such a purpose. Let me assume provisionally that her behaviour is her answer—somewhat in the nature of a compulsion—to the feeling of defeat ; of lack of resistance and adjustment. Its connection with the nature of her disease is there manifest. Her feelings are of such a type that other people, particularly men, were regarded as stronger, hostile and superior. *On account of her safety-tendency and desire for power*, she had from the beginning underlined and grouped in a one-sided way, her own quite normal feelings and forced them into the rôle of a scare-crow. The masculine protest turns against this fiction for reasons of its own safety because this fiction has been evaluated as feminine, as shown by her attitude toward me. *In the mechanism of the masculine protest this activity of her safe-guarding tendency continues to strengthen all her feelings of man's superiority and hostility.* In consequence, her early recollections were full of examples in which the man was the stronger. Her psyche is always under the influence of what might be called an ascending fiction, whose point of departure is drawn with powerful strokes in some such way as the following :—" I succumb, therefore I am too weak ". The desired counter-foil to the above is the end-goal : " I must behave as though I were a man, *i.e.* I must belittle man for I am too feminine and shall otherwise succumb ". The neurosis within these two fictions is staged, its exaggerations and suppressions being determined by the safe-guarding tendency.

Let us turn back. Of what did the patient complain? *She experienced, she said, a feeling as if people were hostile to her, as though she made a bad impression upon them !* This compulsion-idea flowed, of necessity, from the psychic situation of the patient, for it not only brought into strong relief her feminine fiction and thus took the form of a reminder, but also made room for her masculine fiction. She could then discard her feminine rôle and live as far as this was possible in her masculine rôle ; to her mother she could behave as though she were a man. Her mother is the only person with whom she has, since her illness, been in touch and whom she *dominates*, at times reducing her to the point of desperation. The feeling of hostility which animates her is then transferred to others, for "only he fears misfortune who is himself wicked". The marked absence of social consciousness is quite noticeable.

We must remember that other disease-manifestations had preceded her compulsion-idea; for example, her speech impediment and her exaggerated timidity when in the presence of others. This was in fact the first act of her neurosis, the expression of her increased tension when in company. It is as if she were making special efforts to safe-guard herself in speech—in order not to succumb—and were, at the same time, quite capable of constantly keeping before herself the safe-guarding fiction of her weakness in the form of a mechanism related to stuttering. This attitude she was able to maintain until, on account of the attacks of men—the physician, her cousin—*she was compelled in the protection* of her masculine protest *to go further and either fight or run away*. This is the point she had reached in my case, as the above account shows. Analyses of stutterers justify me in making the same inference. Their stuttering is an attempt to withdraw, by means of passive resistance, from the superiority of others. It is based on an intensified feeling of inferiority whose persistent and tenaciously held purpose is to watch, examine and steal marches upon their partner. The main idea is to gain a (decisive) influence by means of a masochistic attitude and to be able in addition to say, "What would I not have accomplished had I not been a stutterer!" Thus do these patients console themselves and evade their own sensitiveness.

I know that many a reader of my earlier works has been puzzled by this point and has asked how any person could, under these circumstances, have developed a masculine protest. The analogy with *passive* resistance (of the patient) ought to clear up this question. In such behaviour, special cases are frequently encountered in which "feminine" and "masculine" lines temporally coincide and effect a compromise, the uninterrupted safe-guarding tendency continuing however to adhere to its upward-tending impulse. This is clearest in the

Messalina types where defeat is felt as victory. Can this really be so difficult to grasp?

Let us go back to our patient. We can now put into their proper relationship both of the trains of thought directed against me. Her pointed remarks, her subjectively aggravated condition, are as much threats against me as her actual threats to absent herself from treatment. The first remind us more of present, the last of earlier disease-manifestations. We are now familiar with the cause of the strengthening of her masculine protest; it is her submissiveness during treatment. She informed me, for instance, that she had dreamt but only remembered *that she woke up after a shriek.*

Such fragments of a dream are well adapted for interpretation. It is much as if the physician had forced an entry into the psyche by means of a large breach in its walls, without having first to overcome minor obstacles. Upon my questioning her as to the nature of her cry, she answered by giving me some recollections going back to her childhood. As a child she would cry frightfully if any of the other children or any people tried to hurt her. On one occasion she had been locked in a cellar and terrified in addition by the information that rats were there. She had also shrieked at the top of her voice in the office of the nose-specialist. I believe that a similar situation had occurred in her dream, *i.e.* she had shrieked during her dream-fiction as though something similar to what we have just mentioned, were going to happen to her.

Every dream can be best expressed by such an introduction as the following: "Granted that . . ." I mentioned this long ago in my smaller studies and I am now in a position to give fuller details. Many points in Freud's interpretation of the dream will be corroborated, other points, on the contrary, shown to be unimportant and misleading. We cannot definitely enough insist that dream analysis was made possible by Freud's work on the dream-content, the dream-purpose and the residue of waking life contained in the dream. Freud's conception that the main function and guiding principle of the dream is to revivify and achieve in the dream, the old wishes of childhood, must however be given up. It served, and could have served, no

other purpose except that of a temporary expedient,
and although self-contradictory and meaningless when
brought into connection with reality, it did nevertheless
fulfil in a masterly way, its purpose of bringing the
dream under the control of ordered thinking. The
principle of wish-fulfilment is itself nothing but a fiction
although marvellously adapted to advance the true
understanding of the dream. What makes its employment as an accessory, seem so self-evident from a logical
view-point, is the wide range of such an abstraction,
allowing space for all psychical impulses. Indeed all
that is necessary is to search for the actual or possible
impulses that lie behind the dream-fragment of a fulfilled
wish. Nevertheless the positing of Freud's formulas has
enabled us neurologists to bring order into the dream-
material and to gain a perspective. It was possible to
apply the calculus to it. (Vaihinger.) The contradiction that the stress seemed to fall upon infantile wishes
called up by analogous complexes of the present as
opposed to the past, that a new contradiction obtained
from past experience had to solve the dream, proved the
untenability of Freud's formulas and forced him to the
creation of extensive fictions. Of these the nearest at
hand was the concept of fixation of incestuous infantile
relationships, and this had to be generalized and distorted into gross sexuality, because the dream fiction
rather frequently operated with sexual analogies in order
to express other relations, just as quite frequently
happens among people conversing in a public-house.

The most striking feature, the protective, anticipatory and safe-guarding elements that cause and are
the contents of the dream, were actually obscured and
forced, in hostile fashion, into the background as soon
as Freud's formula permitted us to apply a calculus to it.
*These features consisted of the protection, anticipation and
safe-guarding aspects that engender and form the content of
every dream. The main function of the dream is the attempt
to safe-guard the importance and superiority of the ego.*
That function according to our views determines the
main character of the dream - work. The dreamer
attempts to gain the masculine line, and protect himself,
like the neurotic, paranoic, artist, and criminal, against
any nascent feeling of defeat. His evaluations of
masculine - feminine come from his childhood, are

individual and, by their contradiction, constitute the main fiction of the neurotic.   The ideational impulses of dreamer and neurotic take final form in analogies, symbols and other fictions based on the contrast of below-above and masculine-feminine.   The tendency is always upward toward the masculine protest, analogous to a turning of the body, to a raising up of the sleeper.

If now we apply these two categories, according to which the dream must be orientated, *the guiding pictures*, as Klages says in his *Prinzipien der Charakteriologie* (Leipzig, 1910), to this minute fragment, namely the motor affect-expression (the shriek), into which we have gained some insight from the statements of the patient, then we obtain the following:—First, the patient is afraid of an act of violence similar to what she had suffered in childhood from a boy and later at the hands of the nose-specialist; secondly, she reacts toward the *anticipation* in the same way in which she acted in her childhood toward any humiliation.   To this is to be added a suggestion given by the patient which had been obtained from me.   I had in conversation, in order to show the difference in the type of psychic reaction of man and woman, mentioned the fact that if both men and women were clothed in woman's dress, we should be able to recognize the woman by the way in which she would behave if a mouse appeared.   The woman would draw her dress about her legs.   A similar idea recurred in the patient's previous recollection of her imprisonment in the cellar with the rats.   Thus in her motor affect-expression, the shriek, there is also present a psychic content:—" They want to imprison me, force me, humiliate me (cellar) because I am a girl ! "   As a counter-attack we find a psychic content responding to the feeling of the feminine rôle, namely, the masculine protest which tells her, " Yell! that people may hear you, that they may refrain from forcing you, that they may free you ! "

If we compare these two reciprocally sustaining trains of thought with the patient's attitude toward me, we discover a second train of thought accurately reflected and brought directly to bear upon me.   The patient "yells", *i.e.* takes up a hostile position to me, protects herself against my " superiority " and declares she wishes " to be free ", *i.e.* absent herself from treatment. Her first train of thought, "I am being over-powered, held captive, humiliated", must therefore have been present in the forgotten dream-fragment. When I made this statement she made no remark, so I continued and insisted, "I must have appeared to you in this dream as the superior man". Her resistance continued and was only slightly influenced by my declaration that in her exaggerated precautions, she was conjuring up unnecessary *fear-spectres*, being afraid that she would succumb to my treatment, a treatment against which she protested by yelling.

Her sense of her feminine rôle, of her possible longing for love, is clearly exaggerated in the interests of her safety and *the libido, against the latter of which she wishes to protect herself* and is consequently falsified. She behaved as if she felt weak in my presence, believing this fiction to be the truth, because thus she felt herself best protected.   Now we understand what her tendency toward "reversing" means :—*the desire to be the stronger one.*

Unfortunately I did not succeed in keeping her under my treatment for more than a few days, a fact that indicates the severity of her disease, her unapproachability and her incapacity for true human relationship.   A year later I was informed that her condition had become aggravated in the foreign country to which she had gone.

X

The Concept of Resistance during Treatment
(1916)

A PATIENT who had been under individual-psychological treatment for two months came to me one day *and asked whether she could not come the next time at four o'clock instead of three.* No matter how insistently patients, in such and similar cases, make their requests, we are justified in assuming that the desired alteration is an indication of intensified aggressiveness, of a masculine protest directed against the physician. We would be wrong and acting in direct opposition to the purpose of the treatment, which is to enable the patient to gain inward freedom, if we did not attempt on such occasions, to investigate the reasons for the request.

The patient claimed that she would have to go to the dressmaker at three o'clock, a rather weak reason, which was only slightly strengthened by the fact that owing to the length of the treatment, the number of free hours was somewhat restricted. As I was not free at the hour she asked, I suggested as a test five or six. This the patient *rejected* with the remark that her mother would be free at five and expected her at a friend's house. So we see here an insufficient reason advanced (for the alteration) and are consequently justified in assuming that the patient is showing a resistance to the treatment.

Freud has repeatedly pointed out that analysis must realize these resistance phenomena which are frequently connected with *transference.* Since according to our view the psychic relations involved in these two questions are different (from those of Freud) and are frequently misunderstood, I shall attempt to discuss them in relation to the above-mentioned case.

What we have first to consider is the particular

point in the analysis of the treatment, at which resistance asserted itself.   In the case we are discussing the
patient had been talking for a few days about her
relations to her brother.   She told me that occasionally
when alone with him she experienced an inexplicable
feeling of disgust.   She had, however, no feeling of
aversion to him and gladly accompanied him to the
theatre.   But she was careful not to *offer him her
arm* on the street lest strangers might mistake her
for his mistress.   She often conversed with him at
home and frequently permitted him to kiss her, a
practice in which he liked to indulge.   Kissing was
one of her most passionate pleasures and at times *she
experienced a veritable kissing-mania.*   Of late she had
been more reserved toward her brother because, *owing
to her acute sense of smell she had noticed that his breath
had a bad odour.*

The patient's psychological relation to her brother is
thus clear enough.   She experiences certain emotions
and plays with certain possibilities *against which she
immediately seeks to protect herself.*   If these emotional
stirrings take the form of female desires (permitting
herself to be kissed, taking her brother's arm, desire for
the society of men), then she confronts them with the
masculine protest, clothing the protest, however, in *an
inconspicuous logical dress.*

What does she do to maintain her masculine attitude toward her brother?   Unconsciously she introduces *a false evaluation,* develops such remarkable
and fine perceptions and prophetic vision that she is
occasionally quite right in her inferences.[1]   The fear of
being mistaken for her brother's mistress only those
will be in a position to understand who have had a
similar attitude toward one of their brothers.   She is
quite right about the odour from her brother's mouth,
although it is rather peculiar that *no one else in the
immediate circle of relations* who are frequently kissed by
him, seems to have noticed it.   Our patient has consequently made a *revaluation* unfavourable to her brother,

---

[1] A maniac may also be in the right.   If I am to correct a lesson, and
this is often to be done with patients *mutatis mutandis,* and discover a real
typographical error, I have the right to point this out again and again.
However, we are concerned with a lesson and not with the pointing out of
a printer's error.

indicating clearly what her object is. Some people would perhaps in this case only hear her "no".[1]

If anyone doubts the likelihood of any indications of sexual love between a brother and sister, instead of calling attention to the extensive data furnished by history and what can be obtained from criminal statistics and pedagogical experiences where they are proved, I would merely insist that *I do not regard them as possessing any great depth*. It seems to me that it is very much a case of a brother and sister playing "father and mother" in the nursery, where the girl by reason of her neurotic masculine attitude, attempts to safe-guard herself in order not to go too far. Her brother has long ceased to be to her merely a brother but occupies the rôle *of the future suitor*. *She lives together with him in a world of fancy* and tries to show *of what she is capable and in what way she is planning to protect herself*.[2]

Her recollections and the surviving emotional traces

---

[1] *False evaluations* whether under or over-evaluations are of the greatest importance in the psychical dynamics of normal life and of neurosis and merit the most detailed study on the part of individual psychology. The "fox and the sour grapes" represent an instructive example. Instead of realizing his own inferiority the fox deprives the grapes of their inherent value—and thus *retains his high spirits*. He is prepared for his *megalomania*. These types of psychical procedure primarily serve the maintenance of "free will" and of personal worth. The same purpose is served by the over-evaluations of *personal achievements* and aims caused by the individual's flight from the pessimistic feeling of his own inferiority. They are thus "arranged" and arise out of an *exaggerated safety-tendency* directed against the feeling of "being below". That the exaggerated masculine attitude of male and female neurotics, utilizes to the full this "arrangement", I have repeatedly shown. The senses of the patient—hearing, smelling, vision, and skin, organic and pain sensations—are over-worked, over-concentrated and made subservient to this safe-guarding tendency so that the patient becomes the judge and the culprit rolled into one. Compare Schiller's epigram : "You are right, Schlosser, we love what we possess and desire that which we do not own ! Only he possessed of a real soul loves, whereas he of a small mind lusts !" When the patient actually understands his attitude he corrects it by bringing his values into harmony with the facts of reality. His adjustment has then begun.

[2] This anticipatory thinking, anticipatory perception with its accompanying safe-guarding tendencies, is one of the *main functions of the dream* and among other things, at the basis of what seems to be telepathic and prophetic happenings, just as it is also the essence of every form of prognosis. The poet Simonides was once in a dream warned by one who was dead, against embarking on a certain sea-trip. He stayed at home and was afterwards informed that that particular boat had sunk. We may perhaps be allowed to assume that this famous poet, who had been so "pointedly" warned against this journey, would probably have stayed at home even if he had not had this dream and this warning.

of past events tell her of what she is capable.   The total
impression the patient receives is the following: "*I am
a girl*, not strong enough to conquer my sexual desires ;
even in childhood I possessed little energy, my fancy
playing with forbidden objects and I was not even able
to control myself (my desires) in my brother's presence !
I am going to be calumniated and maltreated ; I am
going to be sick, to bear children in pain, be conquered,
be a slave !   I must therefore from the beginning and at
all times be on my guard, not succumb to my desires,
not subject myself to a man, indeed *mistrust all men !
To do that I must myself behave like a man !* "   Her
feminine sexual nature becomes her enemy and this
enemy she endows with unbelievable powers and wiles.
*In this way there arises in the emotional life of the neurotic,
a caricature of the sexual instinct which it is really worth
while attacking.*   The male neurotic likewise fears *those
emotions he regards as feminine,* such as tenderness,
desire to subordinate himself to a woman, which make
their appearance in his love-life and he consequently
makes caricatures of them in order to attack them.
From other, non-sexual relations, he obtains analogies:—
bodily traits, former weakness, indolence, listlessness,
and early infantile errors.[1]   All serve as evidence of
the presence of non-masculine, *i.e.* feminine traits and
are confronted by the masculine protest.   That real
accidents are "arranged" and put into effect, that the
defiance attitude enables female patients (this holds for
girls who show defiance of their mother's warnings),
to employ their own female sexual activity in the form
of the masculine protest and enables male neurotics to
avoid the love relation by resorting to feminine softness
and aboulia (in the case of so-called "neurasthenia"),
impotence and fear, all this I have discussed in other
sections of this book.   These 'arranged' and frequently caricatured inner-perceptions find a place in the
woof and warp of the psyche and serve as *warning signs*

---

[1] I had some patients who were always glad to point out the periodicity
of their attacks, thus directing attention to their feminine "nature", but
thereby betraying, in my view, the fact that they had remained under the
influence of a fundamental doubt—"*am I, or am I not, masculine or feminine ?*"
Their theory (of periodicity) calms them : "Every person is both masculine
and feminine !"   When analysed I always encounter some evidence that the
periodicity of these attacks is being used as a means of resistance against the
physician.   But the patient is always implicated in it.

that are to call forth powerfully the masculine protest
and the protections against succumbing.

We have thus come to the conclusion that the
patient hardly runs any danger to-day of committing
incest, and that *in her desire to safe-guard herself she
has gone further than was really necessary*, but that by
so acting *she has served one of the main objects* of
her masculine protest namely, *not* to have her future
life develop along feminine paths or *be dependent
upon men.*

*The depreciation of man is a normal manifestation among
neurotics.* This fact may appear quite clearly, as in
the example above, or it may be so completely disguised,
that some readers seeing my statement would find their
data unable to throw any light on the general validity
of my interpretation. Frequently enough we do discover in neurotics, masochistic and "feminine" traits
and far-reaching tendencies toward subordination and
suggestibility for hypnotism. The hysterical longing
for the great, strong man before whom we can bend
our knee has always appealed to us! How many
of the neurotic patients are inspired with admiration
for their physician and chant hymns of praise to his
honour! They act as though in love. But the obverse
side turns up after a while,[1] for none of them can
stand adjustment. They argue as follows: "What a
weakling I am! I must use all my means in order not
to succumb!" And like a person about to make a
high jump they withdraw a few steps and duck their
heads with increased effort, in order to jump over the
others. One of my patients frequently said that she
was unmoral and was at all times ready to enter into a
liaison. Unfortunately men repulsed her aesthetically.
Another patient who was being treated for impotence,
had been previously hypnotized by a charlatan. Upon
leaving, this hypnotizer had told the patient that if he
would put the fob of his watch around his head he
would fall asleep. The patient was not cured of his
impotence but always fell asleep. He visited many
physicians after this and whenever their medicine or
mechanical treatment were ineffectual, he asked to be
hypnotized, which none were able to do. Thereupon

[1] Cf. my discussion of pseudo-masochism in the "Psychic Treatment of
Trigeminal Neuralgia", in this volume.

at the end of the visit, he took out his fob and showed the physicians how he put himself to sleep. The meaning of his behaviour was: "You cannot even do what a charlatan did; you cannot even do what a fob can!" If the patient, who since that time has become distrustful and interested in depreciating men and women, ever becomes aware of the secret of his psyche, the fob will lose its power.

Whenever I traced *this depreciatory attitude toward the masculine* to its origins, I always found it rooted in some infantile pathogenic situation in which the patient when a child, desired to get the better of his father and either actually attempted or filled his imagination with the various attitudes of offence and defence, to be adopted toward father, brothers and sisters. But it seems also quite clear that the character of the neurotically-disposed child, his exaggerated envy, ambition, and will-to-power, greatly stirs up his desire for domination.

From this view-point it is easy to grasp the double-rôle of the neurotically-disposed child *in his relation to women* and also easy to test it by means of the data obtained. On the one hand, woman—like everything we cannot obtain immediately—is idealized in the most extravagant manner and clothed in all the magic qualities of strength and power. Mythology, folk-tales and folk-beliefs frequently deal with a type of giantess, of female-demon,—as in Heine's poem *The Lorelei*—where the man is represented as microscopically small or hopelessly lost. The neurotic frequently retains *terrifying traces of his infantile attitude*, conscious or unconscious phantasies or protected memories (Freud) and reminiscences of women who towered above him or found their way over him (cf. Ganghofer's biography and similar statements in Stendhal). Later on a feeling of timidity in the presence of women or the fear of remaining tied to them, of not being able to get loose from them, is found expressed in one form or another in the psychical super-structure. Against this compulsory psychic relation which threatens to subordinate a man to a woman, the neurotic directs all his safe-guarding tendencies, strengthens his masculine protest and his ideas of greatness and by means of these safety tendencies, humiliates and depreciates woman.

Quite often two types of female figures appear in his phantasies and in his consciousness : Loreley and (Wismamitras) beloved ; the ideal and the coarse-realistic figures ; the mother (Mary) type and the prostitute (cf. O. Weininger). In other cases either a composite form arises like the real hetaira, or one of the above two types appears very definitely in the foreground (feminist and anti-feminist).

When not more than six months old the child is known to reach out for all objects and is unwilling to return them. Shortly after that, under the pressure of a will-to-power, it seizes hold of people who take an interest in him. Jealousy is the safe-guarding tendency accompanying this desire for possession. If the child is forced to make further anticipatory constructions, (uncertainty as to sex-rôle), then an early sexual maturity or timidness often arises. I have come to the conclusion that *in the relation of the child to its parents, a subsequent neurotic trait is already operative which attempts both to posit, and at the same time protect itself against, a goal of god-likeness.* Passive experiences as such possess no driving force ; they are not causes but merely land-marks, *recognized in each individual perspective of power, employed,* remembered or forgotten. They have obtained recognition because they portray striking manifestations of the dynamics of the neurotic and furthermore, because they can be utilized in the neurosis *as reminders or types of expression* within the frame-work of the masculine-protest. " I am a weakling in regard to women ! As a child I already subjected myself, in the form of love, to a woman ". Reading between the lines this means : " I am afraid of women ". Immediately following this " daemonic " fear of woman, of her " puzzling nature ", her " eternal inexplicability ", her " compelling power ", we find man either resorting to *depreciation* or flight. Psychic impotence, ejaculatio praecox, syphilophobia, fear of love or marriage then supervene. If the masculine protest manages to assert itself and makes sexual intercourse possible, the neurotic feels either the completely disqualified woman, *the prostitute or the corpse,*[1] worthy of his love. *Analysis subsequently discloses the real motive, the belief that these can more easily be controlled.* As another alternative we

---

[1] *I.e.* objects incapable of resistance, of deceit, or domination.

find the masculine protest forcing a man unwilling to face the world, into the rôle of a Don Juan.[1]

I have never met a masculine neurotic who has not in some form or other, laid particular stress upon the inferiority of women and probably, at the same time, of man. The fight against a rival in love arises out of the latter tendency[2] and is primarily envy. The female neurotic even more consistently depreciates both *man and woman.* Our patient, as she is dealing with a male physician, resorts as on other occasions, to a depreciation of the ever reappearing man. This she does all the more insistently if she realizes that he is " superior " to her in knowledge. In the present case her "*resistance*" set in after I had explained to her important facts about the character of her neurosis. She countered with a new protest, " *Because you were correct in so many things* ". But she wished to be in the right! If in her dream or in day phantasies she drew pictures in which she represented herself as frivolous or wicked and entertained thoughts of sexual relations with her brother or with me, this is to be understood as a neurotic exaggeration designed to safe-guard her against just these things. This "*love-transference*" to the physician is consequently fictitious, to be interpreted as a caricature and not to be taken as "*libido*". It is in reality no (real) "transference" but simply an attitude and habit going back to childhood and representing the road to power.

The later development of her disease was typical. The final struggle for the depreciation of the physician began. She knew everything more thoroughly and could do it better than the doctor. Hardly an hour would pass without her attempting by means of objections and reproaches of the most flagrant kind, to undermine his medical prestige.

The means at the disposal of individual psychology suffice amply for eradicating the patient's mistrust against people in general. Patience, prevision, warnings make progress fairly certain for the physician. The progress consists in disclosing to the patient the pathogenic infantile situation in which his or her masculine protest

---

[1] Many (two) women at the same time or closely following each other ; never permanent. Only the sensation of a transitory victory not entailing *any return on their part* entices such people.

[2] Cf. also the corresponding behaviour of the patient in the chapter on " Psychic Treatment of Trigeminal Neuralgia ".

is rooted.   The friendly relation to the physician permits both patient and physician to get a complete insight into the neurotic activity, to realize the falsity of his emotional promptings, the erroneous assumptions made by the neurotic disposition and the neurotic's superfluous expenditure of energy.   From the individual-psychologist the patient learns for the first time in his life, to know himself and to control his over-tense instincts.   To accomplish this it is necessary to do away with resistance against the physician.   The practitioner makes his connection with the patient through vestiges of the group-consciousness that survive in the neurotic or psychically diseased individual.

XI

Syphilophobia

(1911)

*A Contribution to the Meaning of Phobias and Hypochondriac
States in the Dynamics of the Neurosis*

I HAVE rarely encountered a case of neurosis that did
not disclose in a marked manner, a train of thought
indicating a fear of syphilis. Sometimes this symptom
was in the foreground—frequently the only one for whose
sake the patient had come to see me; at other times it
became fused with numerous other symptoms in the
most complicated manner. Generally the patients are
individuals who have never been infected. However,
neurotics who had at one time been infected, show at
times a phobia of this type although they substitute for
it frequently a fear of gonorrhea, lice, vermin, tabes,
and paralysis; or they tremble finally at the thought
of the children they are not for a long time yet
to beget. They exhibit a tremendous interest in this
syphilis-complex, pursue the theme by talking and
reading about it, and not infrequently we see how this
interest manifests itself in drawing and inventiveness.

That people with phobias, and hypochondriacs are
careful, is well known and we would not waste time
mentioning it *if it were not for the fact that they share
this trait with all neurotics*. A thorough investigation
of this condition would demonstrate to everyone's satisfaction that the phobic and hypochondriac symptoms
possess one admirable trait, that they safe-guard their
possessors against danger to an extent making precautions in our sense of the word seem almost superfluous, *for they can be entirely replaced by phobias,* just as
fear is replaced by safe-guards.

There thus arise those portrayals of personal situations which present such great difficulties for the neuro-

logist attempting to understand and analyse them. *Since the phobia springs from the patient's safety-tendency,* protecting him even more than is necessary, he may allow himself the luxury of being careless.   In fact every man possessed of the fear of syphilis can quote instances of the lack of precautions taken.   The psychical connection of this " voluntary ambivalence", as Bleuler would incorrectly say, is hardly suggested by this phrase.   *It is inherent in the dynamics of the psychical hermaphrodism with its subsequent masculine protest.*   The controlling, one might say, watching (Schiller's "sentimental") power of the neurotic psychic life becomes subjected to the following influence: "Look, how careless I can be! I know no limits!   Therefore be careful!"   This is the coercive psychic stirring of the man with phobias, stirrings that he permits to come to the surface either because he is reminded of imprudent acts or because, and this is more significant, *he arranges them on a small scale.*

Belonging to this neurotic arrangement, for instance, is a permanent or transient prejudice against safe-guarding tactics.   In explanation of this "irresponsibility" we often find many apparently inadvised remarks such as that the "safe-guarding measures are of no value!" or "I am not able to use them" and phrases of that kind.

That the objections of the frivolous-appearing neurotic have a certain amount of justification cannot be denied. However, this justification ought to hold for all!   Indeed it is easy to satisfy one's self that the patient with syphilophobia of this type is also quite capable of employing safe-guarding measures.

To this behaviour of the patient the same significance is to be attributed as that I have repeatedly described in my former works :—he is playing with danger, running after punishment in order to entangle himself all the more securely in his own safety-net, to keep more definitely before his eyes both the dangers existing in the external world and his own inferiority.   One of my patients who came to me shortly after being infected with lues to be treated for neurotic symptoms, expressed the above attitude in the following words :—" Now, that I have become infected with lues my fears have become somewhat lightened.   For ten years I have been waiting in fear and trembling for this infection!"   What really brought him relief was the fact that he was now freed from love and marriage. Most of the people with syphilophobia, however, protect themselves immediately against the danger of infection, by safety-measures. They safeguard themselves against every line of contact, far or near, that could possibly be infectious ; they refrain from touching or from drinking out of strange glasses ; shut themselves off from company and use only private lavatories. Belonging to the larger circle of their safety devices we find masturbation, ejaculatio praecox, pollutions and psychical impotence. The possession of *avarice*, for example, renders the path to love extremely difficult. Their *aesthetic* and *ethical principles* attain a tremendous size, their eyes, ears, and noses detect mistakes and confusion everywhere. Girls with syphilophobia flirt continuously but start back frightened from the thought of love and marriage, just as the male patients do. Their explanations are based either upon men's odour, uncleanliness, fickleness, deceit or their unchastity when entering the marriage relation. Not infrequently girls give expression to a fear of being infected by their husbands. Other safety-devices are frigidity, used by women and homo-sexuality and perversions employed by both men and women.[1]

When analysis has disclosed the various interconnections of the symptoms and the patient realizes that his fear of syphilis is a form of retrospective protection, a kind of *hallucinatory excitement*, mirroring the final consequences of an ill-considered step leading to a possibility of infection,[2] this fear, in many cases, then decreases. For the attainment of a definite cure of the neurosis we have in many cases to continue until the

[1] A double psychical mode can be detected in perversions, as I have pointed out in another connection, cf. the chapter on "The Problem of Homosexuality". The first mode consists of perversions, in the main masochistic or pseudo-masochistic in type, designed *to chain down* an individual by personal submissiveness. The second type consists of perversions representing an extreme form of submissiveness, with the object of getting rid of one's partner, of instilling fear into oneself, of fleeing from other partners, from marriage, etc. These are all quite transparent when masochism is confined to the domain of phantasy. Connected with these—in revenge—are often found sadistic utterances and either fancies or feelings of revulsion ; a tendency toward lust of power, sternness.

[2] The hypochondriac's condition is made up of hallucinatory irritations that visualize *the final consequences, i.e. termination in some infection*, anticipatory tabes, paralysis, headache and forgetfulness.

very end of the analysis, which demands a profound grasp of unconscious basic facts and impulses.   The final conclusions to be obtained from such an analysis are the following :—

1. The fear of syphilis is never the only form of safety, but is regularly found with either all or, at any rate, most of the neurotic safe-guarding tendencies.

2. All safe-guarding tendencies are initiated, one might say formally announced, by the appearance of nervous premonitions.

3. The nervous premonitions arise out of the feeling of inferiority and uncertainty due to organic inferiority and developed in childhood from the fear of permanently occupying an inferior rôle, all these feelings being, to a great extent, retained in the unconscious during subsequent development.

The forms of this neurotic dynamics I have discussed in different parts of this volume.   They are connected with the various efforts made by the masculine protest in its reaction to the feeling of femininity and refer to the contrast, to be taken both literally and figuratively and expressed in the relations of the "*above and below*".

The fear of woman stands out definitely as the most prominent of the safe-guarding tendencies encountered among those afflicted with syphilophobia.   The history of the patients generally discloses strong, masculine parents, who by their importance and power oppressed the child and made him partially responsible for his neurosis.   The degenerate children of geniuses furnish the best evidence for this.   The neurotic resorts to *depreciation* of men and women in order to escape from his own feeling of inferiority.

An equally marked and exaggerated craze for cleanliness is also quite apparent and is similarly due to safe-guarding tendencies.   It expresses itself in washing-compulsions, fear of stains, dirt or dust.   It is part of this same tendency to endow both defecation and urination with a kind of ritualistic aspect.   Here *constipation, like all other symptoms, often assumes the symbol of an impulse toward cleanliness and waste of time.*   Organic inferiority, manifestations of the urinary and intestinal apparatus (haemorrhoids, fistulas, hypospadia, enuresis as well as urinary disease in early stages), are frequent and their manifestations are kept in the memory as fear-inspiring reminiscences although likewise used as preoccupations. Phantasy is continually infested with problems—depending upon how early attention has been drawn to them and when checked—of illness, death, pregnancy, childbirth (in men also). It fixes its attention upon eruptions, spots or swellings and employs them symbolically just as it does *thoughts about castration and the smallness of the genitals. The sensation of an unattained and never-maturing masculinity, introduces compensation, extreme exaggerations of domineering, sadistic and erotic impulses.*

An acute *mistrust* of people, the continuous *desire to find fault,* is connected with this *depreciatory tendency* and prevents the development of any permanent friendly or love relationship. An additional obstacle in life is furnished by *the doubts* carried over from childhood and originally engendered by the feeling of inferiority, representing the most prominent form of that primary uncertainty which leads to laziness.

From experiences possessed by everyone, people suffering from syphilophobia derive the conviction of *the exaggerated nature of their eroticism.* This conviction weighs heavily upon their resolutions, evokes the phobias and continually intensifies them. If this fear does not suffice to safeguard the patient then psychical impotence or other safeguards develop. Not infrequently other phobias accompany it such as agoraphobia, erythrophobia, neurasthenic hysterical and compulsion manifestations that disqualify the patient for social intercourse, thus protecting him against love and marriage. On one occasion I witnessed a "combination" including a sneezing-fit in which the patient behaved like the hero in Vischer's *Auch Einer* without having known this novel.

Girls with syphilophobia are found with the masculine attitude fully developed. The depreciation of man reaches the same proportions as the depreciation of women among men.

The significance of the *phobia as a means of safety* is clearly seen in those cases where the patient, if he is on the point of seriously considering marriage, erroneously finds an exanthem or a gonorrhœal flow and takes to flight. Signs of organ inferiority such as para-urethral canals, phimosis, diminutive penis, cryptorchism, small testes and enlarged labia minora are frequent.

Analysis discloses, as so often in the psychology of neuroses, an explanation quite opposed to the viewpoint of the patient. The patient intimates that he is afraid of lues and will consequently refrain from sexual intercourse. But we can prove that *he is afraid of women and consequently " arranges " his syphilophobia.* The hostility against the other sex always breaks through and can be traced back to early childhood. I have already referred to the literary and scientific utilization of this problem (Schopenhauer, Strindberg, Moebius, Flies, Weininger) and shall therefore briefly point out the *ubiquity of the fear of women as expressed in poetry and art.* My attention was called to the poet Georg Engel (*Die Furcht vor der Frau,* and *Der Reiter auf dem Regenbogen*) because of his sharp formulation of the problem, as well as to the very thoughtful work of Philip Frey, *Der Kampf der Geschlechter* (Vienna, 1904).

Schopenhauer expresses himself as follows in his *Aphorismen zur Lebensweisheit:* " Both the knightly principle of honour and venereal disease have poisoned νεῖκος καί φιλία of life. Venereal disease has a much more extensive influence than we imagine at first blush, for it is confined not merely to the physical will but likewise to the moral side. Since Amor's quiver became filled with poisoned darts, a strange, hostile even infernal element has entered into the relation of the sexes in consequence of which a sinister and terrible mistrust permeates it. The direct influence of such a change in one of the bases of all human society, has spread, in a smaller or lesser degree, to the other human relationships ". We are certainly not doing an injustice to the penetrating vision of the great philosopher by bringing his " hostile " relationship to women into connection with his originally hostile attitude toward his strong-minded mother. That Schopenhauer in other respects also approximated to our portrait of the person with syphilophobia is well-known. Let me emphasize *his trembling and astonishment at the potency of the sexual instinct, his hyper-sensitiveness, mistrust* and definitely expressed *depreciatory attitude* in dealings with

men and women. Did he not bestow upon his dog the
name "man"? His negation of life is a negation of
the sexual instinct in the same sense that syphilophobia is. It is the same motif as that found among
our neurotics :—The struggle against the strong woman,
the fear of woman, *the fear of being placed* "*below*".
August Strindberg, one of the most marked of masculine protesters, wrote the following in his *Book of Love*
about the weapons of love : " With what weapons can
woman best defend her petty personality so as not *to
be subordinated to man* and lose her personality?" Let
me in this connection, refer to the man's neurotic fear
of the woman who is "on top" and to the secret wish
of all feminine neurotics, to be "above", facts pointed
frequently out in this book.

I shall now mention a number of *paintings* that have
sprung from the same psychic mechanism. The impulse
perceptible in them is so clearly to be traced back to the
fear of woman, that we ought not to be surprised to discover in them again, all the above-mentioned problems of
phobia. This is more definitely noticeable in symbolic
and stilistic representations A number of the very finest
works are concerned with the Kampaspa,[1] Delilah and
Salomé motif and when regarded superficially, seem to
present the idea of triumph in the abstract or the power
of love. At times, this problem—fear of woman—
becomes even more general and delineates it spatially
(big woman—small man, the woman above—the man
below). That the *Madonna motif* is well adapted for
this theme is easily understood. Among the reactions
to this original fear (of woman), there is also found
the depreciation of woman *since art is predominantly in
the hands of men.*[2] Of decisive importance is the fact
that as in phobia, a whole series of pictures could be
presented taken either from one or a number of artists,
that show the above-stressed safe-guarding tendencies.
This is quite noticeable in the general insistence
on these problems by Rops. The identity of these
with the problems of the neurotic, hardly need any
more proof than my drawing your attention to the

[1] Kampaspa the mistress of Alexander riding on Aristotle.
[2] This is clearly one of the reasons for the superiority of man in art, namely
that the most far-reaching problem connected with painting and sculpture *has
its origin in the psychic impulses of man.*

following pictures : "La Dame au Pantin", "Sphinx" "Cocottocracy", "L'Alcoholiste", "*Mors Syphilitica*". Baudelaire's statement that he could not think of a beautiful woman without at the same time associating misfortune with her, sounds like the text to the above pictures and describes the sensation of syphilophobia. In his *Les Fleurs du Mal* Baudelaire says: "You tread over the dead, O Beautiful One, and ridiculing them, select as your prettiest ornament, fear.   Murder and horror are your loveliest decorations to tell us hypo-critically and ostentatiously of your pride.   You are the moment which barely blown across our path is gone, the flame that barely crackling fades away.   The man who ardently embraces your beautiful body is like a dying man who clasps his own grave."[1]

As has been frequently pointed out the artist is made of the same stuff as the neurotic.   *The uncertainty springing from organic inferiority*[2] accompanies him throughout life ; he never feels anywhere at home ; his fear of action, of tests, stage-fright and of never coming to an end, are as much to be interpreted as safety-guarding tendencies pushed too far, as is the neurotic's pulling back in the case of the fear of high places, or agoraphobia, and his quaking before the most powerful of masculine triumphs, love.   He is not so much afraid of the heights as the depths and *while his greed impels him upward, he is trembling at the idea of being "below"*.   He is saved from a neurosis which he possesses to a certain extent, by his strong and potent social feeling.   His syphilo-phobia is but a small part of the safe-guarding tendency protecting him against falling "below" and for that reason he draws it in most horrible colours.[3]

In practice, from my experience, we generally obtain examples like the following, all of which can be easily understood in the light of what we have said above.

1. A recently and happily married manufacturer came to me one day with the complaint that during the

---

[1] Cf. the discussions in Gustave Kahn's *Das Weib in der Karikatur Frankreichs* (Stuttgart) from which work these quotations have been taken.
[2] Cf. the chapter on "Psychic Compensation" in Adler, *The Study of Organ Inferiority*.   English translation, 1917.
[3] One neurotic showed a pronounced aversion to painting.   He explained it by saying : "Painting arranges all things that are *co-ordinate* as though they stood above another."

last few days he was uninterruptedly tormented by the fear of contracting lues. He could neither sleep nor work; was afraid to sleep with his wife, to kiss her or to make use of the lavatory for fear of infecting her. After detailed questioning it was discovered that shortly before the outbreak of his phobia, he had kissed an unknown girl at the station. He was cured after two interviews, after it had been made clear to him that he was trying to safe-guard himself by means of syphilophobia against any further deviations. His disposition toward phobia was probably not appreciatively influenced by the cure.

2. Dream taken from the prolonged treatment undergone by a physician suffering from compulsion-ideas and frequent pollutions.

"I dreamt that I was present at the siege of Vienna by the Turks, waiting for their defeat and flight. In my dream I knew at what time the defeated Turks would appear before me for I had read it. In order to be of aid I took my revolver and tried with the help of some comrades to take the fleeing Kara Mustapha prisoner. At the appointed time Kara Mustapha appeared with a number of others on black horses. My comrades ran away. I saw myself confronted by an overwhelming power and was on the point of fleeing when I received a shot in the spinal cord. I felt how I was dying".

The analysis showed this *as an attempt at anticipatory thinking* in the dream, concerned with reflections about the contraction and final outcome of lues, tabes and death. The connection of thought led from Turks to polygamy. What the dreamer, a young physician, knew from reading, related to the period of an exanthematous eruption. The horsemen or a black horse ("That is the dark thanatos") is death. The shot in the back means, in addition to tabes, also the experience of being defeated by a man (one more hole!) and the seizing of the gun is the attempt at masculine protest. The masculine protest finally triumphs in a roundabout way by the use of the precaution, "Renounce the prostitute!" In other words, renounce those women who are the only ones to be taken into consideration in our patient's case. As an additional protest-thought we have:—many wives, Turks, harem!—The second dream which I analysed in "Träume einer Prostituierten" (*Zeitschrift für Sexualwisenachaft*, 1908, Heft 2) discloses a similar safe-guarding tendency. Lenau has treated the same problem and in similar fashion in his *Warnung im Traum* :

" No house was now to be seen and frightened he beheld only graves and solemnly beckoning crosses around him. Then she turned toward him in the moonlight to heal him of his suffering ; but she who with grey-blurred countenance clasped him to her breast was —Death."

I shall not give any detailed analysis here. In those cases where a patient shows syphilophobia we can be certain that the fear of women or the fear of men, generally both, is likely to be encountered.

XII

Nervous Insomnia

(1914)

A DESCRIPTION of the symptoms of insomnia will not give any essentially new information. The complaint of the patient will refer either to decreased duration and insufficient depth of the sleeping state or to the time of wakefulness. The main emphasis, and it seems rather trite to mention it, always falls on the insufficient rest and its resultant tiredness and inability to work.

For the sake of accuracy let me state that quite a number of patients complain of the same fact (*i.e.* tiredness, etc.), although enjoying undisturbed or even more than normally lengthened slumber.

The nature of the illness of which insomnia is a symptom can be easily circumscribed. There is no psychic disease and no accompanying group of symptoms in which this suffering is not to be found either of long-standing or intermittent. The most serious forms of psychic diseases, the psychoses, are generally heralded by exceptionally severe types of insomnia.

The attitude of the patient to his symptoms is interesting. He markedly stresses the tormenting nature of his disease and the numerous remedies taken against it which are always of no avail. One man spent half the night ardently trying to conjure up sleep, while another did not retire till past midnight in order to fall asleep from extreme tiredness. Others repeatedly attempt to remove even the gentlest noises or count up to one thousand a number of times, occupy themselves with long trains of thought or experiment and changing from one position to another until daybreak.

In some instances—in milder forms of insomnia—sleeping rules are formulated and adhered to. In one case sleep could be obtained only if the patient drank some alcoholic beverage, took some bromide; if he ate a little or a good deal, early or late at night; after his card-game; if he had company or was alone; had taken neither black coffee nor tea; or on the contrary imbibed one of these drinks. The not infrequent antithetic nature of the conditions propitious for sleeping is a striking fact; all the more so because a fairly large number of explanations are given for their attitudes, some insisting that sexual intercourse is a well-proved expedient, others that on the contrary, abstinence is.

It is easier to snatch an afternoon sleep, but here too there are a series of conditions ("if no one disturbs me", "if I can retire at the proper time", "immediately after eating", etc.). It may, on the other hand, tire a person or cause headache or drowsiness.

If we look over the descriptions given by the patients, we get the impression not only of being in the presence of sick people—especially if we consciously fix our attention upon the effect of the disturbance—but of individuals with diminished, increased or nullified capacities for work, of there being some obstacle in life for which they lack all sense of responsibility.

For the sake of simplicity let us dismiss older examples where alcoholic intemperance or misuse of narcotics have gained control over the patient and engendered new symptons and obstacles. The examination of insomnia due to organic causes does likewise not fall within the compass of this work.

It deserves to be mentioned, however, that frequent use of narcotics aids the patient in gaining the same excuse for increased difficulty of his work as does insomnia. He will get up later, suffer from a feeling of drowsiness, lack of concentration, and waste, as a rule, a good part of the day trying to recuperate from his slumber.

The "harmless methods" on the other hand, have a bad reputation. They either are only efficacious at the beginning of the treatment or not at all. They work initially with those patients who, in all walks of life, are characteristically known by their external obedience and good-natured amiability. The stopping of a successful cure always shows the patient's attitude to the new treatment, as if he wished to demonstrate the uselessness of the physician's endeavours. More obstinate and unwilling neurotics occasionally begin the treatment by insomnia and try *to put the blame upon the physician.* Generally during their anamnesis we discover that they have on past occasions, likewise, employed insomnia as a means and as a sign of increased aggravation of their condition, in order thus to be able to demand that they be spared certain work and to be able to force their own will upon other people.

All that we can infer from the patient's descriptions, or all we ourselves can feel intuitively, indicates the pronounced estimation in which sleep is held. No physician will underestimate the importance of sleep but those who obtrusively force into the foreground self-understood facts should be asked the object of their procedure. What, in the long run, is meant by this marked stressing of sleep, and what here manifests itself definitely enough, is this—that the patient demands recognition of his difficult position. For only if this acquiescence is obtained will he be excused from responsibility in his mistakes of life and be permitted to attach double importance to his success.

If one follow the psychic trial of strength leading to the arrangement of insomnia which develops later into a weapon and protection for the threatened personality-feeling, we soon learn to understand how insomnia has taken its proper place in connection with the endangered situation of the patient. The feeling of the applicability of the means (insomnia) used, the patient obtains from experiences either of his own or others, or from the effect of the suffering inflicted upon his environment and upon himself. We should not be surprised then, if the physician or any other method adopted, are frequently designed to serve no other purpose but that of confirmation, *i.e.* as long as the psychic situation of the patient is unknown and remains unchanged.

Here it is where Individual-psychology can set in. Its therapeutic purpose should be that of bringing the patient to the realization of the true nature of the interconnections of his symptoms and his giving up of his secret desire of not being held responsible for his plans. He will be impelled to assume responsibility, to take definite action or to renunciation, as soon as he acknowledges to himself and the physician that his insomnia

is a means to an end, and when he refuses to see any
mysterious destiny in it. Its coincidence with other
nervous symptoms such as compulsion and doubt, in
so far as their technical employment in the neurosis is
concerned, is clearly visible.

We are quite clear now as to the type of person who
will develop the symptom of insomnia and we can
describe him to the patient with astounding accuracy.
Such a type exhibits lack of faith in his own powers and
an ambitious personal goal. Traits like the over-
valuation of success and of the difficulties of life, of a
certain unwillingness to face life, will never be found
missing any more than the hesitating attitude and the
fear of making decisions. Generally the minor means
and artifices of the neurotic character are clearly manifested, such as pedantry, depreciating tendency and
lust for domination. Occasionally the tendency to self-
depreciation appears, as in the hypochondriac and
melancholic attitude. In short, insomnia may represent
an important connecting link in the chain of every
neurotic's method of life.

Speedy success in treatment is not to be obtained
with any certainty. If such a success is imperatively
required it is possibly best accomplished by informing
the patient directly and tactfully, that insomnia is a
favourable sign of a curable psychic disease. The next
step would be to endeavour, by showing great interest,
to discover the nature of the patient's thoughts at
night and to pay no further attention to the insomnia.
Occasionally insomnia is then displaced by a very deep
sleep extending far into the day—which, like insomnia,
prevents him from accomplishing his task.

The patient's thoughts during his sleepless hours are,
in my opinion, of great significance from two aspects.
They are either a method of remaining awake or contain
the basis of the personally conceived psychic difficulty
for whose sake insomnia has been called into existence.
The latter I shall discuss in the following chapter,
" Individual-psychological Conclusions on Sleep Disturbances ". I always detected the following meaning
in the train of thoughts of a sleepless person, *obtaining*
some object without incurring any responsibility, other-
wise either apparently unattainable or attainable only by
the employment of one's whole personality and conscious

responsibility. This meaning was frequently to be read " between the lines", at other times to be inferred as the purpose, but occasionally appeared quite clearly from the context. Insomnia thus fits easily into the group of psychic manifestations and arrangements that have as their object the construction of a " *distance* " between the imagined goal and the patient, the initiation of an "actio in distans ".

The task of individual-psychology is to describe this "actio", to furnish us with an understanding of the patient's attitude to his world and to demonstrate the connection of insomnia with individual difficulties. The therapeutic and truly valuable part of such a study lies in the fact that it discloses to the patient his fictive, misunderstood and logically contradictory leading idea, and frees him from the obstinate immobility of thought derived from it. At the same time the patient is carefully forced out of his position of irresponsibility and compelled to accept responsibility even for his unconscious fictions. That this gradual clarification is to be attempted only with the kindliest of attitudes on the part of the physician, our school has frequently enough emphasized.

The means for engendering insomnia are comparatively simple and easily understood as soon as the utility of the symptom has once been demonstrated. The methods coincide absolutely with those a person would employ who purposely desired to be sleepless. To mention only a few :—card-playing, paying visits or inviting people to the house ; restless movements in bed ; occupying one's thoughts with business ; thinking of difficulties of all kinds and exaggerating them ; planning, counting, indulging in phantasies ; insistent desire to sleep ; counting the strokes of the hour when awake and permitting them to wake one up ; falling asleep and permitting one's self to be awakened by a dream or by a pain or fright ; getting out of bed and walking up and down the room ; waking up at an early hour. They are always acts that almost anyone would be able to accomplish after some practice if they were at all necessary to free him from responsibility. For example, a patient makes up his mind to get up early the next morning in order to study for an examination. He is terribly afraid that his insomnia may interfere with

his plan which thus proves his sincerity. *He wakes up,
i.e. wakes up at three in the morning,* remains sleepless,
complains bitterly about his mysterious fate and is thus
quite freed from any guilt in connection with his
examination. Is there anyone who doubts the possibility of waking up *at any predetermined hour ?*

More puzzling is the disturbance of slumber through
pain. In my examples it was always a question of
pain in the leg, abdomen, back of the head and the
back. My explanation of the first is that it is caused by
spasmophilic susceptibility induced by unconscious but
planned *over-reaching.* The last I found in people who
were accustomed *to inhaling of air* and who generally
had *scoliolithic curvature of the spinal column.* Incidentally, these anomalies in position play a great rôle in the
symptomology of neuroses and can easily be employed
by unconscious tendencies for engendering pain, particularly in the group of symptoms connected with
neurasthenia and hypochondria. Frequently the patient
can be lifted out of his fixated susceptibility to pain,
provided one has a certain degree of luck, by persuading
him that he has a segmental naevus in his head (a sign
of inferiority).[1] Subsequent orthopedic treatment is important and valuable. Frequently the patient's carriage
tells us of the existence of such an interconnection.

Of much rarer occurrence but very illuminating are
those instances where according to the patient and his
family, sleep can be obtained by the patient's allowing
his head to hang downwards over the edge of the bed,
of making movements with the head or striking it
against the wall. Many people will perhaps regard
as less certain, the method adopted by patients with
purposeful intensified hyper-sensibility who attempt to
prevent every conceivable noise or glimmer of light,
and being almost inevitably defeated, in view of the
impossibility of their task, awake up (that being their
object).

I shall now give a few examples to illustrate my
views. A patient whose illness and conscious behaviour
was to dominate and annoy his wife, began to suffer
from insomnia due to the fact that (as he says), the
slightest noise awoke him. Even the breathing of his
sleeping wife annoyed him. The house-physician

[1] Cf. my *Studie über Minderwertigkeit von Organen.*

thereupon advised him to sleep alone. A painter whose frightful conceit prevented him from ever finishing a painting and placing it before the public, is attacked at night by spasms in the leg, which compel him to jump out of bed and walk up and down his room by the hour. On the following day he is, of course, incapable of work. A female patient suffering from agoraphobia developed in order to dominate her household more effectively,[1] was nevertheless not able to prevent her husband from going to the tavern in the evening. She developed the habit of waking up at night a number of times, frightened and groaning, and annoyed her husband to such an extent that on the following evening, he became sleepier earlier and came home earlier. She thus attained her object. Another patient who was compelled against his will to travel occasionally and who in general wished to prove to himself and others that illness incapacitated him for his profession, interrupted his sleep continually by means of stomach-ache and pains in the back as described above, and slept consequently far into the day, increasing his tiredness and consequently his inability to work in the day-time, by taking sleeping potions. His condition had hardly improved when he discovered two valuable ideas that would in similar fashion, excusably make him incapable of work. He found that riding in the morning was very beneficial for his health and he had himself consequently awakened at six o'clock. Nevertheless he retired at midnight. In order to harden himself for the bad beds in which he slept when away from home, he bought a field-bed and slept very poorly until two in the morning and then crept into his comfortable bed. In both cases the result was inability to work. Another patient wished by conscious exaggeration to make his rich relatives shoulder the blame for the bad state of his business. Although according to him, the cause of his illness they refused to help him. He had learned the trick of pressing his arm, on which he lay when asleep, so hard that it would wake him up. Now that in addition to everything else he had also become sleepless, the guilt of his relatives was self-evident.

The physiology of sleep has, as its main specific trait, the piling up of enervating materials and the flooding of the blood vessels in the brain. There certainly are

[1] Cf. chapter on " Dreams and Dream Interpretation ", in this book.

forms of insomnia caused by primary disturbances of the sleep-regulating mechanisms (painful vascular and kidney diseases, psychic shocks, etc.). Neurotic insomnia is of an entirely different nature. Like other nervous symptoms it helps the nervous expansion tendencies and *to a certain extent this nervous insomnia forces its way through, irrespective of the physiological condition of insomnia.*

APPENDIX

On Positions assumed in Sleep

The individual-psychological methodology thus shows us that the phenomena in sleep are adapted to the individual life-line and as long as these phenomena are, according to the superstitions of mankind, regarded as the effects of powerful causes, they are quite removed from the influence of human caprice and responsibility. We are convinced, however, that the actual and real foundations for dream-building and the desire for sleep, never manifest themselves in an undiluted physiological manner but that they are always understood by the tendency of each individual and utilized and elaborated in the interests of an individual's expansion-tendency. A careful examination based on extensive data will certainly show that the *sleeping-posture* of a person indicates his guiding-line. A few examples follow below. Generally it is possible to tell an individual who has been thoroughly analysed by individual-psychology, what his sleeping-posture is. The following are a few examples. I respectfully invite psychiatrists, neurologists and teachers to increase this list.

1. K. F. sixteen years old, apprentice, suffering from hallucinatory confusion. An examination of his sleep-posture showed that he was accustomed to sleep on his side *with drawn-up arms*, a rather provocative position. I frequently met him in the day with his arms drawn up. His psychic condition showed complete dissatisfaction with his profession. He had wanted to become either a teacher or a pilot. When asked whether he knew how he had developed the habit of holding his

arms drawn up, he stated that that was the way in which his favourite teacher M. had always walked. It was this M. likewise who had made him think of the idea of becoming a teacher, a plan that had to be abandoned owing to the poverty of his parents.

His sleep-posture consequently very clearly indicated hostility to his present occupation and was an imitation of Napoleon arrived at by the circuitous route of the imitation of the teacher who had the same psychical make-up. The obsession of young Kellner, we should remember, was that he was destined to be the field-marshal in the attack on Russia, an idea that in the following year was taken up by other apprentices.

2. S. suffering from progressive paralysis. In sleep he drew himself together covering even his head. From his medical history I extracted the following :—" No megalomania, apathetic, helpless, without initiative."

Let me in conclusion on the basis of personal observations of sleep-postures taken by children, again insist upon the great significance their proper understanding might have for teaching.

XIII

Individual-Psychological Conclusions on Sleep Disturbances

(1912)

A PATIENT who had for a long time been suffering from intermittently recurring attacks of fainting through which his domination over his whole family, particularly over his mother—as analysis showed—was to be achieved, awoke on two successive nights in great fear and was unable to sleep again until three in the morning. The patient's situation was briefly as follows. He was on the point of travelling with his parents to Karlsbad when, on account of some unforeseen difficulties, the journey had to be postponed for a fortnight. The night after this was decided, he woke up in great fright, called his nurse who was sleeping in the adjoining room and through her persuasion, as the patient had foreseen, the mother soon appeared. The patient asked for a bromide that he had been taking for a long time in connection with a former treatment. After being awake from one to three in the morning he fell asleep. The same thing happened the following day. On the first night, while awake, the thought of a type-writer had come into his mind, on the second night his thoughts had, in addition, wandered to the towns of Görz, Budweis and Gojau. He thought of the last as a city but did not remember where it lay. He had had a dream with the following content:—" It seemed to me that we had received news from Karlsbad that my mother's favourite brother had died. I put on mourning and boasted about it ". The analysis of the dream showed that he had once had the wish that his brother, his mother's pet, should die. The transference of the scene to Karlsbad, however, indicates that the father is meant here. He apparently worshipped him but desired his death nevertheless so that he might have his mother, whom he did not love, for himself. This riddle is quite intelligible in spite of all, if we remember that the possession of his mother had become his objective of battle, *the symbol for his domination and will to live ;* that, for many years, all that he did not possess and would never be able to possess, he believed he could obtain by dominating his mother. Every set-back that he experienced he saw in the form of something his mother had taken from him. Since the domination of his mother had become the symbol of domination—all sexual motives being quite absent—he was living entirely under the hallucinatory idea (for it cannot be called by any other name), that if he possessed his mother he would become ruler, kaiser, God.

The type-writer which he thought of during one of his sleepless nights was his brother's property, and the latter refused to let him use it, *even when he wanted it for practice.* Indeed on one occasion when the brother had visited Paris, he took the machine along, just as rather recently he had had his mother accompany him when he went to look for a summer residence.

I do not mean to contend that in order to account for an attack, a number of superimposed *causes of a humiliating nature are necessary.* In the majority of cases, however, this assumption has proved to be true, a fact that often renders a general view of the situation as well as an insight into the interconnection of the attacks with their determining causes difficult. In one case we find : first a disappointed expectation, the postponement of the journey and secondly, the mother's going with the brother—two causes whose inner connection as indications of the favourite brother's superiority over the patient, are quite evident. We likewise discover what the nature of the favouritism shown the brother appears to him to be, and how he reacted to it by means of aggressive acts and death wishes.

By means of his attacks, not dissimilar to epilepsy, he had succeeded in certain cases where he had received a set-back, in having his mother partially pay more attention to him, only however to leave the rather disagreeable fellow shortly after. These attacks became milder after a time owing probably to his realization of their nature. Similar results could be obtained by means of nocturnal attacks accompanied by fear. Indeed he could do more. His mother would have to come to his room at night and stay with him as long as his sensitive and offended nature thought fit. This is what his thoughts connected with the type-writer mean. That is the reason also why he developed his arrangement of insomnia.

That his attitudes had the object of attracting other people to him, can be seen from the unimportant detail that, on the following day, he asked me to come to him instead of his coming to me as usual.

Another justifiable question is the following. Why did he seize upon the arrangement of fear? And why did he come to use a construction like insomnia?

The answer to the first can be derived from the material bearing on the analysis of his personality. In childhood he had been afraid of locomotives and their whistles and would utilize this fear to force his mother to come to him so that he could hide his head in her lap. Apart from this he had always been a brave child. We may therefore surmise that his nocturnal fear was connected with a locomotive. Do we not know that he wanted to travel to Karlsbad and that his brother had gone away with his mother in a train?

During the second of his sleepless nights there came to his mind not only the type-writer but also the town of Görz in Istria and Gojau, a town, as it turned out, near Budweis. He had been in Görz once to meet his mother when travelling from Venice to Karlsbad. On that occasion he arrived in Budweis at 1 o'clock at night, had been compelled to wait two hours at the station and left again at 3, in a sleeping coupé. He fell asleep at 3. Now this interval between 1 and 3 at night was the time during which, on his two sleepless nights, he had suffered from fear. In other words both of his attacks *were repetitions of his journey to Karlsbad* and he thus indicated that a psychic condition had matured in him of such a nature, that he could hardly wait until he would again be travelling *alone with his mother* to Karlsbad. This impatience expressed itself in his incessant complaint about the heat by which he seemed to say, " I must immediately get out of Vienna ".

He could not, at first, think of any place called Gojau. Upon consulting the railroad guide he found that it was a place connected with Budweis by an infrequently used side-line. I am indebted to G. V. Maday for pointing out the thought of death recurring here again,—for this side-line ended in a station called "Black-Cross".

His waking up at 1 o'clock at night, *i.e.* at the exact time when he had been sleepless in Budweis while waiting for the Karlsbad train, demonstrated clearly that in spirit, the patient was, in his sleep, making the journey to Karlsbad that he had made on one occasion before without his mother. This time, however, he was attempting to achieve by means of his infantile "arrangement" of fear definitely connected with insomnia, his personal ambition of making his mother come to his room. His psychic condition might then be described as follows :— "If I didn't have to wait (*i.e.* for my mother to be subordinated to me or for my brother's or father's death), I might—as my brother did—journey along with my mother". His wish for preferment of the kind that had existed in childhood when his mother would put her hands over his ears when the locomotives whistled— this wish went back consequently to a reminiscence (of childhood), just as his sleeplessness was connected with Karlsbad. He would then by means of his fear and insomnia, be able to dominate his mother and perhaps persuade her to take the trip.

Among other things this case can show us how the guiding ideas of the personality-ideal do not rest even during sleep and how, so to speak, they pass transformed into bodily attitudes (*in the dream* into psychic), *in order even during sleep to ferret out tentatively the path leading to the attainment of the guiding-idea.* As in all instances of great uncertainty, the extent of the anticipatory construction is dependent upon personal experience. For ample reasons, the most abstract experiences, those reminiscences nearest to the essence of the idea, are the ones utilized, for they possess the value of *warnings* or *stimuli* selected not because of their proved efficiency during danger but because *they seem to fit* in best with the whole personality. They must, in some way or other, however, be really efficacious for they would otherwise soon be abandoned. This subjective evaluation need not possess the slightest objective significance. All that is necessary is that the neurotic arrangement formed, should lie along the path of the neurotic's fictive goal. In the above case the only thing demanded was that his standing in the eyes of his environment should rise. The patient has forced his mother against her will to serve him. This represented the part of his former God-ideal he had so far attained, in this particular case, part of his former Kaiser complex. (From this point of view we are in a better position to understand the hallucinatory ideas of epileptics and other psychotics who so frequently wish to be Kaisers, the expression of powerful abstractions corresponding to the original guiding fiction.)

The following example illustrates how ungratified vanity may, by means of the more powerful tension of *thought-functioning*, lead to insomnia. The laurels of Miltiades kept Alcibiades awake. Indeed insomnia is frequently found as the result of ungratified vanity. The patient is like a man on his guard.

I hope it will not diminish the interest of the following case if I state that it was a physician who here subjected himself to an analysis. The reason for the analysis lay in the following occurrence which the author relates thus:—

"I was able in connection with the terrible catastrophe of the 'Titanic', to study the way in which it affected me. In my free moments I found myself often talking about the catastrophe and arbitrarily discussing the question, to which I continually returned, whether some means could not have been devised to save the drowning people.

"One night I woke up. Like a true psychologist I put the question to myself why I, ordinarily an excellent sleeper, woke up then? I could not find any satisfactory answer and, within a short time, found myself seriously thinking *how it would have been possible to save the drowning passengers of the 'Titanic'*. Shortly after, about three o'clock, I fell asleep.

"On the following night I again woke up. I looked at the clock and saw that it was half-past two. Transient thoughts about the various theories of insomnia flitted through my brain. One of the theories that occurred to me was that which claimed that, once accustomed to wake up, it was easy always to wake up at the same time. Suddenly, however, I realized intuitively what the nature of my awakening was. *The 'Titanic' had gone down* at half-past two. In my sleep I was a passenger on the boat, had thoroughly identified myself with the terrible situation of the wreck and had now for the second time awakened when the boat was going down!

"On the second night my thoughts likewise travelled in the direction of finding a means of saving one's self in such a situation, of saving one's self and others. At the same time I suspected that *a preventative and preparatory attempt at safety* was involved here that was to serve, at one and the same time, precaution and ambition. I realized without further trouble that the trip to America—an old longed-for goal—symbolized in an imaginative way my struggle for scientific recognition. As I would have acted in the waking state I acted when asleep. I was in search of a method of safety and constructed a most ingenious situation to prepare myself for defence and mobilize my resources :—'*Imagine* yourself in the *greatest kind of danger*—ponder over it! Regain consciousness!'

"It was quite easy to understand that this method of reacting toward threatening dangers and people close to me, must represent my personal attitude. I soon found the connection.

"I am a physician. It is one of my duties *to find methods against death*. From that point — I was on familiar ground. The fight against death had been one of the strongest spurs dictating my selection of a profession.[1] Like so many other physicians I had become a physician in order to conquer death. The occasion for such a guiding fiction is generally derived from some experienced dangerous situation and critical illness.

"I remember a number of occasions in my youth where death had seemed near. I had developed after rachitis, in addition to difficulty in movement, a mild form of spasm of the vocal cords, a condition I later on, as a physician, encountered frequently among children. The glottis would contract during crying and produce a condition of breathlessness and loss of voice, interrupting the crying until the cramp had spent itself when the crying could again continue. This lack of breath is exceedingly uncomfortable as I well remember. I believe I was hardly three years old at the time. . . . The unnecessary fright of my parents and the solicitude

[1] " Ueber Berufswahlphantasien " by Dr Kramer in *Heilen und Bilden*.

of the house physician had not escaped me and filled me, quite apart from the discomfort due to lack of breath, with a feeling that to-day I would like to designate as one of restlessness and uncertainty. I remember further how, on one occasion, shortly after an attack of coughing, the thought occurred to me that, since no remedy had heretofore availed, I might myself rid myself of this annoying trouble. In what manner I had come upon such a thought, whether through suggestion from without or whether it was some idea of my own, I cannot say. However I determined to stop the crying and thereafter whenever I felt the desire to cry, I gave myself a shove, restrained my weeping and the coughing ceased. I had discovered a method against my suffering and possibly, against the fear of death.

"Shortly after—I had become three years old in the meanwhile—my younger brother died. I believe I understood the meaning of death. I stayed with him until he expired and realized when I was sent to the house of my grandfather that I would never see the child again, that he would be buried in the cemetery. My mother called for me after the funeral to take me home. She was very sad and had been weeping but smiled a little when my grandfather in order to cheer her up, made some jocular remark probably referring to the possibility of her having more children. For a long time I could not forgive her that smile and I may be justified in inferring that my resentment indicated that I must quite clearly have realized the awe inspired by death.

"When I was four years old I managed to get under a wagon twice. All I remember is that I woke in pain on a couch without knowing how I had come there. Apparently I had been unconscious.

"When five years old I had pneumonia and was given up by the doctor. Another physician, however, suggested a new treatment in consequence of which I recovered in a few days. In the joy over my recovery the question of my having been on the brink of death was afterwards discussed for a long time. It was from that time on, I recall, that I began to picture my future profession as that of medicine. In other words I posited a goal that I might expect would put an end to my infantile worry and fear of death. It is clear that I anticipated more from the profession than it could give. I should not have expected that any human power would be able to conquer death or the fear of death and left it to God. However life demanded action. Consequently I was compelled when changing the form of my guiding fiction to alter my goal in such a way that it would approximate to reality. I was led to select medicine as my profession in order to conquer death and the fear of death.[1]

"From the phantasy connected with the selection of a profession occurring in a somewhat mentally retarded boy based on similar impressions—the death of a sister, sickness since early infancy, knowledge of death—I found that this boy had determined to become a grave-digger so that, as he told me, he would be able to dig the grave of others and not be buried himself. The rigid antithetic nature of his thoughts, for the boy afterwards became neurotic—above or below ; active or passive ; hammer or anvil ; flectere si nequeo superos Acheronta movebo—did not prevent a middle course from developing, for the recurring infantile fiction passed from a stage of indifference to one of contradiction.

"The following experience dates from the time of my selection of a profession, *i.e.* when approximately five years old. The father of a playmate asked me what I intended to become. I answered, a doctor! The man who had possibly had bad experience with physicians retorted, 'Then you ought to be suspended from the nearest lamp-post!' Naturally this exclamation left me quite unaffected because of the nature of the idea that had dictated my choice. I believe I thought at the time that I would become a good physician to whom no one would be hostile.

"Shortly after I went to a board school. I remember that the path to the school led over a cemetery. I was frightened every time and was exceedingly put out at beholding the other children pass the cemetery without paying the least attention to it, while every step I took was accompanied by a feeling of fear and horror. Apart from the extreme discomfort occasioned by this fear I was also annoyed at the idea of being less courageous

---

[1] For the significance of death in philosophy, cf. P. Schrecker, *Persönlichkeitsphilosophie* (Munich, 1912).

than the others.   One day I made up my mind to put
an end to this fear of death.   Again (as on my first
resolve), *I decided upon a treatment of hardening.*
(Proximity of death!)   I stayed at some distance
behind the others, placed my school-bag on the ground
near the wall of the cemetery and ran across it a dozen
times, until I felt that I had mastered the fear.
After that, I believe, I passed along this path without
any fear.

" Thirty years after that I met an old schoolmate
and I exchanged childhood reminiscences of our school
days.   It happened to occur to me that the cemetery
was no longer in existence and I asked him what had
happened to it remembering the great uneasiness it had
at one time caused me.   Astonished my former schoolmate who had lived longer in that neighbourhood than
I had, insisted that *there never had been a cemetery* on the
way to our school.   Then I realized that the story of
the cemetery had been but a poetic dress for my longing
to overcome the fear of death.   It was to serve the
purpose of showing me, as in other relations of life,
that death and the fear of death could be overcome
and *that some method of accomplishing it must exist. It
had had the effect upon me of some powerful vow,* that in
critical situations I would succeed in discovering a remedy
for it.   Thus did I combat my infantile fears, became
a physician and in this manner do I still ponder over
the problems of the psychical type that attract me as
we have seen to be the case, to a marked degree, in
connection with the ' Titanic ' catastrophe.[1]

" My ambition, has been so definitely fixed by the
guiding fiction of overcoming death that other goals
hardly present any interest.   I may have given the
impression as though ambition was quite wanting in
me in connection with the main human relations!   The
explanation for this double vie, split in personality, as
writers call it, lies in the fact *that ambition after all
represents a means to an end,* not the end, and in consequence it is occasionally employed, occasionally pushed

[1] Another way of overcoming the fear of death is found in Wagner's
Siegfried: " No longer does fear obsess me at the idea of the dusk of the
gods *since it has been willed!* "   Cf. in this connection the psychical mechanism
which I have described as characteristic of compulsion-neurosis (the fiction of
free-will, substitution of external compulsion by one's own etc.), and the work
of Furtmüller, *Ethik und Psycho-analyse,* Munich (1912).

to one side, depending upon the manner in which the anticipated goal can be more easily attained either with or without it."

This short analysis shows the same dynamics that I have proved exist both for the healthy and diseased psyche. Waking up at night proves to be a symbol, a simile of life in which is reflected the past (uncertainty), the present (danger from unscrupulous people), the future (search for a means) and the guiding goal (the overcoming of death).

Sleep may be looked upon as abstraction; its purpose described as enabling the socially conditioned day-thinking, thinking which has been socially adjusted, to obtain rest, permitting the sense organs with their function of social intermediary and their tendency to transcend the purely individual and corporeal, to cease temporarily from functioning. In sleep both the corporeal and psychic life is thrown upon the mercy of a fixed, already prepared psyche belonging to previous periods which have also been well prepared. These preparations seize upon the psychic activities of the previous day and conduct them further onward to the goal toward which they tend. Remnants of conscious ideational processes, such as *the dream*, reflect in hallucinatory fashion, these progressive psychic activities. The dream which is merely an accompaniment as dream-thinking, never the cause of any action—for on account of its abstract and fragmentary manner of expression it is generally not fitted for it—need not be intelligible. Where it is intelligible, where it initiates or seems to initiate actions, where it attracts, repulses, or warns, there it is being directed by some individually prepared tendency. The same is true with regard to what the dream remembers or forgets, both remembering and forgetting being induced by this previously mentioned tendency.

Sleep disturbances belong to the same tendency. Insomnia is safe-guarded so that it may be used as a certificate of illness as in our first instance, whenever it proves itself to be the best fitted means for the attainment of personal superiority and the gratification of one's own will. Those complaints of patients that seem to contradict this interpretation, merely serve the purpose of increasing the prestige the symptom enjoys.

Wakefulness in these cases results from a definitely planned arrangement, even if it unconsciously persists by reason of the mechanism of fright, pain or some arbitrary act of unknown motivation. The accompanying dreams in the form of analysis frequently show the source which the neurotic tendency has either falsely stressed or out of which it has purposely derived the feeling of solicitude for that which is to be confronted. That dreams may be of secondary importance, or even be missing, is elucidated by the second case described. On the basis of extensive material we are justified in interpreting the patient's intermittent insomnia as a tremendous faith in himself, to whom waking thought represents incontrovertible authority. The absence of dreams during the two nights—as the dreamer states— is not at all peculiar. Since his acquaintance with the problems of dream-analysis, he has very rarely dreamt, probably because dreams have lost their value and significance owing to his better preparation for his actions.

In the first case we discern clearly a line of direction that seems somewhat suspicious, a self-depreciatory willingness (epileptic neurosis) to go as far as death if necessary, for the attainment of a vague idea. His transient sleeplessness appears as though he had stumbled on his path, just as the attacks of loss of consciousness were accompanied by marked traumatic lesions. The final course this case will take is not quite transparent, yet as an indication of the rôle of a genuine and an affect-epilepsy it ought not to be passed over. When treated psycho-therapeutically these attacks became amenable to explanation, could be predicted, made milder and possibly even reduced to certain proportions. Once when under observation for a month with the regard to the necessity of a trepanation, the attacks that had occurred regularly every fortnight, suddenly ceased. From my treatment he derived merely an amelioration in the intensity of the attacks, a freer manner and a more sociable character. Shortly before he gave up my treatment, on account of his stubbornness and obstinacy, I had succeeded in proving to him that he was unconsciously working in the direction of developing digestive disturbances. Some days after that he took ill with a long drawn-out icterus. I can give some further personal details of this case. I was informed, at second hand, that he subsequently exhibited frequent attacks of rage, developed deliria of short duration in which he played the rôle of a Kaiser—(this I had inferred from his unconscious phantasies where he had used the Kaiser rôle as a symbol). Half a year after the end of my treatment he died from heart-weakness during a short attack of rage, and not during an epileptic seizure.

XIV

Homo-sexuality [1]

(Lecture delivered before the Jurististisch-Medizinische
Gesellschaft of Zurich, 1918)

IT is in the nature of human association to develop
autonomously certain conditions and rules (Furtmüller)
which we all accept and which at all times we feel as
inherent, real and existing.

The historical data concerning "Greek love" is
extraordinarily complex and tiresome and we must
therefore search for synthetic view-points if we wish
to briefly present the history of the psychological
analysis of homo-sexuality. Perhaps it will suffice,
if to-day, I point out the main points in the views of
the largest of the group—to which scientists and laymen
alike belong. To them the most significant fact in
homo-sexuality is the emphasis on the question of
inheritance, as though implying that individuals come
into the world homo-sexual. The attitudes on this
question are divergent. One group assumes that the
germinal complex—in the case of a masculine homo-
sexual—is decreased in favour of a complex of a
somewhat feminine type ; the second group believes
in certain inherited components, that have been
specifically strengthened, etc.

No one has ever claimed that the inherited feminine
factors, the female-appearing aspect, is any more
prominent among masculine homo-sexuals than are
female traits in a woman, and yet in examining homo-
sexuals we almost exclusively find individuals either
with female tendencies or such as are directed into
female channels, whereas the masculine tendencies
appear to be absent. On the other hand, (normal)
women frequently exhibit masculine tendencies. For

[1] Cf. Adler, *Das Problem der Homo-sexualität* (Reinhardt, Munich, 1917).

the demonstration of these being inherited and not acquired traits the above facts are quite unfavourable. For we may justifiably ask where are the masculine impulses? Let me add parenthetically that, of course, the masculine impulses are not lacking *i.e.* not entirely so, but that they are forced so far into the background by the feminine bearing (of the homo-sexual)— at least in certain clear-cut examples—that this discrepancy, this inward contradiction is particularly noticeable.

A second objection that is equally justified and must be unhesitatingly faced, is the enormously frequent occurrence of facultative homo-sexuality, *i.e.* of a certain number of homo-sexual experiences in the life of an individual, be it in childhood, on long journeys as in the case of sailors and prisoners, in the life of the soldier or in boarding-schools. This facultative homo-sexuality, which many reliable informants assume to be almost a normal manifestation in the life of every individual, does not incline us any the more to attributing a perponderating importance to the factor of heredity.

A second group of scientists assumes a fixation of certain sexual experiences (generally in childhood). The facts seem in one sense to contradict this theory, for we know that such apparent or really homo-sexual experiences in childhood are extraordinarily common and that the homo-sexual experiences described by patients or people accused of indulging in them, turn out frequently to be of so vague a type that we can at best draw no conclusions from them except that it is quite remarkable to notice the extent to which the homo-sexual regards such early experiences as basic for his whole development. The same objection applies to those authors who wish to explain the homo-sexuality by the assumption that such early experiences become fixed.

We feel ourselves compelled to propound another problem and one which is likely to place the questionable nature of this last explanation in an entirely different light. We may rightly ask why homo-sexuals fixate these particular experiences, experiences that we normal people unquestionably also share. That is a problem with which pedagogy is concerned although from another angle. What is it that we customarily imitate? Is not man in the expression of his imitative faculty, quite definitely directed and circumscribed by almost inviolable laws? If we watch young people, children, grown-up people, all of whom show marked tendencies toward imitation, we shall find that no one ever imitates anything that does not in some way fit into his purpose.

Now why does a homo-sexual find the fixation of a homo-sexual experience fits into his nature? We shall have to go back to a time prior to the experience to explain this. In examining particular cases it was discovered that quite apart from any sexual occurrences, these people particularly emphasized the fact that even when they were only two or three years old, they had been regarded as girls, had taken a special pleasure in playing with dolls, spent almost all their time in the company of girls, etc.

Thus the interpretation of a fixation of infantile experience hardly leads us to any understanding of the apparently alterable attitude of some people, an attitude that seems from the earliest years of an individual's existence to challenge the whole nature of our society. By his development, the homo-sexual negates the fundamental principle of the preservation of society and it is hardly feasible to believe that—irrespective of the manner in which he has come to his view-point and his emotional outlook—he should not have felt, noticed and utilized the tremendous resistances that have blocked his path during his homo-sexual evolution. We might say that it is so infinitely more difficult to be homo-sexual than normal that this fact alone should give us a measure of the tremendous expenditure of energy necessary for going through life as such. This expenditure of energy is noticeable in fact in every pervert. It can be observed in the very nature of his deductions, in his attitude toward men, women, toward his experiences. Step by step we can see the preparations he makes for coming to a unified attitude, one out of which it will not be easy to shake him. The mixed cases—of which there are so many and which are really in a large majority—frequently show the homo-sexual development in its various stages and how, only by the expenditure of very special powers, are homo-sexuals able to abandon the normal path and so distinctly circumscribe life that there is left no room for anything but homo-sexuality.

Appealing both to our sympathies and our sense of the comical is the manner in which such an individual in question hypnotizes himself step by step and forces upon himself violently the concept that he is not adapted for normality. His arguments have so little cogency that we must have accustomed ourselves to the language of the homo-sexual to remain patient. I am acquainted with some who in their external appearance are quite normal and who yet emphasize some detail about themselves, such as the fact that their language is not masculine in structure, that their hair-growth is not as strong as in other men, etc. There is no difficulty in corroborating the impression that homo-sexuals have gone to some pains to bring together everything that will give convincing evidence for their belief that they are different from other men.

Our question is therefore to find out from what source has come this ineradicable tendency to disclaim all masculine traits and the desire to gain complete certainty, corroboration and justification for their specifically different emotional and intellectual view-point. As in the case of all manifestations of the human psychic life we can only arrive at an understanding of the situation when we have grasped the meaning of the whole personality, when we have discovered its object and penetrated into its inmost soul, understood the nature of its answer to the demands of communal life. After homo-sexuals tell us of their activities which have possibly brought them into conflict with the law, or which torment and circumscribe them, we find that in other walks of life the normal standard to be expected of a man quite adapted to life—except possibly sexually —is likewise absent. The most salient traits—which appear clearly in the character of a homo-sexual are the following :—*inordinate ambition and extraordinarily pronounced caution or fear of life.*

Starting from these universally encountered facts we may ask ourselves what is going to be the fate of an individual who possesses within his nature two such contradictory traits of character as an ambition that never can hope to be gratified and a cowardice that paralyses this activity as soon as the very first steps have been taken to gratify his ambition. In some form or other every neurotic possesses those two traits although more weakly expressed. We thus find upon further inquiry into the character-physiognomy of the homo-sexual the fact corroborated that he presents us with the clear-cut picture of a neurotic man, whose nervousness does not express itself clearly because, through his homo-sexuality, he has confined his activity within narrow limits of a type that the nervous man only succeeds in developing by means of a neurosis. In this narrow circle nervous symptoms cannot exhibit themselves very well. As a rule the homo-sexual *by excluding the conditions making for difficulties*, succeeds in creating for himself a type of existence to which he is either quite adapted or which he can more easily follow than that of hetero-sexuality, which continually throws him into the current of life and brings him into relation with all the problems, demands and difficulties of social existence. Nevertheless among many homo-sexuals whose sphere of activity has not become too narrow, we encounter some remarkable symptoms. Of these symptoms the prevailing forms are compulsion-manifestations.

In the history of homo-sexual childhood we are struck by a number of manifestations of similar behaviour and similar expression that can easily be connected. One of the most important points of my interpretation is the fact that I have succeeded in demonstrating that it is at all times exceedingly difficult for homo-sexuals *to realize the nature of their sex* and that this realization has taken place much later than in the case of other children. As a rule we find, in these cases, that as children they had a fine complexion, wore long dresses, wore girlish clothes for a longer period than other children, always had girl playmates and that they hardly came into contact with experiences that would emphasize the fact that their sex was different from that of girls. They are already *mistakenly* embarked along the path of a girl's psychic development when, to their astonishment, they are made aware of the fact that they really belong to the other sex. This added difficulty for children, whose ambition is particularly stimulated and whose *caution* hinders them from undertaking any new action, is of extraordinary importance. After that, experiences of a different kind no longer suffice (to dissuade them) and they, on the contrary, utilize these different experiences in order to give strength to the belief that they are different from other children, that a miracle of nature has here become manifest and that they represent a new species. This difference as a rule appears to them in the nature of a *distinction*, a view-point that their ambition of course willingly encourages.

How does ambition come to play so great a rôle among these children? We are not here concerned with children whose development has proceeded along direct lines and not been rendered difficult but, either with children who have developed a feeling of weakness and inferiority from the *position* in which they found themselves, or with those who have been on the one hand, weighed down by the pressure of their environment or, on the other, so petted that a very early desire for being protected in the future against every rough blast of wind, of always occupying first place, takes on an intensive form.[1] This holds for both extremes of bringing-up, for both feed and intensify the child's longing to attain a future in which he will remain entirely untouched by the difficulties of life. This striving and the fear of not succeeding, causes their phantasy to be directed in a strange manner toward the idea of domination and desires of domination and induces them to search for a type of prospective situation in which they need fear danger from no side. If besides the difficulty of recognizing his own sex, the existence of impoverished and bad pecuniary family conditions, or of disorganized relations between the parents, gives the child additional difficulties, they are likely to suggest to him the thought of looking for the consummation of his ambition by a very narrowly circumscribed method. The question that mainly arises is that of his relation to the other sex

Various answers can be given to this. We know that in some cases of homo-sexuality the opposite sex seems to have been completely excluded while in others a number of compromises exist. In all instances however there is a kind of condemnation of the other sex. When a child turns in the direction of homo-sexuality,

[1] Cf. Adler, *Studie über Minderwertigkeit der Organe* (1907).

it is at the same time showing its depreciatory attitude toward the other sex. This is but the same mechanism looked at from another angle. Each manifestation calls up the other so that both lines are bound to meet at some point. We must consequently regard them not separately but in their inter-connection. If on account of the aggravated nature of the infantile situation an ardent ambition has developed, the latter will quite clearly not be able to last unless carefully protected. The coalescence of these traits of character are impossible because a specific attitude developed not only in the adult life but even in early childhood, can be perceptible in bodily movement and more particularly in the attitude assumed toward life. To understand this we need take into consideration but one fact, that these characteristics are not so definitely apparent in safe-guarded situations. The attitude of the homo-sexual toward life will always be a *hesitating one*.

Homo-sexuality has a number of different aspects. In some fashion or other and in varying degrees, a homo-sexual will be found to be antagonistic to social life, to have changed his occupation, to have begun later and finished earlier. His entire life flows along as though regulated by some brake-mechanism. The power required for operating this brake, he must himself produce again and again.

First Case.—A man in the thirties, belonging to the most aristocratic circles, well-built, with muscles of an athlete. He has admittedly a less pronounced growth of hair on his face than the normal man. He informed me that his brothers were likewise not distinguished for their hair-growth, although this had not been true of his father. His father, an immigrant, had come from a region well-known for the fact that the race of people inhabiting it possessed a meagre facial hair-growth. This trait of which the patient had spoken to physicians and which he had persuaded himself was a proof of his hereditary homo-sexuality, he himself could demon-strably trace back to a racial peculiarity. Yet this seems in no way to have affected his attitude. This in itself must suffice to demonstrate the nature of the purposive ingenuity employed by the patient to prove his contentions. We must not think of his action as prompted by any evil intent but rather as exhibiting

that unconscious deceit possessed by neurotics, to which
they continually come without realizing it, through
their ever present caution in life. This is therefore
more in the nature of naughtiness than of consciously
dishonest purpose. He was the youngest of three
brothers. All the children were very strictly super-
intended. Until the age of ten he had never associated
with girls. His brothers were the only members of his
family with whom he had been in any way intimately
connected. He was the youngest. This last factor is
not without significance for the psychology of the
youngest child is extraordinarily complicated and interesting. There are two traits in particular which
always distinguish youngest children, traits found in
such different proportions that such children seem,
for example, often to exhibit contradictory characteristics. The first trait is the sensation of oppression
due to their small size. They always appear under
pressure and can always be recognized by the fact that
they wish to be bigger than they really are. They are
always intensely affected by events and words referring
to their smallness and which might possibly hurt their
vanity. We know in what way the fairy-tale stresses
the rôle of the last-born and of the particular temperament ascribed to him there. He is always at work—
he is the one that possesses the magic boots, etc. This
it is that makes plausible the phenomena that some
well-known historical personages whose rapid progress
is most markedly apparent in art, were very frequently
last-born children. We can speak here of *position-
psychology*. The position of youngest under the pressure
of ambition spurs him continuously on and he is always
desirous of accomplishing more than those around him.
This happens however only under propitious conditions.
Sometimes, on the contrary, the difficulties and obstacles
that confront the youngest child are frequently the cause
for his loss of faith in himself and of his development
of special caution and resignation. This caution may
even be expressed to some degree in the features. In
army reviews during the war I was able to pick out
those who were last-born children. Their features
reflected either a restless and trembling ambition or
the desire to break loose.

Our patient stated further that he had been pushed

aside by his older brothers, although he always wished
to be in the foreground ; that he was continually throwing challenges to the others and that, in short, he was
swayed by a more than normal ambition.   On the other
hand he stated that he never cared to take any risks,
thought over every situation a hundred times and became
a prey again and again to doubt and trembling.   The
family supervision was a particularly careful one so that
any premature knowledge of the nature of sex can be
excluded.   At the age of ten he was put into a convent
school where he remained in the exclusive company of
boys.   I know that this convent school is strict and
narrow.   When his sex-instinct began to exhibit itself
more definitely he was not at all clear in his mind as
to the meaning of sex nor of his particular sex-rôle.
Girls appeared to him as something puzzling and unintelligible.   In addition he had been taught that any
yielding to sexual instinct was a heinous crime.   When
later on despite everything, matters became clearer and
he had learned more about sex from his comrades,
masturbation was the only path left open to him.   This,
it is true, he also regarded as a sin, but looked upon
it as the lesser of two evils, for in this case he was at
least harming no one else.   From the point of view of
the community this attitude is quite erroneous.   Kant
has propounded the question why masturbation should
be regarded as something sinful.   To me it seems that
the nature of general normal human feeling, the nature
of the differentiated social consciousness, of love of
one's kind, makes each individual regard masturbation,
which is a form of anti-social sexual gratification, as
wrong even if we have to accept its existence as in the
cases mentioned above.

In the above example we should particularly stress
the fact that on account of his social position, as an
aristocrat of very exalted position, his life had to a
marked degree to be an isolated one.   He associated
with few people, and from the beginning he had been
educated for the life of a land-owner.   As a matter
of fact there is nothing in his whole life that could
be regarded as an indication of initiative.   He had
graduated under very normal conditions from the
convent school and taken over his parent's estate.   He
was not an evil-intentioned individual and has never

harmed anyone. He has always remained exactly
where he was placed or where a rigorous destiny
had put him. We become aware of the "distance"
firmly-adhered to, separating him from the life of the
community and its demands and present in his homo-
sexuality likewise ; and we find with regard to the question of sex a defective activity, although it admittedly
is often more strongly expressed than here.

Then suddenly a real event happens. He marries.
His wife was an orphan belonging to a family of
high station. Shortly after his acquaintance with
her he confessed to his homo-sexuality. As is so
frequently the case with girls, she was attracted by
the task that seemed to present itself of playing the
rôle of saviour ; and so she married, well aware of
all the conditions and limitations. The marriage
was a thorough failure. He turned out to possess
complete psychic impotence. Behind this psychic
impotence lay of course his incapacity for application to any task. People of this kind, incapable of
devotion either to a particular task or individual and
always interested in maintaining their reputation, are
always at some distance from actual life. Our patient
was in a psychic stage of development in which he
shrank back from any further test of his worth. He
now had an estate and a wife, and refused to recognize
any other demands of life. His subsequent policy was
to reject all further demands by proving his homo-
sexuality and his neurotic troubles to constitute an
illness. He could feel quite guiltless as regards his
wife for he had confessed everything to her and she
could not justifiably reproach him. Because of the
situation in which she was placed, she was now
obliged to be at his disposal as friend, helper and
secretary. He had made no promises to her. Here we
consequently have a situation as far removed as possible
from the bustle of the world, one that we might have
surmised, from what we knew of his childhood, our
patient would seek to attain. We may assume on the
basis of many other manifestations in his life and on
that of other neurotics, that his purpose not to participate
in life of the group was firmly rooted and that it is to be
regarded as his ideal solution of life. Supported by the
fact that he had arrived at an ideal solution he came to

N

the physician full of caution and ostentatious secrecy,
the same causes that he had used to excuse himself
from associating with his fellow-men lest they immediately recognize a homo-sexual in him; for homo-sexuality
appeared to him a stigma.

In all these cases that view-point is also important
which insists that homo-sexuals stress their delinquency
with pride[1] unless certain circumstances prevent its
expression. Even the compulsion-ideas and compulsion-
acts coincide with a mood of the patient's that seemingly
rejects them and to whom they appear unintelligible.
From the previously attained view-point this attitude
shows some fundamental differences although psychologically the difference is not very great.   A sexual
compulsion idea propelled by the sexual instinct must
seek some outlet, and if that outlet is still possible and
made easier by the nature of the patient's activity, then
compulsion-ideas must in some fashion be intelligible
to him, for otherwise he would be turning aside from his
goal of gratification.   Quite a number of homo-sexuals
find something unintelligible and mysterious in their
thoughts and phantasies and try incessantly to fight
against them.   The analogy of homo-sexuality with
compulsion-neurosis is thus fairly well established.

Second case :—

In scientific literature for reasons probably connected with jurisprudence, masculine homo-sexuality
is mainly discussed. The same basic principles can be
shown to exist however in the case of female inversion.

The patient, the elder of two children, was 25 years
old. She was 4 at the time her younger brother was
born. Upon his birth all attention was transferred to
him and she was pushed into the background. Out of
this fact afterward developed an over-powering ambition.
Her family life was sombre, her father a man of violent
temper and her mother improvident. The rather intelligent girl noticing what was happening in the family,
was revolted by the idea of marriage, withdrew herself
from the company of her father, finding him merely a
brutal, bad-tempered man. She attempted to extend

[1] Cf. Pindar, *Fragment* 123 (*ed. Christ*). "He who is not inflamed with
love for the youth Theoxenes has a heart of stone. Condemned by Aphrodite,
he strives arduously to gain money or is driven along that cold path which ends
in his becoming a servant to female effrontery."

this idea to have it include her brother, in order thus to convince herself that all men were brutal. She therefore withdrew from association with both of them. Her life naturally then became exceedingly isolated. She experienced no desire to play and was exceedingly unpleasant in her relations to her playmates. However, her ambition gained for her the sympathies of her teacher. The family decided to let her study. At the age of ten she witnessed a servant give birth to a child. Her disinclination to and terror at the feminine rôle were markedly increased by this sight. As puberty approached she began to brood to an unusual degree and fell a victim to drink. So here again we find an expenditure of energy necessary to force the patient out of the groove of normal life in which, as the child of wealthy parents, she had been brought up.

Her definite transformation into the homo-sexual phase took a considerable length of time. She had become acquainted with a female homo-sexual of her native place. It was only two years after she had met this girl, however, that one day, after a violent quarrel with her mother, she went in a spirit of revenge to live with this homo-sexual and from that time on she continued to live with her. She had always kept at a distance from men, except for a young man, a relative, of peculiarly repulsive figure and ugly features. With him she became more intimate, carried on scientific and social discussions and occasionally allowed him to take her out. He appeared to be absolutely safe. This extreme caution proved her misfortune, for one day she admitted to him her homo-sexuality and he thereupon endeavoured to persuade her to marry him. They married and separated after four weeks. She proved to be impotent if we may use that expression. The matter became public and the mother with whom the girl had always been on terms of intense enmity, asked me to undertake the treatment.

The patient discussed her inclinations with me and her ambition to do something in science. Her aversion for the female rôle was so clear-cut that it could not possibly be misunderstood. She attempted to make herself impossible in society. Whatever the nature of the work proved to be she always found some way of discontinuing it. This idiosyncrasy was rooted in an erroneous infantile evaluation of the demands of life, demands she exaggerated because of her pessimistic outlook and her fear of not being able to fulfil them, a fact reflected in her low estimate of women.   The dangers of normal sexual life appear to homo-sexuals, when seen through their pessimistic spectacles, extraordinarily great and we must regard it as natural that they recoil from all undertakings that would lead to an acquiescence in the (true) sexual rôle.   Their attitude is that of people desirous of interfering with the flight of time and normal development.   We know the reasons but inverts do not, and they fight against recognizing them.   They accept as true what we know to be error and are fortified in their stand by the mistakes of an apparently scientific, specialistic and lay literature that tells them that their belief in the unalterability of homo-sexuality is right.   The psychic atmosphere in which homo-sexuals live, build their phantasies and act, renders them *irresponsible*.   The possibility of their ever becoming amenable to the intervention of society is, however, by no means excluded.   It seems to me that the most important thing in any attempt at a cure is, after all, the recognition of the logical demands of life and this is felt even by patients and at the very least enables them to develop great secrecy and causes them considerable excitement on those occasions when they are pursuing their *idée fixe* or following their enthusiasm. The voice of the community, that must always show its disapproval of homo-sexuality, is announced in this fact.

XV

Compulsion Neurosis

(Address delivered November 1918 before the Gesellschaft der Aerzte, in Zurich)

ALL who know the state of mind of the compulsion-neurotic will have realized that such a person is struggling along lines of activity *removed from those of normal human expression.* Worry and torment are never absent in the compulsion-neurotic.

It is astounding to find patients who have never been in touch with medical literature, call the promptings of compulsion-manifestations by a term that both science and philosophy have taken over, namely an imperative. Philosophy, strange as it may appear, is frequently found to employ the same expressions and possess the same conceptions as the neurotic.

The forms which compulsion-neurosis generally exhibits are washing-compulsion, prayer, masturbation, ethical ideas of the most manifold kind, brooding, etc. From the view-point of a systematic subdivision of the field, compulsion-neurosis could be considerably extended, for we find the same mechanism in the symptomology of enuresis nocturna, nervous refusal of nourishment, hunger-compulsion, perversion, etc.

The symptoms of compulsion-actions have been neglected in the literature of the subject.

I am personally acquainted with three cases of the compulsion.

Let me first mention the now unknown romanticist von Sonnenberg who from early childhood till the age of puberty suffered from the symptoms of prayer-compulsion. He was an obstinate, ambitious and unrestrained boy, frequently at odds with his environment. At an early age religious ideas manifested themselves. This latter symptom generally appeared during the hours of instruction and in consequence *either the instruction would be interfered with or interrupted.* Jean Paul has also described in *Schmelzle's Journey to Flaez* a number of compulsion-acts. During the childhood of the hero of the story, the latter was at times seized with the necessity of shouting "Fire," a fact that easily led to panics. These and similar symptoms are remarkably frequent and lead at times to marked disturbances in public life.

In the third case, found in Vischer's *Auch Einer* the entire point of view of the hero is built upon his sneezing and sniffling compulsion.

It is particularly characteristic of compulsion-neurosis that all such acts possess as an introductory stage, what might be called the struggle of the patient against the environment. In this introductory phase he is subjected to sensations of oppression. All writers on the subject specifically mention that the patient is fully aware of the senselessness of his compulsion-symptom.

Like all maxims and views found in the literature on neurosis this statement must be taken with a grain of salt. Some patients stated that they had experienced a feeling of deliverance and satisfaction at the manner in which their symptoms behaved because these were rooted in their whole nature and thus demonstrated both their justification and necessity. Previous to this stage of an emotionally determined decision in favour of the symptom, there is found a tremendous tension in the psyche that may have been in existence for months or for years. We are thus justified in assuming that the position taken by the patient only serves to loosen the symptom as if in his professed struggle against the compulsion-act he wished to appropriate to himself the right of producing the symptom. We must likewise not forget that the nature of the patient's method of argument is arbitrary for he is judge, plaintiff and defendant rolled in one.

Compulsion-neurosis presents a fairly complete disease-picture and exhibits the basic traits of general neurosis. Inter connections of the most manifold type exist. The transition to the neurasthenic complex is of very normal nature. If we carefully observe such a compulsion-act as air-inhalation which is far more frequent than generally assumed, then its connection with a large number of neurasthenic, stomach and intestinal disturbances will soon become apparent. Its relations to hysteria are just as frequent and in war-neuroses analogies with hysterical tremor, paralysis and spasms were indeed widely known. Not infrequently indications of either slight or severe paranoidal mani-festations are found in compulsion-blushing. The connection with anxiety-neurosis is shown by the fact that when the compulsion-symptoms are suppressed their place is taken by anxiety. Often the compulsion-neurosis either passes into alcoholism or morphinism or is connected with them. The connection with impulsive insanity, compulsion-impulses toward criminality, with compulsive self-accusation and moral insanity, all result in special neurotic physiognomies. A large number of relations exist with such apparent bad habits, as *e.g.*, certain forms of laziness, pedantry, waste of time and particularly tormenting and hypermoral conceptions, fanaticism for truth, etc.

In one sense every individual shows in his psychic constitution traits that call to mind compulsion-neurosis and which, developed along many different lines, lead occasionally to disturbances of a definite type. For instance, exaggerated faith in supernatural help which in certain individuals permeates their whole life and activity. And then again, conditions about which normal people might easily give us information such as counting of syllables, reading signs of firms, counting windows, etc., all of which appear quite senseless.

Between compulsion-neurosis and neurotic doubt an extraordinary connection exists.

The psychic interconnection of all these manifesta-tions should bring home to us the danger of becoming lost as in psychology, in the study of differences that cannot be measured.

There are a number of proofs for the correctness or approximate accuracy of a neuro-psychological view-point.

One test is the following. In the absence of the family physician a neurologist might be called in to examine a patient. He must not allow himself to be enticed into asking leading questions nor into making methodical inquiries, yet he must proceed in such a manner that light can be thrown upon the whole personality of the patient.　　And this he must do without previous consultation with the family physician.　　The physician generally sees the connections that emerge from the questions and answers of the patient during the examination although the latter has not the slightest notion of what is happening.

This method is of course not free from criticism and a further test as to the correctness of our interpretation of the symptoms is consequently necessary.　　It is best to put on one side the question of symptoms, which is, of course, the real reason for the treatment, and concern one's self exclusively with the personality of the patient. Attempts should be made to obtain information about him, to penetrate into his nature, his purpose in life and his attitude toward the demands of family and society.　　A fairly sharply-outlined conception of his character will then soon emerge.　　The examination will soon prove that the patient possesses a number of traits that can then be fused together into a composite picture.

We shall first of all find that we are not concerned with individuals to be thought of as exclusively passive, for a certain degree of activity will be present.　　This can be detected in the fact that they do not keep themselves completely in the back-ground.　　As a rule they have passed examinations and have learned something. They are, however, all on the threshold of some definite decision in life—love, marriage, the selection of a profession, the coming on of age, etc.

After drawing a conclusion from the sketch (of their lives) furnished from the direction of their character-lines, after traits of marked sensitiveness and an attitude we might call unapproachability have been demonstrated to exist, after we have shown patients to possess little love of neighbour or humanity, few friends, and an ambition so noticeable that they are conscious of it themselves, then we are in a position to visualize concretely how these individuals answer the demands of life with a kind of warding-off gesture.

As in other neuroses we may here speak of a *positional-disease* in contradistinction to a dispositional disease as some authors assume.　　Frequently the family influence weighs down so heavily upon the patient that it forces him either into latent or open opposition.

An attitude of hostility is then manifested in connection with every demand made by society.

If we were to put the question to the patient, " *What would you do if you were quite well?* " he would almost certainly name that particular demand of society that it might be assumed he was trying to evade.

Second-born sons, girls in families of boys, boys in families of girls, are with astonishing frequency subject to compulsion-neurosis. The second-born is practically always in a position which brings closer to him than to others (either through error or by favourable events) the temptation of fighting with reinforced energies for recognition within the small family circle.

The third test for the correctness of the results obtained consists in the direction-lines that we have shown to exist in the inner nature of the patient, letting us see that the symptoms are necessary, opportune and in some form or other utilizable. There is, of course, not the slightest necessity for assuming any causal dependence, for the patient is not, for example, bound to his symptom as would have to be the case causally. It looks more as if the patient were letting himself be enticed and mislead by his symptom. In fact we are dealing with a human deviation so near to all of us that we can sympathize with it.

This error in the psychic structure of the patient arises from his more or less pronounced pessimistic outlook, built on a feeling of inferiority and it quite automatically *produces in him the temptation to turn back as soon as society makes demands upon him.* Such a fact also proves that any alteration of the patient's real nature can come about only *by explanàtion.*

Let me explain the above inter-connections by means of two cases.

Case I deals with a young woman who had been forced into marriage against her will by a somewhat strict father. She had always been serious, ambitious and markedly conscientious, her conscientiousness to be explained by the fact that her father, whom she regarded as the most definite personality in the family, laid weight upon this particular quality. She was the only girl in a family consisting of three boys and told me quite spontaneously that she keenly felt *her secondary position.* Her duties were concerned with household matters and there she was under the care of a somewhat cantankerous, complaining mother.

She showed little resistance to her (enforced) marriage. It had been a Catholic marriage but had been annulled after two years on account of certain offences of her husband. Shortly after that she became acquainted with a man with whom she soon fell in love and to whom she was married according to the Hungarian rite. This marriage met with the disapproval of her mother-in-law. Then came the war. She had had a boy by her first marriage and with the child she was compelled to join her step-mother while her husband was in the army. She thus found herself shortly after her marriage, in a position from which with every fibre of her being she wished to free herself. For this new situation called into life again a feeling of defeat such as she had known when living with her own mother. Her mother-in-law's criticisms were very severe. About that time a book of Prof. Förster's fell into her hands, wherein she read that the marriage relation was under all conditions undissolvable and that divorce was a crime against morality.

After that she from time to time had the feeling, accompanied by depression, that she ought really to return to her first husband. The depression itself was constant. It was one of those cases of compulsion-neuroses where manifestations of depression occur which in turn feed the compulsion-idea. The significance of the compulsion-idea lay in the fact that it furnished her with a certificate of illness and obtained through it certain privileges that as a matter of fact her ambition most coveted. She was then freed from criticism, could put the care of her child, *i.e.* the household duties upon which she definitely looked down, in the hands of her mother, and soon found herself the centre of attention in the family and possessed of a number of fictive advantages, which any ambitious young woman might regard as some sort of a recompense for all the disadvantages that had been her lot in connection with her brothers.

If anyone doubts the correctness of *the goal of superiority* I postulate in all neuroses, let him make the following test. Let him, for example, look for the purpose of the symptom or compulsion-idea such as this woman's belief that she had committed a sin. What

is the real ulterior notion behind this thought? Her
conscientiously religious father had never developed
such an idea.   In other words, the daughter is insisting
that she is more conscientious and more religious ! She
was an extremely ambitious person and one whose
ambition had never been gratified because it *could* never
find fulfilment in a new situation, or, for that matter,
considering its nature, in any situation.   She really was
indulging in a revolt that took the form of passive
resistance, a type of behaviour that can be shown to
exist in every neurosis.   She disqualified herself for the
performance of her proper work *by positing a compulsion
of her own making in place of that of society and of life* and
so *preoccupied*, she pushed aside all the demands of
society and of her immediate family circle.   It can in
all cases be shown *that the greatest enemy of such patients
is time*.   She must waste her time, for the very existence
of time constitutes a demand in the form of—" How are
you going to use me "?   *To waste time* the patient devised
an extensive system of correspondence with clergymen
and moralists, and depressions with their forced appeal
for sympathy from her environment.   She shrank back
before the fulfilment of the duties her second marriage
entailed, because she wished in particular to evade the
criticisms of her second mother-in-law.

Case 2.   The patient is an unusually able and
ambitious person.   He had in childhood already felt
his incapacity to face life, and this had definitely differentiated him from his comrades.   He had never had
any idea about his future life or of marriage.   We
may conclude, considering the *natural development of
such ideas*, that this was not merely a case of such
thoughts being absent, but of a decision not to have an
occupation and not to marry, resolutions that are
frequently found in children.   The patient was unusually ambitious, but, as this *evasion* proves, lost
confidence in himself.

He had been carefully brought up by his parents.
His father was a markedly honourable person.   The
patient had in his childhood already suffered from
being placed in uncomfortable situations that had
wounded his pride in his moral conduct.   He had been
detected by his father in a white lie and this had followed
him throughout life.   Not long after this event, compulsion-ideas in the form of an intense *feeling of guilt*

manifested themselves. His suffering made his whole environment feel uncomfortable and his family tried to mitigate it. For months at a time he brought accusations against himself on account of some erroneous information he had given ; brooded a whole year over inconsequential matters ; informed his parents of everything and then went to his teacher and informed the latter that a year before he had given an incorrect piece of information.

He passed his examinations and graduated from a high-school. Then *when he was about to face life* and pursue some occupation, he was prevented by a severe illness. Not only did his consciousness of guilt persist, but it compelled him to kneel down publicly and repeat prayers to himself. Then he consoled himself with the hope that people would regard him not as a fool but as an extraordinarily religious man. It was upon such an assumption that he prostrated himself in public.

His illness seemed to disappear as soon as he was told to look about for some other profession. He went to another city. There, after lengthy preparations, he threw himself upon the ground in front of a shrine to the Virgin and, in the presence of a large number of people, made accusations against himself and confessed his sins publicly. He was put under confinement and then taken home by his father.

After some amelioration in his condition he began to study for another profession. Then one day he suddenly disappeared. He was found in an insane asylum to which he had sought refuge until he got better. *There, freed from all demands*, his condition improved. His self-condemnatory ideas gradually disappeared into the background. They were, as a matter of fact, concerned with utterly unimportant questions, and although they still terminated with an imperative necessity of kneeling down and praying. He felt himself, however, now capable of making some resistance. The physician advised him to return home and *take up some kind of work*.

On the same day he suddenly appeared, absolutely naked, in the common dining-room.

After a considerable period of time he left the asylum in a greatly improved condition and pursued his studies further. On every occasion, however, on which he was confronted either with a self-imposed task or one imposed from without, he fled to the insane-asylum and stayed there for some time. He was regarded as a man with excellent knowledge of his own subject, thus showing that he was not merely passive, but really in advance of his colleagues. He himself, however, was entirely under the ban of his own incompetence. His greatest ambition was to be superior to others, particularly to his older brother. His illness permitted him to feel somewhat gratified ; did he not hold so much *in reserve !* He could for this reason always be permeated with the thought of what *he might have accomplished had not this fatal neurosis befallen him,* consumed so much of his time and caused him such endless trouble and worry ! From the above we may draw legitimately the inference that his intense ambition led him on into a disease that proved his salvation, just as under similar conditions, people seize upon a narcotic, upon alcohol, morphine, and occasionally even enter politics.

To build up such a life upon purely intellectual lines is impossible. Consequently he employed all his abilities and feelings in the construction of his disease arrangement.

He was now satisfied if he only proved merely superior to the members of his smaller circle of acquaintances. This can also be inferred from the nature of his compulsion-idea, "I am better than the others for I feel myself guilty where others are incapable of it. I am more pious, virtuous, more conscientious than all the others put together, including my father."

As he wished to be the first in a small circumscribed group, not the first in society, not along the main paths of life and not by means of the exertion of all his powers, he was content with his own personal opinion and with the simulation of superiority.

The tendency toward a goal of superiority is found in all neuroses and is the driving force of compulsion-neuroses. It is never absent. Nevertheless the symptom of compulsion-manifestation is adapted only for neurotically disposed individuals whose life-line lies in proximity to the demands of society. The outburst of a compulsion-neurosis would then, just as a revolt, prevent complete devotion to society's demands.

Conclusion

When in a mood of anxiety, worry and torment, compulsion-ideas, compulsion-speech and compulsion-acts appear in the form of "an imperative intuition." The frequency of these neuroses is well known but is even greater than generally assumed to-day, that is, if we interpret the neurotic compulsion as a symptom-picture of the neurosis and it is not made to appear curtailed by an unjustified method of subdividing it. As a literary example let me quote the delightful biographical sketch of life written by the now forgotten romanticist, Sonnenberg, who was suffering from melancholia when he died ; secondly, Vischer's *Auch Einer*, and the figure of Schmelzle drawn by Jean Paul. Enuresis, compulsion hunger and sexual perversions belong unquestionably to this group.

The generalized statement of some authorities that the essential traits in the compulsion neurosis consist of the patient's realization of the senselessness yet inevitableness of his acts, does not always hold. Occasionally, on the contrary, the patient emphasizes the purposeful nature of the compulsion and its correspondence with his character. The significance of this stress on the senselessness of the phenomenon does not lie in the place where the scientists look for it, *i.e.* as though constituting a proof of the unhampered intelligence of the patient, but rather because it secures a certificate of illness for him. It lies in the fact that it underlines the inevitableness of his acts in spite of all efforts, in the establishment of a condition of frightful suffering, and the piling of additional loads upon him that lead finally either to a partial or *complete exemption from our normal duties.*

The lines of demarcation between the neurasthenic, hysterical and fear-neurotic complexes are often vague. Alcoholism, morphinism, etc., are closely related; impulsive insanity, instinctive activities, compulsory self-accusations and certain stereotyped features and disturbances of psychic nature show a similar psychological structure. Manifestations of normal psychic life conduct us to the utilizable basis of the compulsion-phenomenon. Certain types of habits, exaggerated principles, misuse of truth and of morality are psychologically of similar structure. The connection with a mood of doubt interfering likewise with any progressive movement is also close.

The explanation of compulsion-neurosis according to the individual psychological method discloses the unconscious purpose of the patient *to unburden and free himself by means of a diseased compulsion from the compulsion due to* the necessary demands made by society:— to construct a subsidiary field of action in order to be able to flee from the main battle-field of life and fritter away time that might otherwise compel him to fulfil his individual tasks.

The only test for the correctness of the psychological demonstration of our views must be a proof that the patient has been planning to withdraw himself from the demands of life or at least to obtain some mitigation of the responsibility for his decisions or his actions, by the use of means other than those of the compulsion-neurosis, *i.e.* quite independently of pathological manifestations, and by the employment of excuses, evasions, and pretexts.

The treatment should consist in clearing up the nature of the facts, in removing of erroneous notions dating from childhood, in frank discussion and treatment of the exaggerated ambition, and lastly, in isolating the patient's self-love and hyper-anxiety tendencies.

XVI

On the Function of the Compulsion-Conception as a Means of Intensifying the Individuality-Feeling

(1913)

I

In a general way I might claim that in every compulsion-neurotic there inheres the function of withdrawing from external compulsion, so that he may obey only his own compulsion. In other words, the compulsion-neurotic struggles so definitely against the will of another and against every foreign influence, that, in his fight against these, he comes to the point of positing his own will as sacred and irresistible. The following is a very instructive case. A woman, forty years old, complained *of not being able to do any housework* because she had lost the knowledge of performing even the simplest things. She was consequently under the compulsion of repeating to herself all the things *she had to do.* She then was able to perform her tasks. If, for example, she had to place a chair at the table she would first have to say to herself "I must place the chair at the table!" Then she would succeed. The patient (in other words) had first to replace an external will, the obligation to do (female) house-work, by her own will in order to do anything. Those who remember Furtmüller's delightful work on Ethics and Psycho-analysis know this mechanism to be one of the pillars of ethics. It represents also one of the main pillars of compulsion-neurosis and enables the patient to prove his semi-godlikeness where all other influences appear nullified. Let me briefly mention also how the working-compulsion enables a person to demonstrate the uncleanliness of his environment, how the masturbation-compulsion prevents the influence of the sexual partner, how the prayer-compulsion appears, in the most peculiar manner, to place at the disposal of the person praying all heavenly powers. " If I did not do that ; if I say or do that ; if I do not say that prayer, and say those words ; such and such a person will die." The meaning becomes immediately clear as soon as we state the positive formula : " If I do this or leave it ; if I let my will work ; then this person will not die." Thus the patient obtains an illusory proof, just as if he were lord of life and death or like a deity.

On this subject we may further add that excessive doubt and neurotic anxiety represent means utilizable in the neurosis and permit the patient to adhere to his life-line, to thwart every outside influence (on his profession and attitude) and every outside expectation. Compulsion, doubt and fear will always be found to represent these safe-guards in the neurosis, that are to enable the patient to appear on top, masculine and superior, as I have shown in the previous chapters.

II

A patient aged 35, suffering from apathy and compulsion-ideas, and always in doubt as to her practical abilities, disclosed herself on the first day (of the treatment) as an art enthusiast. The deepest impression made upon her by any pictures were (1) the self-portrait of the ageing Rembrandt, (2) Signorelli's frescoes of the Day of Judgment and (3) Giorgione's Three Ages (also known as The Concert).

We see the patient's interest fixed on old age and the future, and we may assume that we are dealing with a person who believes that she is only with difficulty maintaining her balance, a person obsessed by fear, and to whom it appears that any loss whatsoever is likely to plunge her into serious deviations. She must therefore be a person who is trying to pass from an insecure position to one of comparative equilibrium, for which reason her artifices, *i.e.* her neurotic symptoms, appear necessary.

And yet all must be lost—youth, beauty, power, influence ! Only two ways are left open, either reversal and search for a new life-line ; and this makes her feel the illness arising from her former position to be a disturbing element. This path is bound eventually to take her to a nerve-specialist! Or she may intensify her symptoms and her prominence in order to gain power. Such patients are generally sent to a physician by their families.

Any position that is tenaciously adhered to through pedantry, fear and compulsion, merely indicates in a neurotic patient an old feeling of insecurity. We may indeed, in the above case, have to assume that this woman who, when first told that she was dissatisfied with her feminine rôle, denied it, had nevertheless arrived at her neurosis by means of the masculine protest.

She told me the next day that the society of Vienna was quite exhausting to her, that it was easier to rest in the country. The connection permits us to infer that this tiredness represented a purposeful arrangement with the object of indicating that any future transference of residence to Vienna was unfeasible.

If we connect the explanation of both these days we obtain the following picture :—an unusually ambitious woman who always wished to play the main rôle, is not content with her rich fund of abilities, but trembles at the idea of not being able, as she grows older, to hold her own in the upper society of the capital. She looks busily into the future in order to anticipate her dethrone-ment, and from the impressions she is able to utilize, and the ever-present difficulties of life, she weaves an emotionally steeped belief that she is not adapted to practical life, *i.e.* not adapted to the rôle of an ageing housewife.

She must therefore succeed in evading either by neurosis or neurotic symptoms—in this case by means of compulsion-ideas or by a feeling of helplessness and tiredness—a truth that she posits unconsciously, for she assumes that age degrades a woman, makes her merely man's helper, an article of luxury, to an even more marked degree than in youth. Instead of indulging in extensive discussions let me provisionally give as proof of my contention the fact that this woman, the nearer she felt herself to the rôle of a woman, all the more definitely refused "to play the game". She became frigid and retired for four days during her menses.

On the second day she told me the following dream :
"On your table Wilde's *Dorian Gray* was lying. Inside
the book there was a large piece of white artistically
embroidered silk. I asked myself how this piece of silk
came to be in the book."

The first part of the dream contains a corroboration
of the aggravated cause of her present condition, like
the portrait of Dorian Gray beginning to age. White
silk, silk embroidered curtains and similar things have
particular value for the patient. "A book on my table ;
a book written by me." Her precious things, her
treasured possessions in my book! This astonishes
her. The thought arose in her mind whether I was not
going to write about her fear of old age.

Her old attitude of reserve interposed as a utilizable
method of increasing her distance from the physician.

The necessity of intensifying the neurosis is caused
by numerous factors :—the struggle against her feminine
rôle, *i.e.* the over-evaluation of the masculine (artistic)
profession ; the depreciatory attitude toward the house-
wife ; natural events such as marriage, love, old age,
and discussions of all kinds that threaten her ideal of
superiority. The neurosis is made up of individually
utilized and recognized psychic and bodily artifices
through whose interaction the fiction of being exceptional, of power and of free-will, can be preserved. The
exclusion of all external demands was given by the
increase in power due to the certificate of illness.

XVII

Neurotic Hunger-Strike

THE fear of eating begins as a rule at the age of seventeen and almost always with girls. Its adoption is generally followed by rapid decrease in weight. The goal, to be inferred from the whole attitude of the patient, is the rejection of the woman's rôle. In other words it is an attempt by means of an exaggerated abstinence—as is so generally the case—to retard the development of the female bodily form. One of these patients painted her whole body, in addition, with tincture of iodine in the belief of inducing decrease of weight in that manner. At the same time she repeatedly impressed upon her younger sister the importance of eating and was always inciting her to eat. One patient finally reduced herself to a weight of twenty kilo and looked more like a ghost than a young girl.

In all these instances we are dealing with girls who as children had already tested the value and significance of the "hunger-strike" as a means of attaining power. In every developed neurosis this pressure upon the patient and upon the physician is always present. By doing this everything is at once centred about her and her will dominates the situation in every respect. We can now understand why patients of this type lay so much value upon the nature of the food and why they must safeguard this evaluation by means of a "fear arrangement." This process of nourishment cannot be stressed too much, for its over-evaluation permits them to logically pursue their goal to rule over others (like a man! like a father!). It is only then that they feel the right to criticize everything for they have now arrived at the point of view which allows them to make efforts to look down upon the cooking skill of their mother, to dictate the choice of foods, to insist upon punctuality in meals, to force people at the same time to direct their attention to them and to solicitously inquire whether they are not going to eat.

One of my patients changed her attitude after some time, and insisting suddenly upon the importance of eating, began to crave and devour huge quantities of food, a behaviour that evoked the same solicitude from her mother. She was engaged and apparently desired to marry as soon as she was "well." However she obstructed the progress of her female rôle by all sorts of nervous symptoms (depressions, outbursts of rage, insomnia) and particularly by resorting to continual "fattening cures," thus developing into a monstrosity. She continually consumed bromide and declared that without it she felt worse ; she complained at the same time of marked bromide acne, which disfigured her just as much as her excessive fatness. (Nervous constipation, desire for defaecation, tic, cutting of grimaces or compulsion-neurosis frequently serve the same purpose.) Many patients attain the same goal by eating in public and fasting in private. The enormous importance of hunger-strike in melancholia, paranoia and dementia praecox, where by means of negativism the will of the environment is rendered impotent, is well known.

The artifice of ' To and Fro' is analogous to many other neurotic arrangements. By means of it the symptom of "frittering away time" is developed. This is quite intelligible when it is remembered that the patient through "fear of making a decision"—in the above instance, through "fear of his partner"—has decided upon the "hesitating attitude," "retreat" or suicide. The importance of the nourishment is first over-evaluated and then we have the fear of the taking of nourishment so that finally, as might have been expected, there is no other alternative but that of either adopting the hesitating attitude, of a truce, or of retreating before the normal demands of society. In this behaviour we see definitely reflected the old infantile feeling of inferiority in connection with the demands of life. Other "artifices of the weak" are easily enough detected. Impulses toward revenge are always present just as is the exercise of tyranny over the other members of the family.

XVIII

Dreams and Dream-Interpretation

(Lecture delivered in September, 1912)

THIS is an age-old problem that can be traced back to the cradle of mankind. Fools and wise men have tried their hands at it and kings and beggars have attempted to extend the limits of their world knowledge by dream interpretation. How does the dream arise? What does it do? How are its hieroglyphics to be deciphered?

Egyptians, Chaldeans, Jews, Greeks, Romans and Teutons listened eagerly to the mystic language of the dream and in their myths and poems, we find indicated many traces of their arduous research for its understanding, for its interpretation. We hear them repeatedly insist as though obsessed ; the dream can disclose the future ! The famous dream-interpretations of the *Bible*, the *Talmud*, Herodotus, Artemidorus, Cicero, and the *Nibelungen-Lied*, impress upon us with undeniable certainty the conviction that the dream is a peering into the future. Even up to the present day the idea of obtaining knowledge of the unknowable is always brought into connection with reflections upon dreams. That our rationalistic age externally repudiated the hope of unveiling the future and laughed at such attempts is intelligible enough and it is this attitude that has made any occupation with the problem of the dream open to ridicule.

In order to circumscribe our field let me insist that I do not hold the view that the dream is a prophetic inspiration, that it can unlock the future or give knowledge of the unknowable. My extensive preoccupation with dreams has taught me one thing, that the dream like any other psychic manifestation comes into being through powers inherent in each individual. At the very threshold of any investigation there appear problems indicating that the possibility of dreams being prophetic was not easy to posit and that dreams are more likely to confuse than clarify the situation. The question to be asked clothed in all its difficulties is :—Is it really impossible for the human mind, within certain definite limits, to look into the future?

Unbiased observations lead to the strangest results. If the question (of the dream peering into the future) is put directly, an individual will generally deny it. But let us not pay any attention to mere external words or thoughts. If I were indeed to question the other portions of his body, (*i.e.* not his mouth or brain) for example, his movements, carriage, his actions, then we would receive quite a different impression. Although we deny the possibility of looking into the future, our whole manner of life is such that it betrays exactly to what an extent we would like to obtain certainty with regard to future events. Our behaviour clearly shows that, right or wrong, we do adhere to a possibility of obtaining knowledge of the future. Indeed it can further be shown that we would not be able to do anything if the future complexion of things—either those we desire or fear—did not determine the direction to be taken, furnish us with the incitement to act and disclose to us both the evasions and obstacles. *We continually act as if possessed of fore-knowledge of the future, although we realize that we can know nothing.*

Let us start from the petty things of life. If I buy something I obtain an anticipatory sensation, taste and pleasure. Frequently it is only this steadfast belief in an anticipated situation, with its pleasures and inconveniences, that makes me act or refrain from action. The fact that I am open to error will not deter me. On the other hand I refrain from acting in order, *if doubt develops*,[1] to weigh two possible future situations without coming to any decision. If I go to bed to-night I do not know that on the morrow when I awake there will be daylight, but I prepare myself for it.

But do I really know it? Do I know it in the same sense as I know that I am standing in front of you? No, my knowledge is of an entirely different order. It is not to be found in my *conscious thinking*. Yet its

---

[1] The function of doubt in life and in the neurosis is, as I have shown, always to obtain a cessation of aggressiveness, to evade decisions and to conceal this fact from one's self.

traces are indirectly in my bodily attitude, at my command. The Russian scientist Pawlow was able to show that in the stomach of animals when they *expect* a certain food, the juices necessary for digestion are secreted *as though the stomach had fore-knowledge of what foods it was to receive.* That means, however, that our body must be operating, like our mind, with some knowledge of the future if it wishes to play its rôle and be adequate ; that it makes preparations as though it could foretell the future. This reckoning with the future is as in the last-mentioned instance quite foreign to our conscious thinking. Let us however ponder on this question ! Would we ever act if we *consciously* grasped the future? Would not reflection, criticism, the constant weighing of pro and con constitute an insuperable obstacle to what we really desire to do, to act? *Our apparent knowledge of the future must consequently remain in our unconscious.* A condition of diseased psychic make-up exists—it is common and expresses itself in manifold ways—extreme doubt, compulsion-brooding, *folie de doute*—where the inward suffering actually drives the patient *into the only path* for properly safeguarding his importance and his feeling of individuality. The painful examination of one's own future prospects so prominently emphasizes its uncertainty and the anticipatory thinking is so definitely of a conscious kind that a set-back follows. The impossibility of knowing the future either consciously or with certainty fills the patient with indecision and doubt and thus every one of his activities is interfered with by considerations of a different character. The contrast is given by that mania which manifests itself where a secret and otherwise unconscious future goal expresses itself impetuously, overwhelming reality with evil intent and enticing the conscious self to irresistible assumptions in order to protect the pathological self-consciousness from making mistakes in its co-operation with society.

That conscious thinking plays but a minor rôle in dreams hardly needs proof. Similarly the critical faculty and the contradictions brought about by the inactive sense organs are also inoperative. Is it conceivable that the expectations, wishes, and fears connected with the given situation of the dreamer should manifest themselves undisguisedly in the dream ?

A patient had been brought to the hospital after he had taken ill with a severe attack of tabes ; his mobility and sensibility was in consequence of his disease markedly limited and he had in addition become blind and deaf. As there was no means of communicating with him, his situation was indeed a very remarkable one. When I saw him he was continually demanding beer and abusing the nurse in all sorts of obscene language. His real strivings, as well as his method of enforcement remained untouched. If, however, we were to imagine one of his sense-organs as functioning it is evident that not only his statements but likewise his thought-connections would have taken a different turn. The non-functioning of touch during sleep is felt in many ways particularly in the displacement of the realm of action and in the *less hampered emergence of a goal.* This necessarily leads as compared with the waking stage, to an intensification and stressing of conation and in content to analogical but more sharply outlined characterizations and suggestions. These latter, however, in consequence of the dreamer's caution may be accompanied by restrictions or obstacles. Even Havelock Ellis (*The World of Dreams*) who offers other explanations mentions this problem. Looked at from other view-points we can understand why in the case of the above patient, as in dreams, only an understanding of the true situation of affairs could bring about a *rationalization* (Nietzsche) and a "*logical interpretation*".

Nevertheless the direction of the activity and therefore the *anticipatory, prescient function of the dream* is always clearly discernible ;[1] it foreshadows *the preparations developed in connection with actual difficulties encountered by the dreamer's life-line,* and the safe-guarding purpose is never lost sight of. Let us attempt to trace these lines by an example. A patient with a severe case of *agoraphobia,* who had taken ill with hæmotropia, dreamt the following as she lay in bed incapacitated from pursuing her duties as a business woman :—

"I enter a shop and find the girls playing cards."

In all my cases of agoraphobia I found this symptom used as an excellent means of forcing upon

[1] First described in Aggressionstrieb 1913 (Cf. *Heilen und Bilden*), in Chapters vii, x and xi of this work, and in *The Neurotic Constitution.*

the environment, relations, husband or wife, employees, certain duties and dictating laws to them like *a kaiser or deity*. This tyranny is accomplished by preventing any person from being absent or withdrawing from business on such excuses as attacks of anxiety, dizziness or nausea.[1] I always in such a case think of the similarity of this attitude to that of the Pope, *the deputy of God*, who regards himself as a prisoner (in the Vatican) and who by this very renunciation of his personal freedom, intensifies the worship of the believers and forces all potentates to come to him (" The journey to Canossa ") without their being able to expect a return visit. The dream of my patient occurred at a time when this trial of strength had already become manifest. The interpretation is simple. The dreamer put herself into the future situation in which she would be out of bed and on the look-out for transgressions of rules. Her whole psychic life is permeated with the conviction that without her nothing could possibly be in proper order. This conviction she adheres to in other phases of life, for she *degrades everyone and tries pedantically to improve everything*. In her ever-wakeful distrust she is always endeavouring to discover errors in others. So thoroughly is she filled with experiences emphasizing mistrust that she really developed greater acuteness in detecting mistakes than others. She knew exactly what employees would do if they were permitted to? She also knew what men do when they are alone. "All men are alike!" For that reason her husband always has to remain at home.

Unquestionably considering the nature of her preparations she will, as soon as she recovers from lung-trouble, discover quite a number of omissions in her business, which is situated right near her home. She may even discover that the employees have played cards. The day after her dream she had the servant bring her the cards and on some pretext or other, had the girl-employees called to her bed-side repeatedly in order to give them new directions and to supervise them. In order to obtain light on the future she only

---

[1] Cf. *Adler*, " Beiträge zum Organischen Substrat der Neurosen " (*Oesterr. Aerztezeitung*, 1912, Hefte 23 and 24), and an excerpt from the medical history of the above-mentioned patient in the chapter on " The Rôle of the Unconscious ", in this book.

has to ferret out in her sleep-consciousness, in consonance with her over-strained *goal of superiority*, some fitting analogies and to take literally and seriously the fiction of the *recurrence of similar*[1] *manifestations in individual experiences.* Indeed in order to prove herself to have been in the right all she need do is, after her recovery, to increase the standard of her demands. Mistakes and omissions would then certainly be found to exist.

As another example of dream interpretation, I would like to use the dream of the poet Simonides as handed down by Cicero, a dream interpretation that I have already used to develop a part of my theory of dreams (cf. the chapter " On the Concept of Resistance "). One night shortly before embarking on a journey to Asia Minor Simonides dreamt "a dead person whom he had piously buried warned him from taking the contemplated journey." After this dream Simonides discontinued his preparations for the journey and stayed at home. According to our experiences in dream-interpretation we may assume that Simonides was afraid of this journey, that *he used this dead person*[2] who was under obligations to him, *to frighten and protect himself* by the thought of the horror of the grave and by presentiments of meeting a frightful end. According to the narrator the boat capsized, an event that probably presented itself to the dreamer's mind on the analogy of other shipwrecks. If the boat had really arrived safely at its destination what would have prevented superstitious natures from assuming that it would have gone down had Simonides not heeded the warning and been on board?

We find consequently in dreams two types of attempts of pre-interpreting, of solving a problem, and

---

[1] The deeper knowledge of this "fiction of similarity" one of the most important assumptions of thought and of the causality principle, I owe to my friend and collaborator A. Häutler.

[2] I intend further on to discuss in detail the employment of such very broad emotion-provoking reminiscences that *serve the purpose of* inducing affects and their consequences, cautious actions and at the same time, loathing, dizziness, anxiety, fear of the sexual partner, fainting and other neurotic symptoms. Much of these I have discussed in my book, *The Neurotic Constitution*, and have been able to reduce it either to a likeness (*e.g.* incest-likeness, crime-likeness, godlikeness, megalomania, smallness-mania) or what I have described as a "junktim." As far as I know only Prof. Hamburger has arrived at even approximately similar results. For a detailed description of this neurotic "arrangement", cf. the chapter "On Individual-psychological Neuroses", in this book.

of initiating what the dreamer desires to put into a given situation. This he will seek to accomplish along lines best adapted to his personality, his nature and character. The dream may depict a situation which is anticipated in the future as already existing, (the dream of the patient with agoraphobia), in order in the waking state to put this arrangement into effect either openly or surreptitiously. The poet Simonides apparently employed an old experience to prevent him from travelling. If you firmly believed that this is an experience of the dreamer, that it is his own interpretation of the power of the dead man and that it is his own situation that demands an answer as to whether he is to go or not, if you take all these possibilities into consideration then you get the unmistakeable impression that Simonides dreamed this dream in order to give himself a hint that he could clearly and without hesitation remain at home. We may assume that even if he had not had this dream our poet would have remained at home. What then about our patient with agoraphobia? Why did she dream of the carelessness and disorderliness of her employees? We may detect in her behaviour the following assumptions: "When I am not present everything goes to pieces and as soon as I regain my health and take charge of affairs I shall demonstrate to everyone that nothing can get along well without me." We may consequently be certain that upon her first appearance in the shop she will discover all sorts of derelictions of duty and of carelessness for she will be looking about, argus-eyed in order to show her superiority. She will probably be able to prove she was right and that is why she anticipated the future in her dream.[1] The dream therefore like character, affect and the neurotic-symptom is arranged by the dreamer in accordance with a predesigned purpose.

Permit me now to interpolate here a discussion so that I can meet an objection which very likely has

---

[1] It may be surmised that Simonides who as a poet *yearned for immortality* was according to this dream possessed of a fear of death, whereas the patient with agoraphobia pursuing her fictive goal of domination, had a queen ideal. Cf. also for the first, "Individual-psychologische Ergebnisse über Schlaflosig keit" (*Fortschritte d. Medizin*; Leipzig, 1913), where, among other things, the relation of the infantile fear of death to the choice of a medical profession is emphasized.

occurred to many of you. How am I to explain the
fact that the dream attempts to influence the future
complexion of things when most of our dreams appear
so clearly to contain unintelligible and often enough,
stupid and meaningless matters? The importance of
this objection is so distinctly felt that most of our
authorities have looked for the essence of the dream
in these bizarre, unoriented and unintelligible manifestations and have tried to explain them ; or stretching
the unintelligibility of the dream-life they have denied to
them all importance. Scherner and Freud in particular
among the newer men must be given the credit of
having attempted the interpretation of the mystery of the
dream. Freud in order to give a foundation to his dream-
theory, according to which the dream represents a kind of
revelling in infantile unfulfilled sexual wishes, regarded
this unintelligibility as a purposive distortion, as though
the dreamer in spite of the restrictions imposed upon
him by civilization, did nevertheless desire, in phantasy
at least, to gratify his forbidden wishes. To-day this
view has become as untenable as that of the sexual
basis of neurotic diseases or the sexual basis of our
civilization. The apparent lack of intelligibility in the
dream is to be accounted for primarily by the circumstance that *the dream is not a means* for the attainment of a future position but an accessory phenomenon,
an indication of power, a sign and a proof that both
body and mind are making an attempt at anticipatory thinking and at anticipatory groping in order
to justify the personality of the dreamer in connection with some approaching difficulty. In other
words we have here a synchronous movement of
our thought, one running in the same direction as the
character and the nature of the personality demand and
expressing itself in a difficult language which even
when understood, is not at all clear. Yet this language
indicates the direction toward which the path tends.
As necessary as is intelligibility for our waking
thought and speech, preparing as it does our actions,
so superfluous does it become in the dream, for the
dream is to be compared with the smoke of a fire
which but points out to us in what direction the
wind lies.

On the other hand the smoke may serve to tell

us that a fire is to be found in a certain place and experience teaches us to infer the presence of wood from the fire and from that the fact that something is burning.

If we break up a dream into its constituent parts and if we can discover from the dreamer what these individual parts mean then a moderate expenditure of industry and a certain degree of penetration will indicate to us that behind the dream exist forces at work striving toward a given goal. This direction is adhered to by man in other aspects of life besides those of the dream and is conditioned by his ego-ideal and by those difficulties and inadequacies felt by him as oppressive. From this view-point then, which can rightly be called an artistic one we obtain a knowledge of man's life-line or, at least, of part of it and we get a glimpse of that unconscious life-plan by means of which he strives to dominate the pressure of life and his own feeling of uncertainty. We also get a glimpse of the detours he makes in the interests of this feeling of insecurity so that he may avoid defeat. We have the right to employ the dream as much as any other psychical manifestation and just as much as the whole life of man, for the purpose of drawing conclusions concerning his position in the world and his relation to other people. *In dreams all the transitional phases of anticipatory thinking occur as if directed by some previously determined goal and by the utilization of personal experiences.*

We thus arrive at a better understanding of the initially unintelligible details found in dream-structure. The dream rarely gives a presentation of facts—and even when it does, this is conditioned by a specific trait of the dreamer—in which recent happenings or pictures of the present occur. For the solution of an undecided question simpler, more abstract and infantile comparisons are at hand, comparisons frequently suggesting more expressive and more poetical images. For example, an impending decision may be replaced by an impending school examination, a strong opponent by an older brother, the idea of victory by a flight to the sky, and a danger by an abyss or a fall. Affects that play a rôle in dreams always arise from preparations and anticipatory thinking, and from the protective devices for the actually threatening problem.[1] The simplicity of the dream scenes—simple in comparison with the complex situations of life—represent to such an extent the attempts of the dreamer to find some outlet by excluding the confusing multiplicity of powers present in any given situation, that he is willing to pursue a guiding-line that resembles these simple situations. Just as a pupil who does not understand a teacher's question, for example, often looks quite bewildered when asked with regard to the propulsion of energy, "What takes place when you are pushed?" If a stranger were to enter the room, as this last question was asked, he would look at the teacher with the same lack of comprehension that we exhibit when told a dream.

Lastly, the unintelligibility of a dream belongs together with the problem first discussed. There we saw that *in order to obtain protection for an act we require a belief in the future that is steeped in the unconscious.* This basic attitude for human thoughts and actions, according to which an unconscious guiding-line leads to a personality ideal within the unconscious, I have discussed in detail in my book *The Neurotic Constitution.* The construction of this personality ideal and the guiding lines leading to it contain the same cognitive and emotional material as does the dream and the emotional processes that lie behind it. The same necessity that forces one kind of psychic material to remain within the unconscious presses at the same time so heavily upon the thoughts, pictures and auditory impressions of the dream that the latter, *in order not to endanger the ego's unity of personality* must likewise remain in the unconscious, or better, must remain unintelligible. (Think, for example, of the dreams of the patient afflicted with agoraphobia). What she tried to achieve by means of her unconscious personality was the domination of the environment. If she could have understood her dream then her despotic strivings and actions would have had to give way to the criticism of her waking thoughts. But as her real desire was to rule, her dream must remain unintelligible to her. From this point of view it is also possible to understand that psychic illness and all forms of nervousness become

---

[1] These may gain tendentious strength from the dream picture if this is necessary for the sake of safety.

untenable and are bound to improve if we succeed in bringing into consciousness and blunting the over-strained goals of the neurotic.

Let me now show partially how, with the help of the patient herself, the interpretation of a dream was conducted. The patient came under my treatment on account of irritability and suicide-mania. I wish to stress particularly the fact that the analogical aspect of the dream-thought is always found to be prominent in the supposition [1] with which the dreaming individual begins. The difficult nature of the situation lay in the fact that she was in love with her brother-in-law. The dream follows :—

A Napoleon Dream.[2]

"I dreamt that I was in the dancing-hall, wore a pretty blue dress, had my hair dressed nicely and danced with Napoleon."

"In this connection" (said the patient) "the following occurs to me :

"I have raised my brother-in-law to the rôle of Napoleon *for it would otherwise hardly be worth while* taking him away from my sister (*i.e.* her neurotic nature is not at all fixed on the man but on the desire to be superior to her sister). In order to cover the whole matter over with the mantle of righteousness and further, in order not to give the impression as though I had been instigated by revenge because I had come upon the scene too late, I have of necessity to imagine myself as the Princess Louise so that it appears quite natural for Napoleon to divorce his first wife Josephine in order to take a wife of equal rank.

"With regard to the name Louise, I had been using it for some time. On one occasion a young man asked for my Christian name and my colleague knowing I did not like Leopoldine, said simply that I was called Louise.

"That I was a princess I dreamt frequently (guiding-line) and this is indeed my most intense ambition,

---

[1] Cf. Vaihinger, *The Philosophy of As If*, whose theory of knowledge is in complete agreement with my beliefs on the psychology of the neuroses.

[2] Napoleon, Jesus, Jeanne d'Arc, the Virgin, as well as the Kaiser, father, uncle, mother, brother, etc. are frequent compensation-ideals of the intensified lust for superiority and represent, at the same time, the directive and emotionally-steeped preparations of the psychic life of the neurotic.

which in dreams permits me to construct a bridge over the gulf separating me from the aristocrats. Furthermore this illusion is calculated to make me feel, when awake, all the more painfully, the fact that I was brought up away from home and that I am alone and thrown upon myself. The sad thoughts that come over me, enable me *to behave harshly and cruelly to all people* who have the good fortune to be connected with me.

" As far as Napoleon is concerned, let me point out that since I am definitely not a man, I want to bend the knee only before such as are greater and more powerful than all the others. Incidentally this would not prevent me from stating that Napoleon was a burglar (burglar-dreams). Then again I should only bow before him and not really submit to him, for I would like to hold the man by a string, as is to be inferred from another dream—and then, and then I would dance.

" Dancing must be a substitute for many things to me because music exerts a tremendous influence upon my soul.

" How frequently during a concert was I seized with the intense longing to run over to my brother-in-law and almost suffocate him with kisses.

" In order not to allow this desire for a stranger to rise up before me, I must throw myself passionately into dancing or if I have no partner, remain seated with compressed lips and stare gloomily into the distance in order to prevent any one else from approaching me.

" *I did not wish to succumb to love,* and yet in my opinion balls and love belong together.

" I selected the blue colour because it is most becoming to me and because I had been actuated by the desire of making a good impression upon Napoleon. I had now the desire to dance, something I formerly was not able to do."

From this point on the interpretation might proceed much further and finally disclose the fact that the unconscious life-plan of this girl had as its purpose the will to rule, a purpose now altered and weakened to the extent that she no longer regards dancing as a personal humiliation.

I have come to the end. We have seen that the dream represents a subsidiary psychic manifestation as

P

far as action is concerned, but that as in a mirror it
may betray *events and bodily attitudes* that are related
to subsequent acts.   Is it therefore to be wondered at
the folk-soul at all times with the infallibility that holds
true of all universal feelings, accepted the dream as a
pointing toward the future?   A very great man, one
who united within himself the focal points of all the
sensations of man, Goethe, has expressed the dreamer's
"glimpse into the future" and the help and strength
flowing from it in a wonderful ballad.   The count
returning to his castle from the Holy Land finds it
empty and desolate.   At night he dreams of a dwarf's
wedding.   The conclusion of the poem is :—

"And were we now to sing of what happened later
on, then all the noise and riot would have to cease.   For
what he saw so nicely in miniature, he became acquainted with and enjoyed on a larger scale.   Trumpets
and the jingling, ringing peals of music rang out, and
rider, chariot, bridal throngs, all approached and bowed
before him, an innumerable happy lot.   Thus it was
and thus it will ever be."

The feeling that this poem of the dreamer is directed
toward thoughts of marriage and children is quite
sufficiently stressed by the poet.

XIX

On the Rôle of the Unconscious in Neurosis

(1913)

OUR understanding of the individual problems in the psychology of neuroses is so definitely bound up with the individualistic mode of approach that it may be maintained that *every working-hypothesis also built up out of individual experiences, furnishes us with a picture of the breadth of view-point and the limits of knowledge possessed by the analyst.* This is so manifestly true that it explains why observers come to different views, evaluations and hypotheses ; why it is that one school of thought either emphasize or minimize one point, and another another ; why the significance of certain data escapes some and unimportant details are given special significance by others. He who insists on adhering to a well-formulated doctrine cannot easily be shaken,[1] unless he becomes aware of its inner contradictions. In general he behaves like a nervous patient who refuses to make any change in his life-plan until he has become aware of his unconscious ideal of greatness and has given it up as unattainable.

In contrast to other writers I would like to stimulate the reader to test (my views) and to apply my interpretation to the following discussions. Psycho-therapy is an artistic profession. Self-analysis—important only for the understanding of one's own life-line—is comparable, in a way, to a portrait by one's self. It can give us no guaranty that the analysis is " unpredjudiced ", because this portrait is obtained by the employment of the unfortunately limited means of personality (or of two personalities) and because the individual's perspective does not allow either one's self or others to be viewed in any but an individual manner. To apply

[1] Cf. Furtmüller, *Psycho-analyse und Ethik.*

personal, *i.e.* types of argument different from the customary in science in the evaluation of psycho-therapeutic views, is an unjustifiable nuisance, explicable only because of the newness of our subject and which will surely not continue to exist for any length of time.

These afore-mentioned limits of individuality are not so disturbing an element in psycho-therapeutic practice. If the neurotic has gone to pieces under the pressure of reality the physician can teach him to come to terms with both reality and society. The impact of patient and physician always prevents the neurotic from living in his fiction. While the patient is imagining himself to be fighting for his superiority the physician can demonstrate to him the one-sidedness and sterility of his attitude.[1]

One of the greatest difficulties in treatment is the fact that the patient, although he may possess the proper insight into the nature of the neurotic mechanism, still partially maintains his symptoms. This he does until another of the neurotic artifices is disclosed, perhaps the most important namely, *that the patient makes use of the unconscious in order to be able to follow the old goal of superiority* and his old preparations and symptoms in spite of his recognition of them. Having established this fact we find ourselves again in the presence of that type of explanation of the neurotic life-plan discussed and commented upon in my book *The Neurotic Constitution.* The neurotic psyche in order to be able to attempt the attainment of its over-strained goal must have resort to artifices and stratagems. *One of these artifices is to transfer the goal or the substituted goal into the realm of the unconscious.* If this "moral" goal is hidden away in some experience or in some phantasy, then he may to such an extent, fall a victim to amnesia, either partially or completely, that the fictive goal becomes lost to view. The patient and, incidentally the critic, can attain the same object, if he overlooks the fact of a firmly maintained reminiscence, a symptom or phantasy transcends itself purposively.

It is but another method of expression, flowing logically from what I have established above, if I insist that this same goal or remnants of experiences and phantasies connected with this goal, are to such an

---

[1] Cf. the chapter on "The Concept of Resistance", in this book.

extent and in such a form accessible to consciousness that they aid and do not prove an obstacle to the attainment of a personality-ideal. The biological significance of consciousness, as well as the significance of the above-described participation of consciousness, lies in the fact that it renders possible actions directed to the attainment of a unified life-plan. This view is particularly in accord with the important teachings of Vaihinger and Bergson[1] and point to a quality of consciousness that has developed out of the instincts and has adapted itself to purposes of aggression.

The conscious conception responding to the over-strained neurotic ideal is, therefore, *as far as its conscious quality is concerned, an artifice of the psyche*, as analysis of over-evaluated ideas, of mania, hallucination[2], indeed of all psychoses, clearly discloses although, it is true, *the plan of operation* does not become conscious. Every conscious manifestation of the psyche points, in the same way, to the conscious fictive terminal goal, just as the unconscious impulse does, if rightly understood. The cheap method of talking of " cortical consciousness " can only deceive persons who do not know the connections. The frequent antithesis between the conscious and unconscious impulses is only an antithesis of means. For the purpose of heightening the feeling of personality or for the attainment of the goal of god-likeness, it is irrelevant.

The final purpose and all its over-strained form-transferences must remain in the unconscious if, by reason of its marked contrast to reality, it renders action in the direction of the neurotic guiding-line impossible. Where the quality of consciousness is necessary as a method of life, as the protection of the unity of the personality and as the protection of the personality-ideal, it will appear both in the most fitting form and extension. Even the fictive goal, even the neurotic life-plan can partially become conscious, if such a procedure is calculated to produce the heightening of the feeling of personality. This is particularly true of the psychosis. When, however, the neurotic goal might nullify itself by coming into direct opposition

---

[1] P. Schrecker, *Bergson's Philosophie der Persönlichkeit.* Recently these facts have been prominently stressed by Furtmüller and W. Stern.

[2] Cf. the neurological discussion of Berger's *Hofrat Eysenhardt*, in this book.

with the feeling of the community, then its life-plan is formed in the unconscious.

These conclusions based on the contents of neurotic manifestations, attain theoretical confirmation in one of the inferences that flows from the fundamental doctrines of Vaihinger, regarding the nature of the *fiction*, even though he does not put it in words. In a magnificent synthesis this brilliant thinker takes the nature of thinking to be the means of conquering life, thought seeking to attain its purpose by means of the artifice of a fiction theoretically valueless but in practice an essential idea. It was essential to have a profound conception and clarification of the nature of the fiction, in order to make us thoroughly acquainted with the artifices of our thinking, a conception that is certain to transform our whole view of life. In its very "discovery" there is entailed the further inference that the guiding fiction of psychic life also belongs to the unconscious and that its emergence into consciousness might for its purpose be in part unnecessary and partly injurious.

Psycho-therapy can begin here by bringing into consciousness the guiding ideas of greatness, thereby rendering their influence upon active life impossible. Bearing this in mind we shall show, in the following, that it is only *the unconscious* guiding idea of personality that makes the complete neurotic system possible.[1]

1. The niece of one of my patients gives her employer (my patient) notice. My patient is worried feeling that she is irreplaceable although before that she had not thought highly of her. She complained that she would not be able to manage alone, yet doubts whether she can employ any other person. Her husband is out of the question ; her companion but a parrot. We seem to hear the words, "Only I, I, I ! What would happen if I were not here?"

The woman suffered from agoraphobia. In other words she cannot go out. Indeed how can she go out if she always had to be behind the counter? She safeguards herself by means of her agoraphobia, in order to stay at home and demonstrate her irreplaceability. She has pains in her legs. Takes 3-5 grains of aspirin. She frequently wakes up at night in pain, takes a

---

[1] The contrast between the view of Freud and these other writers is clearly manifest.

powder, and thinks of her business tasks. This happens a number of times every night. She suffers from pain so that she may think of her business even at night. The patient's strained ideal of importance, to be a man, queen, always first—is only effective as long as it remains in the unconscious. Reminiscences of childhood reminding her of the more fortunate rôle of the boys, are in consonance with her present view of the inferiority of woman.

2. The dream of a girl, twenty-six years old, who came under my treatment on account of outbursts of anger, suicidal thoughts and truancy.

"I seemed to be married. My husband was a dark man of medium height. I said, 'If you do not help me in the attainment of my goal I shall resort to any method, even against your will.'"

The unconscious goal of the patient's childhood had been to change herself into a man (cf. Caeneus, Ovid).[1]

She had not been unconscious of this goal in childhood although it did not have the significance for the little girl that it possesses for us. Perhaps it might be better to say that its psychological and social meaning could not have been clearly grasped by the child. This goal expressed itself, however, in unusual, exaggerated wildness, in an almost compulsive craving to put on boy's clothing, to climb up trees, to select the rôle of the man in children's games and to assign female rôles to boys—this in order to maintain the principle of metamorphosis.

Our patient was an intelligent child and soon recognised her guiding-fiction to be untenable. Then two things happened first, she changed the form of her fiction which now became—"*I must be petted by everyone!*" This, reduced to her line of power-craving, meant—"I must dominate everyone, draw everybody's attention to myself." Secondly she forgot her original guiding idea, *so that she might thereby continue to hold it*. This artifice of the psyche is exceedingly important. I need hardly insist that it is never a case of the suppression of sexual impulses or "complexes" in the unconscious but simply a question of having the will-to-power that arises out of the personality-ideal become unconscious, that it concerns fictions that must to such

[1] *Met.*, xii.   This valuable reference I owe to Prof. Oppenheim, of Vienna.

an extent be adhered to in the individual's interests, that they are unable to be employed, tested or minimized.   In this way does the personality ideal safeguard itself in order not to be dissolved and so that the absolutely necessary unity for which, above everything else, the patient has striven be not lost.   *And this he attains by concealing his fictions, by withdrawing them from consciousness.*

3. Dream of a patient who came under my treatment because of attempts at suicide, uselessness, clumsiness, sadistic phantasies, perversions, compulsion-masturbation and persecution-ideas.

"I informed my aunt that I was now finished with Mrs P.   I knew all her good and bad traits and I enumerated them.   My aunt answered : 'You have forgotten one trait—her lust for domination.'"

The aunt was an efficient, somewhat sarcastic woman. Mrs P. had toyed with the patient to the extent of making him wild.   She showed him by her attitude that she despised him, repulsed him and others yet after a time made advances to him again.   Naturally enough the humiliations affected the patient most.   Just as is the effect of defeats for most neurotics, these humiliations were merely excuses for adhering all the more to this relationship in order to induce, if possible, some change in the situation and either to dominate it or unnecessarily chain himself.   The irritated, intensified feeling of inferiority searches for some hyper-compensation and is a typically neurotic trait.   Such patients for instance never free themselves from people who have defeated them.   Once having understood this trait the whole secret of the neurosis lies exposed before us.

In the scientific literature on the subject similar traits are utilized for masochistic purposes.   In my chapter on *The Psychic Treatment of Trigeminal-neuralgia* I have already cleared up this confusing error.   We may only speak of pseudo-masochistic traits.   For, like sadism, *these aid the aspiration for superiority and occasionally appear antithetic, ambivalent, but this is true only as long as we are ignorant that both forms of life tend equally toward the same goal.*   They are of antithetic nature only to the observer, but not to the patient, or from the stand-point of a properly understood neurotic life-plan.

The patient had always possessed a remarkably strong tendency towards analytical examination of the world and of humanity. As so frequently happens this trait developed from a marked depreciatory tendency. The analytical neurotic almost literally acts according to the maxim : *Divide et impera!* He breaks up the often delightful interconnections and obtains a worthless mixture of schedules. *Ecce Homo!* But does this really represent the man? Does this represent the real, living psyche?

The patient would like to be sarcastic like his aunt. However, all he possesses is backstairs humour and he never finds a ready answer. To this "hesitating attitude", it is true he owes his life-plan which forces him always to answer in such a way that his "opponent" —*and everyone is his opponent*—is annihilated ; or either not to answer at all or inadequately so that both he and his family get the impression that it is necessary to treat him gently and to help him in every way.

The day before his dream the patient had been under the influence of a conversation with his older brother with whom he had never felt himself capable of coping. His brother promised that he would try again to help and obtain a position for him. To prevent such promises of his older brother had always been the patient's speciality. And it became necessary to put him under treatment because he had attempted to commit suicide shortly after he had thanked his brother for getting him a position. One day, when his brother scolded him for his shabby clothes, he dreamt that he was wearing a suit over which he had poured ink. When the psychical situation of the patient is known then his dreams are intelligible without any great necessity for analysis. We see here that the thoughts and anticipated acts have as their object, to deprive the brother of his importance, to nullify his influence and his achievements surreptitiously and secretly. *Yet, in spite of all, our patient feels himself to be a moralist and idealist.*

His tendency to depreciating his brother operated under cover, one might say in the unconscious. *Nevertheless it accomplished more than it would, were it consciously realized, because the influence of the community-feeling is made impossible.*

Where this tendency came from is easily explained. It is a product of the patient's over-tense ideas of greatness. But why does it operate in the unconscious? In order to work at all! For the personality-ideal of *the patient* would feel such a conscious depreciatory and accusatory wish to be in the nature of a detraction, *would have a feeling of inferiority.* So he resorts to detours, to traits characteristic of clumsiness and helplessness, traits that represent the craftiness and refinements of a well-tested feeling of inferiority in professions and in life! So likewise the attempt and the recent threat of suicide is a method of increasing the pressure upon the brother.

From the above we draw the very important practical conclusion that we must regard the neurotic action as though it were obeying a conscious *goal.*[1]

And we may provisionally say that *the unconsciousness of a fiction,* of a moralizing experience or of a reminiscence develops as an artifice out of the psyche whenever the personality-feeling and the unity of the personality is threatened by its coming into consciousness.

"Do not forget the lust for power!" is my warning to the patient. In the dream I am placed in the same line as the aunt, and the brother with Mrs P. all of whom were superior to the patient. This transformation of two men into women is the result of that impulse toward depreciation about which I spoke above. But the patient is already warned in the dream, through the words of his aunt, *i.e.* my words. That had up till then been my task and the most important task a psychotherapeut possesses. The present stage of the neurosis is consequently the following :—The patient reacts to the humiliation inflicted upon him by his brother by depreciating his brother. And then he suddenly calls himself to order as in other cases I have done.

The next day he wrote a letter to his sister ; a letter he had hesitated to write. For the first time he openly complains of his brother's arrogance. At the end, it is true, he added that she should keep the contents a secret. Thus open fight still seems difficult for him because it would disclose his secret lust for power.

[1] This view-point is based particularly on the realization *that the patient must proceed along teleological lines.*

XX

Life-Lie and Responsibility in Neurosis and Psychosis

A Contribution to Melancholia

(1914)

THIS essay is essentially based on the belief that all psychogenic diseases, which we reckon as belonging to neuroses and psychoses, are symptoms of a higher kind and consequently constitute the technique, representation and products of individual life-lines. The detailed proof I reserve for another essay. However it is impossible even here not to take into consideration this provisional assumption. In doing so I gladly acknowledge my indebtedness to the views of some well-known scholars. To mention but one psychiatrist, Raimamn has pointed out clearly the connection between individuality and psychosis. The development of psychiatry likewise shows the progressive blurring of boundaries. Ideal types are disappearing both from literature and practice. Let me also mention here the " unity of neurosis " upon which I have laid emphasis. In general it may be said that we are approaching a point of view to which individual psychology has made important contributions. That view-point is that the neurotic methods of life seize with an apparently unalterable regularity, based upon individual experiences, upon the means of a utilizable neuroses or psychoses, in order to triumph.

Psychological results of individual psychology are well adapted to corroborate this view-point. For they suggest as one of their final results that the patient is constructing an inner world of his own on the basis of a defective individual perspective in definite contrast with reality. Nevertheless this perspective which dictates his attitude to society, is from a human point of view easily understood and is in other connections quite general. We frequently call to mind individuals who in life or in poetry have skirted around such an abyss. Up to the present there is not the slightest proof that either heredity, experience or the environment *necessarily lead* to a general or specific neurosis. This etiological necessity, which is never free from personal tendencies or personal connivance, exists simply in the rigid assumption of the patient who thus safeguards his neurotic or psychotic inference and with it the integrity of his disease. He might be able to think, feel and act in a less etiological manner if he were not impelled onward upon this journey by his goal, by that imagined final scene. However it is a categorical command of his life-plan *that he should fail either through the guilt of others and thus be freed from personal responsibility*, or that some fatal trifle should prevent his triumph.[1] The essentially human nature of this longing is strikingly manifest. The individual helps along with all the powers at his disposal and thus the calming hypnotizing safeguarding currents of the *life-lie* permeate the whole content of life. Every therapeutic treatment and certainly every clumsy and tactless attempt to tell the patient the truth, deprives the patient of the very source of his irresponsibility and must expect to encounter the most violent resistance.

This attitude which we have so often described originates in the "safeguarding tendency" of the patient and exhibits his inclination to resort to detours, truces, retreats, tricks and stratagems as soon as the question of *socially necessary decisions* comes up. The analyst is well acquainted with all the excuses and pretexts used by the sick man in order to evade his tasks or his own expectations. Our contributions have thrown a clear light upon these problems and exposed them to view. There are very few instances in which the attribution of guilt to others appears to be missing. Among these instances, the disease-pictures of *hypochondria* and *melancholia* force themselves most upon our attention.

I should like to raise the question of the "*opponent*" which can be employed as a very useful guide in making the nature of the psychogenic disease picture more transparent. The solution of this question no longer

---

[1] Cf. the chapter on " The Problem of Distance."

exhibits the psychogenically diseased individual in his artificial isolation but in his socially determined system. It is easy to understand from this fact the belligerent tendency of the neurosis and psychosis. What might otherwise be regarded as the termination namely, the specific disease, now takes its proper place as a means, a method of life, a symptom indicative of the path taken by the patient either to attain his goal of superiority or to feel his right in possessing it.

In many psychoses and also in neurotically-diseased individuals the attack as well as the accusation fall not simply upon one person but upon a number of people, occasionally upon the whole of humanity, hetero-sexuality or the whole world - order. This behaviour is unusually clearly apparent in the case of *paranoia*. The complete withdrawal from the world which means, of course, *at the same time, condemnation of it*, is expressed in *dementia præcox*. In a more concealed fashion and limited to only a few persons do we see the struggle of the hypochondriac and the melancholic. Here the viewpoint of individual-psychology allows us a sufficiently wide field of vision for understanding even the artifices used in these cases. Thus, for example, when an ageing hypochondriac succeeds in freeing himself from work in which he fears disappointments, at the same time forcing some relative to take charge of his house and make sacrifices for him. The "distance" to the decision—in this case his literary talent—is sufficiently great not to be overlooked. He emphasizes this "distance" by resorting to an unusually effective agoraphobia. Who is at fault? He was born in the revolutionary year (1848) and insists that this is a hereditary stigma. His digestive disturbances represent in the *enumeration of the means* he adopts (Stern) important aids to his lust for dominating his environment. This lust for domination is thus incited to increased work. These disturbances *are caused* by air-inhaling and purposive constipation.

A craftsman fifty-two years old has an attack of melancholia one evening when his daughter before going out on a visit, forgets to take leave of him. This man had always insisted upon his family looking up to him as the head of the family and forced definite services and strict obedience upon them by means of his hypochondriacal troubles.   His   neurotic   stomach   could stand no restaurant food.   His wife was consequently compelled when he went upon his vacation, " necessitated by his condition of health," to prepare his food in a kitchen which she rented in the country.   The fact that he was ageing he attributed to the " unfilial " actions of his daughter and he regarded it as an indication of weakness.   When his prestige was threatened, his impending melancholia was to bring home to his daughter her guilt and to show his family the full significance of his capacity for work.   Now he had discovered a way of acquiring and enforcing that prestige which he seemed to have failed to obtain in the world in spite of his achievements.   He was thus on the road to *irresponsibility* if for any reason his personal rôle should fail him.

A manufacturer twenty years old, was as he grew older, subject every two years to a fit of melancholia which lasted a few weeks.   As in the case mentioned above, he also began to take ill when through, an unfortunate event, his prestige *was threatened*.   He also neglected his work and frightened his family, who were dependent upon his work, by continual complaints about impending poverty.   The situation he thus called into existence resembled in every detail an overwhelming of his environment.   All complaints and criticisms stopped in his presence, *he was freed from the responsibility for his reckless adventures* and his importance as the maintainer of the family became clear to everyone.   The stronger his melancholia became, the more bitterly he complained, *the higher did he rise in value*.   He became well when the resentment against his adventure had disappeared.   Subsequently, his melancholia always recurred whenever he found himself in a financially insecure position and on one occasion because of the intervention of the tax officials.   His condition always improved as soon as his troubles were over.   It was quite easy to see that he was carrying on a policy of *prestige-attainment* within his family, seeking safety in his melancholia whenever discussions on vital matters came up.   In this way he could excuse himself and also relieve himself of any responsibility if anything went wrong and if everything ended well, receive *increased recognition*.   Our example thus shows clearly the symptom of the "*hesitating attitude*" we have described and also the creation of "*distance*" wherever a decision is to be taken.

Before I enter upon a description of the last-mentioned example of melancholia, let me attempt to define more sharply from the view-point of individual psychology the mechanism of melancholia and to throw some light upon that aspect in which it is in marked contrast with paranoia. If we once admit the social-conditioning and the belligerent attitude of melancholia we shall easily discover what it is in the goal of superiority that hypnotizes the sick man. The path he takes in the beginning is certainly rather strange. For instance, he minimizes himself, *anticipates* situations of intense misery and, identifying himself with them, acquires a feeling of sorrow and the outward expression of being completely broken up.[1] This seems a contradiction of his affirmation of a goal of greatness. As a matter of fact his exhausting physical weakness became in his hands a rather fear-inspiring weapon for securing recognition and escaping responsibility. For anyone to be able to achieve a true melancholia is, to my mind, something in the nature of a work of art except that, of course, the creative consciousness is wanting and *that the patient's attitude represents a condition with which he has been acquainted since early childhood.* Tracing it back to his earliest childhood we find that this attitude is in reality an artifice, an automatically conditioned method of life, taking the form of a rigid life-line when he is passing through a period of uncertainty. *Actually this consists in the desire to force his own will upon others and in safeguarding his prestige by threats of becoming ill.*[2] He bends all his energies with their accompanying bodily and psychic possibilities, towards the achievement of this purpose. He disturbs his sleep, his nourishment, his stool and urinary functions so that he may lose strength and prove that he is ill. He is quite willing to follow this course to its logical conclusion of suicide. An additional proof of the

---

[1] Just as, for example, the actor in *Hamlet*. "He weeps for Hecuba! What's Hecuba to him or he to Hecuba that he should weep for her?" In his complaints the psychotic individual betrays in much the same way as the neurotic, the nature of his "*arrangement.*"

[2] Often the melancholic type of procedure shows itself to be either incidentally or predominantly *the revenge impulse* of impotent rage.

aggressive nature of melancholia is furnished by the occasional appearance of the murder impulse and by the frequent presence of paranoiac traits. In these cases the attribution of guilt to others becomes prominent as for example in the case of the woman who believed herself to be suffering from cancer because her husband had forced her to visit a relative suffering from that disease. Summarizing we may say that the difference between the melancholic and paranoidal attitude seems to consist in the fact that the melancholic feels himself to be guilty whereas the paranoiac accuses somebody else. To make the matter clearer let me add that these individuals resort to this procedure *only if they find no other method of establishing their superiority.* We might incidentally point out that both these types represent universal human traits and as soon as we look for them they will be seen to have an extensive distribution.

The psychical susceptibility to psychoses is frequently diminished by the fact that the goal of superiority[1] possesses even greater strength. The asserted impossibility of correcting "maniacal" ideas is partially true but flows logically from the compelling nature of the goal. We were able to show above how the psychotically diseased individual protects his personality-feeling at all times by creating "distance" which he attains by the subterfuge of a life-falsehood. In order to cure his neurosis it is necessary for the patient to "*temporarily*" weaken his guiding ideals. A success running counter to his symptoms will only then be really efficacious if the patient is disposed to let himself be healed or if he is able gradually and unnoticed to slacken the rigidity of his goal. As far as we can see the maniacal idea commits no mistakes. It is under the compelling influence of the guiding idea and fulfils its ultimate purpose which is to make itself irresponsible and protect the ego-consciousness by the creation of "distance." *A logical examination hardly touches the mania because in its capacity as a well-tested modus vivendi et dicendi, it fulfils its purpose and because, moreover, the patient runs for protection to his limited appreciation of that communal sense of reality which we all share.*

[1] I am not here considering the intermediate conditions ranging from marked incapacity for fixing attention to idiocy produced *by inactivity of the reasoning powers*, of long duration.

The melancholic individual we have just been describing betrayed the whole arrangement of his illness in a dream which he had at the very beginning of the treatment. He had become ill when removed *from a place where he occupied the principal position* to one where he would have to prove his worth. Twelve years before, at the age of twenty-six, under similar circumstances he had also had an attack of melancholia. His dream was as follows :—

"I am at a pension where I eat my mid-day meal. A girl in whom I have been interested for some time, serves the meals. I realized suddenly that the world was coming to an end, and at the same time the thought occurred to me that I might now be able to rape the girl, *for I could not be held accountable.* However, after I had committed the rape it became evident that the world was not going to end." The interpretation is simple. The patient wishes to evade all decisions relating to love because he is unwilling to shoulder the responsibility. He has often toyed with the idea of a world-catastrophe (enemy of mankind). The dream, in a sexual disguise, indicates that he would have to believe in a world-catastrophe in order to be able to conquer, for in this manner a sense of irresponsibility could be created. His final act (the rape) shows him on the way to the attainment of his goal through a fictitious arrangement, an "as if", a provisional testing of a method of attack which consists in doing violence to others.[1]

We are now in a position to examine the guiding line of the patient. He shows himself to be a man with no trust in himself, and *one who does not expect to succeed by a direct line of attack.* We should therefore expect to find from the facts of his early life and from the study of his present melancholic stage, that he is going to attempt to attain his goal along some circuitous path. We may also assume that he is going to create "distance" between himself and the direct approach to his goal. Perhaps we are even justified in assuming that should he have to decide he will lean toward an "ideal situation" because in such a situation, confidently anticipating a threatening catastrophe, he

[1] Cf. *Dream and Dream-Interpretation*, in this volume and the author's dream-theory in his *The Neurotic Constitution.*

will himself be free from all responsibility. He will only regain his confidence, it may be assumed, when certain of victory. *This idea obtained from the dynamics of the dream coincides with the view expressed above about melancholia.* Now this attitude, be it remembered, is typical, to a certain extent, for the majority of mankind and is frequently encountered among neurotics. It is part of the essence of the specific power, the singleness of the guiding superiority - belief and the defective connection with the logical demands of life, when irresponsibility and its related ideas are driven into the realm of the psychotic. To account for this we might provisionally assume a special degree of stubbornness and an unsocial craving for domination in our patient, although he denied possessing these traits when asked.

Let me now mention a few of this patient's reminiscences. Once in boyhood when dancing he fell down pulling his dancing-partner down with him and losing his glasses. Before raising himself he reached out for his glasses but carefully held his partner down with his other hand, a fact that led to an unpleasant scene afterwards. In this occurrence we may already detect his unsocial attitude, his tendency to violence. His customary means of enforcing his will are also clearly perceptible from other childhood reminiscences. For example, he remembers lying on the sofa and weeping for an unconscionably long time.[1] He did not know how to account for this last reminiscence. His older brother, who corroborated the patient's stubbornness and will to dominate, informed me quite spontaneously when interrogated, that his younger brother (our patient) had on that occasion forced him by his incessant crying to surrender the whole sofa to him.

I cannot discuss in detail here the manner in which the patient disturbed his sleep, his nutrition, his nutritive and excretory functions, how he lost strength and thus gave proof of being ill. Nor can I dwell on the manner in which by positing unfulfillable conditions and guarantees he attempted to demonstrate both to himself and to others the hopelessness of his condition ; nor how he felt the steps taken by his family and the

---

[1] I have discussed the purposive moulding and survival of childhood reminiscences in *The Neurotic Constitution*, and in a paper delivered before the congress of psychotherapy at Vienna in 1913.

interference of the physician as an additional affront. He went so far as to deny to himself all ability and all possibility of making a living, in that way forcing his family and his friends into his service and into his power, using them then in connection with attempts to make his business superiors more amenable to his wish, which was that he should be transferred to a place where he could again play the rôle of master. His hostility was therefore directed against all the officials under him, and it took the form of interfering with all their demands. His plan was to pass from a condition of irresponsibility to one of violence. Then having finally attained his goal he would allow himself to be convinced that the world was not coming to an end.

In my book, *The Neurotic Constitution*, I found the necessary conditions for the development of mania, to judge from selected cases, to be the following :

1. An intensified feeling of uncertainty and inability to face an imminent decision.

2. The mechanism is a marked deflection from and devaluation of reality. (Among other things this means a denial of the value of rationality as a function of society.)

3. Intensification of the guiding-line leading to the fictive goal of superiority.

4. Anticipation of the guiding ideal.

With regard to its bearings on melancholia I would like to add to this last trait, the fact that the sick man tried to approximate to this well-tested picture of a helpless weak, needy child for he discovered from personal experience that it possesses a great and most compelling force. His attitude, symptoms and his irresponsibility are formed with them in mind.

Psychiatrists insist that the essential character of psychosis is to be found in the absence either of a motive or at least of an adequate motive, for an act. This manner of presenting the problem is almost incomprehensible. The problem of "motive" we individual psychologists are well aware of and it is never absent from our discussions. The vital rôle assigned to-day to individuality and character in modern psychiatry is a real sign of progress, and leads directly to our own problems.

We must remember that the most important question for the sound or the diseased psyche to answer is not the where-from? but the whither? For it is only after we are acquainted with the impelling goal and with a knowledge of its direction that we can attempt to understand its various movements, movements which we take to be in the nature of individual and special preparations.

According to the Viennese psychiatric school melancholia is defined as follows (Pilz, *Spezielle gerichtliche Psychiatrie;* 1910) : " *The essential trait of melancholia is a primary (i.e. not induced by external circumstances), depression in the nature of sadness and anxiety accompanied by thought interference* ". It is a natural conclusion from our view to lay stress upon those motivations caused either by the nature of the goal or by those special guiding lines that we interpret individualistically. This motivation is synonymous with the disguised activity of melancholia. In melancholia we find in complete form the " hesitating " attitude and the " progressive advance backwards ", both conditioned by the " fear of taking a decision ". Melancholia is thus an attempt, a contrivance for conducting in a round-about way what we have designated as the "remnant" and the "distance" of the individual, to its true goal of superiority. As in all cases of neurosis and psychosis this is accomplished *by the voluntary assumption of the "cost".* Thus this illness resembles an attempt at suicide in which it frequently actually terminates. Thought interferences, speech-disturbances, stupor and bodily carriage enable us to visualize concretely the " hesitating attitude " which as intentional disturbances of social functions, *point to a decreased community feeling.* Fear at all times serves the purposes of security, a weapon of defence and a proof of illness, and paroxysms of rage and the raptus melancholicus break out occasionally in the form of expressions of a fanaticism of weakness, an indication of disguised emotions ; maniacal ideas point to sources of purposive phantasies which both furnish and "arrange" the patient's affects in the interests of his illness. The mechanism of anticipation and absorption in the rôle of a person about to perish is unmistakable. The illness always seems to be most intense in the morning *i.e. as soon as the patient enters upon the activities of life.*

The experienced observer has unquestionably not overlooked the "*belligerent attitude*" of the melancholic individual.   Pilz, for example (l.c.), shows among other things, that the conscience-qualms of the sick man often have as their consequence the bestowal of senseless gifts or of testamentary provisions.   We object only to the phrase "senseless".   An apparently passive psychosis *is always teeming with feelings of hate and with tendencies toward depreciation.*   The sick man, for that reason, after having satisfied his desire to punish his family, is seized with the proper conscience-qualms accompanying his act, so that he may be freed from responsibility.

The previous history of our patient shows very clearly that all persons afflicted with melancholia belong to a certain type who are not intensely interested in anything, who easily become uprooted and who easily lose their belief in themselves and in others.   Even when quite well they exhibit an attitude of ambition, of hesitation ; they recoil before responsibility or they construct a life-falsehood whose content is their own weakness and whose inference leads to a struggle against others.

XXI

Melancholia and Paranoia

(1914)

Individual Psychological Results Obtained from a Study of Psychoses

PRELIMINARY remarks :—*The following are the forces conditioning neuroses and psychoses discovered and described by me :—infantile feeling of inferiority ; safeguarding tendencies ; automatically tested methods ; characteristic traits, affects, symptoms and attitudes taken toward the demands of communal participation ; the employment of all these methods for the purpose of an imaginary increase of the feeling of personality as against that of the environment ; the search for a circuitous method and for the creation of " distance " between themselves and the expectations of the community in order to evade both a true evaluation of life and personal responsibility and accountability and finally the neurotic perspective and the purposive, at times insane devaluation of reality.* All these facts led me and a number of other investigators to posit some principle of explanation, a principle that has in a very wide sense proved itself both valuable and essential for an understanding of neuroses and psychoses.[1] The above - mentioned mechanisms are described in detail in the author's books *The Neurotic Constitution, Studie über d. Minderwertigkeit von Organen,* and the present work.

My later conclusions about the mechanism of psychosis can be put in the following way. There are first the three essential meanings of mania already emphasized ; the anticipatory and hallucinatory representations of a wish or the fear whose purpose is to secure safety ; the purposive devaluation of reality and the resultant heightening of the ego consciousness. To

---

[1] Bleuler strangely enough speaks deprecatingly of the fact that " people attempt to explain everything thereby." To me and to others its value consists just in this fact.

these should be added two more of great significance ; the struggle against either the immediate or the larger environment and *the transference of the scene of activities from the main sphere of action to a subsidiary one.*

All these five conditions of mania stand in a logical and psychological relationship to one another.

In the statements that follow, prepared for the Congress of Psychology and Psychiatry, which was to have met in Berne in 1914, and which I now print unchanged, I shall attempt to present the psychological structure of melancholia and paranoia in accordance with the above conclusions.

I. *Melancholia*

Attitude and life-plan of individuals disposed to melancholia ; outbreak of the disease and the struggle against the environment ; transference to subsidiary sphere of action from fear of taking decisions that might bring about humiliation.

1. Melancholia develops among individuals whose method of living has, from early childhood, been dependent upon the acts and the aid of others. Defective activity and manifestations of a non-masculine type are predominant. Such people are generally found to limit themselves to the society either of their family or of a small persistent circle of friends ; always try to rely upon others and are not even above forcing others to submit to them and to accommodate themselves to them by making exaggerated references to their own inability. That their tremendous egoism in times of prestige worship like that of our own, occasionally brings them external success does not in any way contravene our statement. The fundamental questions in their own life, their progress, development, even their adherence to their own spheres of action, these they either evade or approach only hesitatingly, especially if difficulties present themselves. The typical manic - depressive on the contrary can be broadly characterized by the fact that he begins every act enthusiastically but loses interest very soon after. This characteristic rhythm which holds for their movements and attitudes when they are well is intensified and reinforced during the period of their illness by call-

ing up maniacal ideas and by their ostentatious and purposeful elaboration.

Between these two forms lies intermittent melancholia whenever the patient's fluctuating belief in his success is called upon to ward off some demand of life (marriage, profession, society).

2. The whole life-conduct of the "melancholy type" shows its presupposition and starting point to be a fictive but all-permeating stand-point, a melancholic perspective rooted in infantile psychic life, a perspective according to which life resembles a difficult frightful game of chance in a world full of obstacles and in which the majority of men are hostile. We recognize in this attitude of antagonism to the community-feeling an intensified sense of inferiority, one of the contrivances that lie at the basis of the neurotic character as described by me. When protected by their special aggressive tendencies which are transformed into traits of character, affects, preparations and acts (crying !), these people feel themselves able to cope with the facts of life and they try when "sane and healthy" to achieve a reputation among a small number of friends. By letting their subjective feelings of inferiority take a concrete shape they are in a position to insist from childhood either openly or secretly, upon an increase in their "disablement grant".

3. From the incessant attempts made from early childhood to gain prestige it can be inferred that their self-assessment is quite low and yet all their actions seem to suggest—and these disguised hints disclose the psychical affinity with paranoia—that some neglected opportunity for an extraordinary development had somehow been missed. They indicate familiar unfavourable circumstances (as the source of their failure) or betray in their maniacal melancholic ideas the ineradicable assumption of super-human, even divine powers. It is on such an assumption that are based the complaints in which the sick individual bewails, in what really represents *a disguised idea of greatness*, the terrible fate which will overwhelm his family when he is gone ; or he speaks in a self-accusatory way about his part in the destruction of the world ; in the outbreak of the world-war or in the death and ruination of certain people. Often there is found in this enforced complaint about his own

unworthiness, a warning reference to real material and moral dangers for his family circle and that of his friends and an equally marked stressing of the personal significance of the patient. Such then is the goal of victims of melancholia and with such an object do they accuse themselves openly of all kinds of inferiority and *take upon themselves ostentatiously the blame for all failures and errors.* The success of their behaviour is such that, at the very least, they become the centre of attention of their limited circle and are able to induce those individuals who feel obligated to help them to increased activity, to note-worthy sacrifices on their behalf, and always to make advances to them. On the other hand they themselves have become freed from even the slightest feeling of obligation or tie, a condition fitting well into their ego-centric guiding-ideal, for this ideal causes them to feel every connection with others, every adaptation to others or the interference of others with their rights, as an unbearable compulsion and as a serious loss of personal prestige.

Together with these self-accusations and self-reproaches we always find disguised references to heredity, to parents' errors in bringing them up, and to wilful lack of consideration on the part of relatives and superiors. This accusing of others — another phenomenon related to paranoia—can be deduced from the initial melancholic situation. To give examples ; if for instance an outbreak of melancholia occurs in a younger daughter when the mother has decided to go on a lengthy journey with the elder daughter, or if a business man is suddenly afflicted with the disease after he has been persuaded against his will to come to certain decisions by the decisive vote of his partner.

References like the above, to melancholia, body anomalies, etc., serve also to establish the fact that, according to the patient, we are here dealing with an unalterable and incurable disease, this of course enormously increasing its importance.

Melancholia thus like every neurosis and psychosis, helps the patient's object of heightening the social value of his own will and personality, at least in his own opinion. Its special compulsory nature, among individuals of infantile mentality, is due to the pressure of a deeply felt dissatisfaction and a feeling of inferiority which objectively considered is unjustifiable.   It is an incomprehensibly great payment that these people make for a behaviour in the difficult crises of life which, after all, is inherently consistent.   Their sensitive ambition which spurs them on persistently, although with secret trembling, to seek superiority, forces them likewise to retreat or waver before the more important social tasks.   By means of systematic self-restriction they thus reach a subsidiary track represented by a circle of friends strictly limited, and by tasks to which they adhere until threatened by what appears to them a change fraught with difficulties.   Then the scheme that was constructed in childhood, never revived and which has always remained untested interposes itself and they minimize their own importance in order to gain power through weakness and illness.

4. The most prominent offensive weapon of the melancholic type which he uses for raising his position and which he has employed from childhood on, consists in complaints, tears and depression.   He shows his weakness and the necessity for helping him in the most agonizing manner so that he may either force or mislead others to aid him.

5. These patients obtain in their own way, the appearance and conviction of irresponsibility for their lack of success in life, because they repeatedly insist upon the unalterable nature of their weakness and their lack of external help.   The psychic affinity with the phobic and hypochondriac type is clearly discernible.   However it is characteristic of melancholia that with the object of a more powerful attack and because of a more extensive feeling of inferiority, the realization of inferiority disappears and all criticism of the maniacal ideas is excluded, by means of a marked anticipation of an inevitable tragedy and a determined absorption in the imminent danger.   The categorical imperative of melancholia is "act, think, feel in such a way as if the horrible fate that you have conjured up, had already befallen you and was inevitable".   The main presupposition of melancholia-mania is to possess *a prophetic insight, to be like a God.*

It is only by following up this recognition that, when measured in terms of the common bond of the pessimistic perspective, the interrelation between neurosis and

psychosis becomes clear. To take simple examples:—
In enuresis nocturna it is "Act as though you were in
the lavatory"! Pavor nocturnus : "Act as though you
were in great danger". So-called neurasthenic and
hysterical sensations, conditions of weakness, paralyses,
dizziness, nausea, etc.: "Imagine you have a circlet
around the head, something sticking in your throat;
that you were on the verge of a fainting-spell ; that
you could not walk ; that everything was in a whirl
around you ; that you had eaten some bad food ", etc.
    It is always a question of effect upon the environ-
ment. This is true, as I have already insisted for
some time, in case of "genuine epilepsy", in which as
if in pantomime, death, impotent rage, manifestations
of poisoning, warding off danger and defeat, are represented. The nature of the material presented is
dependent upon the organism's possibilities often deduc-
ible from inherited manifestations of inferiority (cf.
Adler, Studie üb. d. Minderwertigkeit v. Organen, 1917),
and they begin to play a rôle as soon as they are able
to benefit and to be of benefit to the higher ideals of the
neurotic. In every case, however, either the patient's
symptom or the attack signify that he has withdrawn
either from the present, (by means of anticipation) or
from reality (by absorption in his rôle). The success
of this withdrawal is probably most definitely expressed
in genuine epilepsy. One of the commonly recurring
features of one of the types seems to be the fact that the
patient is the last-born (occasionally a person followed
at a long interval by another child) ; an asymmetrical
lower displacement of the right side of the face ; increase
in the protuberance of the parietal bone and traces of
left-handedness.
    The psychosis discloses, corresponding with the
more determined attitude of the patient who is on the
point of giving up all honest strivings, a more marked
withdrawal from the world and a more extensive
depreciation and overwhelming of reality.
    6. In the psychosis as in the neurosis, the intensified
reference to the unchangeability of the weaknesses and
sad destiny awaiting us, prove to be necessary in new
and apparently difficult situations, professional decisions
and tests of all kinds devised with the object of developing hesitation or abandoning a certain course, as in the

rather complicated instance of *stage-fright.* The investigator must be very careful not to over-emphasize his own impression of the difficulties of the situation. For what guides the man afflicted with melancholia in his fears, what makes his maniacal ideas "incurable" is not the lack of intelligence or logic, but the lack of desire, the methodical unwillingness to apply this logic. The patient will feel and even act illogically if he can only in this way, and only by means of mania, approach nearer to his goal and heighten his personality consciousness. Anyone who attempts to tamper with his mania appears to him, consequently, as an enemy and he therefore regards all medical measures and attempts at persuasion as directed against his position.

7. It is one of the peculiar traits of the melancholic type that it succeeds in establishing its disease-picture by continuing old well-constructed preparations and that, by freely expressed, intensified reference to its own weakness, it extends the compulsion of continuous and useless helping and the solicitude of the environment. The uselessness of every external pacification after melancholia has manifested itself, is not the result of any lack of logical deduction but flows from the unbendable purpose of the sick man to increase the shock to his environment to the highest degree, to limit the action of all concerned and deprive them of all their prospects. A cure will take place, depending upon the degree of confidence in life still remaining in the patient, as soon as he has enjoyed the satisfaction of having demonstrated his superiority. Promising results have also been obtained by tactful reference to real connections made with no suspicion of posing as superior or a desire always to be in the right. The prophecy when the termination of any melancholic arrangement will take place is certainly not any easier than to foretell when a child will stop crying. Hopeless situations, an unusual degree of lack of interest in life evidenced from early childhood, provocations, and an ostentatious lack of respect on the part of the environment may lead to attempts at suicide as an extreme act of revenge for activity continually directed against one's own person.

The fear of lack of success, anxiety, competition, or expectation of not being able to cope any longer with

society or the family, force this type in case of sub-
jectively-felt trouble, to resort to anticipating their ruin.
The melancholic view-point growing out of this self-
absorption, which by reason of its purposive achievement in waking life and dreams always becomes more
and more deeply rooted, in its influences upon the
whole organism, is the continual motive for a poorer
functioning of the organs. If carefully done the
functions of the organs, the carriage, sleep, muscular
strength, heart-activity, intestinal manifestations, etc.
can be prognostically evaluated. The psychological
connections militate against the etiological interpretation
of Abderhalden's discoveries in psychosis. From our
view-point they must represent definitely conditioned
manifestations or simply intensified symptoms, appearing in psychosis, of an inherited organ inferiority.
We must, among other things, emphasize the fact that
organ inferiority may represent the final stage of an
important basis of etiologically significant infantile
inferiority feelings.

8. Organs, in so far as they can be influenced, come
consequently, under the power of the melancholic goal,
adjust their functions to the need of the whole situation
and thus help to establish the physiognomy of clinical
melancholia (heart, body-carriage, appetite, stool, urine
activities, trend of thought). In so far as they obey
compulsory stimulations they are forced into a melancholic mood. Or it may be that the function remains
approximately normal but is felt by the sick person to
be diseased and is complained of. At times a disturbance and an irritable condition are induced by the sick
man by means of a clear and meaningless behaviour
(by sleep disturbances, by enhanced inducing of stool
and urine activity).

9. In the last case as well as in connection with the
acceptance of nourishment, the patient often shows a
series of disturbances automatically induced and which
then follow systematically and methodically without
sufficient self-criticism. These manifestations as well
as the patient's exhaustive demands on the functions
of his organisms and his erroneous evaluation of a
fictive norm lacking in him, indicate his purpose of
visibly procuring a real proof of illness.

10. The acceptance of nourishment is restricted by

the calling up of thoughts suggestive of disgust or anxious suspicions (poison) and besides, like all other functions, is under the pressure of purposive melancholic self-absorption ("as if nothing were of use, as if everything must end badly"). Sleep is disturbed by compulsory brooding, by thinking of not sleeping and also by resorting to distinctly purposeless means. Stool and urinary functions can become diseased either by contrary influences or by making continual claims upon them, in some cases by producing a condition of irritation in the respective organs. Heart-activity, breathing, the attitude of the diseased personality, the tear-glands occasionally, come under the pressure of the melancholic *fiction* tending to a ceaseless self-absorption in a situation of despair.

11. A closer view, one that is made possible only by means of an individual psychological synthetic approach, shows the melancholic attitude to be *the picture of a condition* which may appear, at the same time, an offensive weapon among people who find themselves in the *position* described above, people in whom we otherwise might expect angry perhaps raging and revengeful outbursts. The early acquired *deficiency of the social activity* conditions that peculiar attitude of attack which, resembling suicide, proceeds from an injury inflicted upon one's self to a threatening of the environment or to acts of revenge.

Occasionally in raptus melancholicus or suicide, which always represents an act of revenge, the affect to be expected is clearly manifest.

12. The presupposition of all activity, the concealed reference to the importance of one's own person, expressed in the demand for the subordination, in the claim upon the services of others, is never absent. Since the insistence upon the guilt of others is likewise always present, the melancholic attitude thus establishes the fictive superiority and irresponsibility of the sick man. By reinforcing the last-mentioned traits (insistence upon the guilt of others), paranoiac nuances are enabled to force their way into melancholia.

13. Since his fellow-man merely serves him as a means for heightening his own personality-consciousness (the pose of friendship and attentive interest is at his disposal as well as disease), the melancholic individual recognizes no limits to the extension of his tyranny over

others, robs them of all hope, and will proceed either to suicide itself or the thought of suicide if compelled *to surrender his main object of being freed from the demands of others*, or actually commit suicide when he comes upon invincible obstacles.

14. In other words an outbreak of melancholia represents the ideal situation for individuals of this type whenever their position is threatened. The question why, nevertheless, he does not enjoy this condition, is unnecessary. The fact is, that melancholia does not permit any other mood to arise and since the patient's object is success, there is no place for any feeling of joy that might interfere with his compulsion-attitude of depression.

15. Melancholia vanishes as soon as the patient has attained, in some manner or other, the imaginary feeling of having regained his superiority and a protection against possible misfortunes by a proof of illness.

16. The attitude of persons who are likely to succumb to melancholia is one of distrust and criticism of society from childhood on. In this attitude likewise we can recognize as one of the primary assumptions a feeling of inferiority with its compensation, and a cautious search for superiority in spite of all statements to the contrary.

II. *Paranoia*

1. Paranoia attacks people whose attitude toward society is characterized by the fact that after a fairly mild upward tendency of their activity or life-line they come to a halt at some distance from the goal that either they or their environment had expected, and that then generally by means of extensive intellectual or, at the same time, active operations in an imaginary struggle directed against self-created difficulties, they obtain an unconscious excuse for either covering up or justifying, or indefinitely postponing, their possible or anticipated defeat in life.

2. This attitude both *in toto* and in individual questions is prepared early in childhood, tested, blunted and protected against the most serious objections of reality. That is why the paranoiac system possesses, to a greater degree than other psychoses, definite

methodical traits and can be influenced only at the
beginning and under propitious circumstances.   In
paranoia neither the communal feeling nor its function,
the "universally valid" logic of reality, is ever entirely
destroyed.

3. One of the presuppositions of this attitude is
shown to consist in a profound feeling of dissatisfaction
with life, felt to be unalterable and which compels the
patient to try to conceal his lack of success both to himself and others in order not to wound his pride or self-
consciousness.

4. To this activity always present and perceptible—
as a rule of a belligerent type and, owing to the nature
of its devices, directed toward a goal of superiority—
is due the fact that the break-down generally takes
place in later years.   The maniacal idea thus likewise
obtains traits of an externally more mature type.

5. This activity whose goal is that of an ideal of
superiority, must in its development, automatically lead
to an *attitude of criticism and hostility toward the patient's
fellowmen*, an attitude that in the last analysis, is directed
against others, against influences and situations behind
which humanity as such is suspected of being concealed.
In this way others are made responsible for that part of
the patient's over-emphasized plans that did not succeed.
In paranoia the anticipation of the goal of superiority
(megalomania) also serves to put on a firm basis the
feeling of superiority and permit the patient to evade
responsibility for failure in society by creating secondary
regions of activity.

6. In the paranoiac's attitude we find reflected the
hostile attitude toward his fellowmen which goes back
to earliest childhood.   This flows automatically from
his active striving for universal superiority which finds
expression in the form of the idea that he must be given
consideration, in the persecution-mania and megalomania.   In all three of these situations the patient
pictures himself as the centre of his surroundings.

7. In the pure form of paranoia, to be taken into
consideration only as a boundary case, there is consequently always an upward tendency, which is brought
to a halt by the creation of the mechanism of the mania.
This is true also of dementia praecox where *the fear of
life* and its demands seem to be greater and which con-

sequently manifests itself earlier. On the boundary line can be noticed cases of zyclothymia, hysterical aboulia, depressive manifestations of a neurasthenic type and conflict-neuroses (cf. *The Neurotic Constitution*) which show a more marked repression of a temporary kind, following an initial aggression. Dynamically the behaviour of psychogenic epilepsy, chronic alcoholism, morphinism and cocainism, shows great affinity with the above. The differences seem to exist in the more tenacious and intermittent repression of the latter after more extensive activity or a lower degree of connection.

8. Both in the forward as in the backward movement of the psychotic wave, a hostile belligerent trait often ending in suicide, is clearly recognizable. Indeed psychosis may be regarded as the intellectual suicide of an individual who feels himself unequal to the demands of society or of attainment of his own goal. In his backward movement there is discoverable a secret *actio in distans*, a hostility toward reality, while the forward movement indicates its inward weakness at the time of its exaltation.

9. The self-evaluation of the paranoiac is intensified to the point of similarity to the deity. It is built up on a compensatory feeling of inferiority and shows its weakness in its speedy renunciation of being able to fulfil the demands of society, the surrender of plans, the transference of the field of action to the domain of the non-real, in the marked tendency toward constructing paranoidal excuses of a *preoccupational* nature and in the insistence on accusing others. The patient clearly lacks faith in himself and his mistrust and unbelief in men, and in the knowledge and ability of men, force him toward the construction of cosmogonic and religious ideas of government as well as to the inherent contrast of these phantasies to the general views. These are all necessary to enable him to get his balance and his additional ballast.

10. The ideas of the paranoiac are very hard to correct because the patient needs them just in this particular form if he is to establish his point of view, the attainment of irresponsibility as an excuse for his lack of success, and if he is to force his activity in society to become arrested. These ideas permit him,

R

at the same time, to adhere to his fiction of superiority *without necessitating a test* for he can always ascribe the blame to the hostility of others.

11. If melancholic passivity is an *actio in distans* for coercing others to subordinate themselves, the purpose of the paranoiac's active phantasy can, on the other hand, be said to consist in obtaining *a time-consuming pre-occupation* and an excuse that will relieve him from responsibility for his lack of success.

12. In contrast, melancholia is, at least externally, based more on the guilt of others than on that of external circumstances.

13. Every discernible outbreak of paranoia occurs when the patient finds himself in a dangerous situation where he feels his demands for a social position definitely lost. This happens as a rule when on the eve of some undertaking, during its course, or when anticipating either a demotion or the coming on of old age.

14. The final condition results from the intermediate creation of a preparatory mania-mechanism by whose action the patient's feeling of responsibility is destroyed. His feeling of importance is, however, increased by means of his self-identification with his persecution mania, his respect-demanding mania and megalomania. This mechanism represents a compensatory activity that has grown out of his expectation of depreciation and develops in the direction of the "masculine protest" just as we have shown in the case of the psychology of neuroses (cf. *The Neurotic Constitution*).

15. The construction of maniacal ideas can be traced back to childhood where, in an infantile fashion, they are connected with day-dreams and phantasies relating to situations of humiliation.

16. The paranoiac attitude gives both the soul and body its adequate position in the mania system. Stereotyped expressions, attitudes and movements are associated with the guiding idea and incidentally are also found abundantly on the confines of the disease and in dementia praecox.

17. Melancholic traits are frequently intertwined with those of paranoia. In particular do we find that complaints about poor sleep, deficient nourishment tend when subsequently amplified, in the direction of ideas of persecution, poison and megalomania. This last

path is at times, taken only to emphasize the special nature of the patient's disease.

18. Hallucinations are connected with marked self-absorption in the rôle to be played and represent both encouraging or warning admonitions. They occur whenever the patient's will-direction is to be regarded as final and yet he is not to be held responsible. These admonitions are to be taken as analogies like the dream, need not be intelligible to the patient but should be characteristic of the policy he wishes to adopt on certain definite problems. Both hallucinations and dreams thus prove to be *contrivances for objectifying those subjective impulses to whose apparent objectivity the patient unconditionally surrenders himself* (cf. dream theory of the author in the chapter on "Dreams and Dream Interpretation" in this book, and in his *Neurotic Constitution* l.c.). The coercion toward irresponsibility prevents the will from being under one's own direction and substitutes in its place apparently strange faces and admonitions.

19. We must add to the above the fixing of the mania-system by means of a purposive, *i.e.* a favourable selection of reminiscences, and *an evaluation of experiences as viewed from their final object.* From our view-point the tendency of this establishing of a system and its vital necessity owing to the nature of the goal-positing, emerges quite positively. (This goal consists in an order for retreat; an arrangement of non-responsibility; that of the guilt of others and the concealment of the personal and evident collapse.)

20. Our attitude thus shows that paranoia makes its appearance at the point where normal human beings lose their courage, where more susceptible natures commit suicide or querulously complain about others, and where the more aggressive types by cowardly avoiding the demands of life, turn to crime or alcoholism. Only people well prepared for adaptation to society maintain their equilibrium. Occasionally we encounter mixtures of the above tendencies.

21. The *single-handed* struggle of the paranoiacally disposed individual to conquer, results in every person being treated as an enemy or as a figure in a chess game. A feeling of real good-will toward his fellowmen is absent as much in the paranoiac as in all those affected

by neurotic and psychotic diseases. Such a person is never a dependable participant in the life of society and enters into normal human relationships (love, friendship, occupation, society, etc.), with an incorrect attitude. This anomalous attitude arises from a low self-evaluation and an over-evaluation of life's difficulties. This it is that misleads him into the creation of an arrangement like neurosis and psychosis. His hostile attitude toward society is, in no sense, inherited or ineradicable but merely a tempting outlet in an extremity.

22. Paranoia rarely disappears because it manifests itself just at that part of the life-line where the patient suspects his *inevitable* collapse will occur. However, quite senseless subjective exaggerations are amenable to correction in the beginning, and on such occasions the disease may be cured.

23. The attitude of a person predisposed to paranoia, already exhibits in childhood an active aspect which brings the person quite easily to a halt before difficulties. We often discover in the life of a patient frequent interruptions of an apparently puzzling nature, of the direct line of development. All enterprises that retard progress (including therein frequent changes of occupation and vagabondage), are in reality coercions of the guiding idea which demand that *time be wasted in order to gain time.*

Love of domination, insufferability, lack of fellow-feeling, absence of love relations or the selection of a few docile persons are regularly recurring manifestations in the person's life. He is recognizable by his querulous and unjustly critical nature.

APPENDIX

Excerpts from the Dreams of a Patient with Melancholia

An official forty years old is transferred to another bureau. Thirteen years before that he had developed signs of melancholia on a similar occasion. As on the earlier occasion he found himself incapable of performing the necessary duties. Incidentally there appeared certain thoughts in which he hinted at the responsibility of others for his condition. According to him he was neglected and difficulties were put in his way. We have, in short, as is almost always the case in melancholia, the path leading to paranoia vaguely suggested. He asked me for poison in order to escape his torments. No matter what the event was he always succeeded in seeing its worst side. Insomnia, digestive troubles, uninterrupted depression and extreme fears of the future increasing from day to day, allowed us to diagnose the case with certainty.

Above I have shown why melancholia is to be regarded as a " remnant problem " where the sick person, to prove his illness falls back upon the device *of accusing and depreciating himself* in order to escape taking a definite decision. Our patient, for example, will, in his own way, either try to circumvent a success unfavourable to his plans or weaken it by proving himself to be ill or finally, by having his success interpreted as a part payment for an imagined deficiency transcending everything the world has hitherto known. There is always present the compulsory demand that he be assisted by others whose kindness is to be taken advantage of and they themselves incited to making greater efforts in his behalf by the patient's insistence upon his illness. Interpreting this situation in its infantile meaning we come to the picture of the weeping child. The following are the earliest childhood reminiscences of this patient:—He pictures himself as a little boy lying on the sofa and weeping. When eight years old, an aunt strikes him ; he runs into the kitchen yelling, "You have deprived me of my honour!" With this special contrivance, *i.e.* to shatter the nerves of bystanders by weeping and complaining (to overpower?) he now faces every new situation. Let us not overlook the fact that this contrivance is only intelligible if we assume that we are in the presence of a very ambitious man, one however, who does not believe in himself to the extent of imagining he would be able to attain his goal of superiority by direct methods. It is quite apparent how—and this belongs together with the above—under the pressure of his secret idea of godlikeness he would like to be freed from the responsibility of his achievements in real life so as not to put his god to a test. This explains his " hesitating attitude " and his unconscious arrangement of the "remnant" and his "distance" from the goal of superiority which he is afraid of losing whenever a new situation arises.

In the first week of the treatment, the patient dreamt his dream of the world catastrophe narrated in chapter 19. If you remember we also found there the mechanism of melancholia. He posits the possibility of a complete lack of responsibility interpreted in his own sense and discloses himself as a strong person, in phantasy playing with the fate of the world like a god. When everything is about to end he may do anything.[1] Is not the same sentiment present in his "You have robbed me of my honour"? When he underrates himself may we not have the continuation read, "Now I am going to approach with my strongest move"? Is not suicide in the air here and is not depression being employed for the purpose of extortion?

All must submit to his will! That is the object of his melancholia. The following is a second dream: "A girl I saw on the street comes to my room and gives herself up to me voluntarily". What is behind this dream? Simple enough. How far removed am I removed from open aggressiveness! There must be a magical power that compels everyone to submit to me! Like a sleight-of-hand performer he helps things along by a threat of world destruction and by the influence of his depression.

A third dream exhibits the arrangement of his depression. "I find the work easy in another post which I had refused. Everything is pleasant and in the best of order". In other words "Where I am not present there I shall find happiness".[2] This is an assumption suggested by his attitude so that he may make the present situation appear painful. To disprove it is impossible, for if he chooses to imagine himself somewhere else we are dealing with an unfulfillable condition. Unquestionably could we transport him to that place he would discover some other subterfuge.

[1] *Freeing himself* at the same time *from the community feeling.*
[2] This is the last line of Schubert's famous song "*Der Wanderer*" (Translator).

XXII

Individual-psychological Remarks on Alfred Berger's
Hofrat Eysenhardt

(Lecture, 1912)

Introduction.—Dr Francis von Eysenhardt was born a few years before the outbreak of the revolution of 1848 in Vienna. His youth coincided with the reactionary period of the early fifties of the last century and he entered the criminal division of the royal courts of justice at a time when the old absolutist Austria was being transformed into a modern state.

Eysenhardt's success was due primarily to his own extraordinary abilities. He succeeded in uniting within himself the qualities of the old officialdom with the demands the new spirit made upon the state officials. At an opportune moment he showed the nature of his own political opinions by insisting that an unconditioned loyalty to the emperor was essential.

His reputation as a criminal lawyer of ability and his brilliant oratory combined to make him very popular. He was made attorney general to the dismay of the criminal world and of advocates. After a number of years he again became a judge and was made presiding officer of the jury courts. His intellectual gifts and his prodigious memory astonished everybody. He was occasionally criticized for showing partiality. Unconsciously he seemed always to be interested only in obtaining a conviction, and the severity of the punishments that were meted out when Eysenhardt was the presiding judge horrified everyone. Yet in his case everyone felt that the impossibility of influencing him in any way was but the expression of a strict sense of justice which he would apply to himself as well as to others. It was regarded as but a just reward for his services that he received the highest judicial position in the giving of the country and was made hofrat.

Eysenhardt, it was said, was destined to become the minister of justice in the next ministry.

Both the external and the private life of Eysenhardt had not been of the usual kind. He had no friends, not even acquaintances. Whole days would elapse during which he would speak no other words than those demanded by his official position. His nature was reserved, unfriendly and shy. These traits were due in great measure *to the frightfully strict and even cruel bringing up that he had received as a child.* His father had been accustomed to punish him with a whip for the slightest error, and in this way the child's feeling for revenge was definitely fed. The cruel treatment at the father's hands came to an end when young Eysenhardt, with the little money he had saved, bought a revolver and threatened his father with it. In his youth he exhibited a somewhat abnormal sexuality; he never associated with respectable girls and was a frequently seen visitor of disorderly houses. His father, it became known, had on one accasion whipped him unmercifully when the young boy had bought *a pair of lady's gloves for himself.* When alone Eysenhardt would cover *these gloves with tender kisses.*

Thus Eysenhardt spent his life despised, feared and admired at one and the same time, in spiritual and intellectual isolation, conscientiously fulfilling his official duties. Suddenly a remarkable transformation took place within him. His outward appearance, in all respects old-fashioned and known all over Vienna, changed, and he appeared one day with his beard trimmed in elegant fashion, instead of the short, rather bristly full-beard, and with new and modern clothes. But it was not only his external appearance that had changed. His hard sombre nature seemed to have received an illumination from within which was pleasantly reflected in his outward form and character. This change was interpreted to mean that Eysenhardt would soon receive a high, if not the highest post in the judiciary. The assumption was perhaps not quite erroneous, for Eysenhardt himself expected promotion. He remained in this almost exalted frame of mind for about three weeks until an important event brought this, possibly the only happy period of his life, to an abrupt end. *A tooth fell out!* This sign of oncoming age found him utterly unprepared, and exerted a frightful influence upon him. The disturbance in his nervous and psychic life refused to right itself, and he was constantly *troubled by doubts* as to whether his intellectual capacities were not likewise showing signs of waning. His usually unshakable nature was now filled with vague fears of impending danger.

When the anticipated ministerial crisis did not bring him the post of minister of justice this had the effect of an electric shock upon him. He found himself thinking continually of the reasons for which he had been passed over. At the same time he began to busy himself intensively with his own ego, something that was quite new to him. He was no connoisseur of human motives and feelings. He possessed only the remarkable gift of being able to extract from the evidence collected, all the criminal processes that led a man step by step to commit a crime. This he then knew how to present marvellously and dramatically. He never recognized in the criminal a fellowman, a person related to himself. Since he had become psychically ill, however, he began to change. His conscience began to annoy him ; he suffered from hallucinations at night, and on one occasion there appeared to him in such a hallucination a person whom he had sentenced very severely for child-rape, a man named Marcus Freund. In all the hallucinations in which persons appeared to him whom he had prosecuted, he was the defendant and they were the accusers. From the first time Marcus Freund appeared to him he was unable to rid himself even in day-time from the thought of this man, and so he finally decided to go through the whole case again *to convince himself* that Marcus Freund had actually been guilty. However he delayed and delayed until one day he heard accidentally that Freund had died, that he had died on the very night upon which he had first appeared to him. After that his collapse became more pronounced, and he imagined that the rest of the world was occupying itself with the case of Freund to the same extent that he was. *Hand in hand with this break-down* of his steel-like personality, the elementary sexual instincts of his nature seemed to become more manifest. In his own home this inward collapse of the man had hardly been noticed. The appearance of this new tormenting *compulsion-idea* had pushed into the back-ground the feeling that he was losing his intellectual capacities, and in consequence his mind became freer and capacity for work greater. He succeeded in pulling himself together once again when he was nominated to preside over a very important espionage case. The notification of his nomination was sweetened by the confidential hint that he had only been passed over in connection with the post of minister of justice because he was to be reserved for this exceedingly intricate espionage case. Eysenhardt seemed to be his own self again and forgot all about Marcus Freund.

However the evening before the last day of the final session of the espionage case something happened which drove him to suicide. The cause of this catastrophe was never entirely cleared up but it was brought into relation with the espionage trial and in which the wife and daughter of the accused, *the latter a girl under age, played a rôle*. There was also the story of a nocturnal adventure in which a police agent found Eysenhardt in a place of ill repute, a very unpleasant situation for him at the time. Eysenhardt left the following note:

" In the name of his Majesty the Emperor !

" I have committed a terrible crime and I feel myself unfitted either to hold my post any longer or as a matter of fact to live. I have sentenced myself to the most severe punishment possible and shall within the next few minutes carry it into effect myself ".

EYSENHARDT.

We cannot begin our discussion any better than by first paying our respects to the psychologist and thinker, Berger.

We long ago answered in the affirmative the question whether the analysis of a work of art for the purpose of discovering the main-springs of human action is justifiable. The only important question to be discussed is simply the general nature of the tact to be employed, and it is of course quite impossible to come to any complete agreement about it.

With regard to the life-history of Hofrat Eysenhardt, there is another important reason for calling this novel to the attention of psychologists, namely its truth to life produced not merely because based upon an historical personage but due likewise to the creative imagination of an artist-psychologist who has more than once given proof of his intuitive knowledge of the human soul.

I would not at all be surprised *if every psychologist took Berger's creation* to be either a corroboration or an after-experience of their own teachings. *For everyone sees only what he can understand* and tries to bring his knowledge to bear upon the investigation of the human soul and of art, just as Steinherr brilliantly points out in Berger's book.

We have no desire to tamper with the marvellous out-pourings of our poets and thinkers and shall therefore attempt merely to determine, through their creations, to what an extent we are on the right path and how much of their work can be understood by reference to the working methods of individual-psychology.

Our field of inquiry leads in the same direction as that opened by Berger's art. We always concern our-selves with striking characters and try to trace back to childhood and even further, the beginnings of every act. We are interested in the striking *transformation of personality* and endeavour *to grasp* the manifold thought-connections and forms of expression of man *in their entirety*.

The thorough survey of the phantasies of children regarding their future professions which we owe to psychologists of our persuasion has taught us in the same way as have our experiences with neurotic people, that the choice of a profession despite many provisos, is likely to show the inmost essence of the *fictive life-plan*, and that this choice of profession is *under the dictatorship of a deified and dogmatic concept of personality*.[1]

We shall direct all our attention to the inter-relation of *personality and neurosis*.

From this connection, if we are interpreting the neurosis correctly, there flow *those fundamental and abstract guiding-lines* of the human psyche which enter into the creation of a character of unusual personality, *whether he be a creator or a destroyer of cultural values, a normal man or an unfortunate carrier of psycho-neuroses and psychoses.*

The scientific judgment and prejudices concerning the

---

[1] That it represents in a way the essential fulfilment of a deeper-lying "formal" impulse to move (instinct?) cf. Kramer, *Berufswahlphantasien* in *Heilen und Bilden.*

psychological structure of unusual men which have been held so far, will find excellent corroboration in the description of Eysenhardt.

The poet has created his hero so carefully and so completely that we may cheerfully follow in his steps without even pointing out warningly that the *attraction of a work of art arises from its synthesis* and that the analysis of science profanes and destroys this synthesis.

Having now drawn general attention to the book, our task is to attempt a grouping which will give us an understanding of the dynamics of the life expressed in our hero so that we may, in part, obtain a support and also some useful formulas for a knowledge of man and also mould our practical activity *with a view to education, self-control and cure.*

Let us begin with Eysenhardt's bodily traits. We are told of his slender shoulders, his bossy forehead, his bushy eyebrows, of the tardy appearance of his moustache, his jaundiced complexion, the blueish rings around his eyes, and of his stomachic and biliary disorders. Clinically this seems to be the picture of a man who has preserved *old traces of rachitis, inferiority-manifestations of the digestive tract and a suggestion of a degeneration of the secondary sexual characters as is so common with neurotic people.*

It has frequently enough been pointed out that this group of body manifestations with its accompanying consequences, pains and inadequacies, misdirects people into making an infantile self-evaluation whose final result produces *a feeling of inferiority and uncertainty.*

The situation of the youthful Eysenhardt, an only child with a tyrannical father, must have conduced markedly to the intensification of what Janet calls " sentiments d'incomplètude ".

In order to meet life squarely and to gain security the psyche of such children must exaggerate, by way of compensation, the normal contrivances, *set its idea of personality higher* and affirm it more dogmatically. Such children pursue their path *toward a god-head they have themselves created* and which then as god, devil or demon, apparently directs their steps.

Their will and desires become more expressive and aggressive, their actions more secretive and cunning ; lust to dominate, envy, cruelty, avarice, flare up and the *preparations* for life are more carefully and precisely made.

I prefer to follow Berger's description.
Eysenhardt is an ambitious man, a truckler and a person of officious patriotism. He is hard and courageous, plays the rôle of a saviour of society, exceedingly skilful, possessed of great gifts as a talker, a great memory and marked intellectual capacity. His curiosity and desire for information and his acute perceptions would have made him a detective genius. He is lonely, egotistical, keeps all the old forms and loves the sharply outlined and clear-cut paths in carriage, attitude, habits and thought. No one is indifferent to him ; he is either hated or loved.

Gottlob Steinherr, a disappointed climber, but not inferior to Eysenhardt in originality, knows Eysenhardt's ideal of personality of the older time when the latter's ambition had expressed itself more directly and more openly. *He infers that Eysenhardt represents a case of the change of criminal and anti-social instincts into legal ones. He assumes that his guiding-lines are brutal sexual instinct and unlimited self-complacency ; he wishes to dominate men, even to enslave them, and to possess women.*

Let us recall the facts we know : *An exceedingly ambitious fictive personality-ideal in danger of being destroyed by his father.* He learns to understand his environment and the necessity of an apparent submissiveness to power and yet threatens his father, one day, with a revolver. His personality-concept had unquestionably borrowed many traits from his tyrannical father, but had then developed far beyond it and had learned to avoid a strong opponent and oppress a weak one. *His sexual behaviour does not represent the cause of his actions but merely an analogy. His aggressive attitude becomes hesitant* and extends in regard to women no further than the glove. The strong woman, the domineering woman, Dion's fury (Plutarch) fill him with terror. He elevates the prostitute to the rôle of lady and dreams of the conquest of a child. *He might easily have become a homo-sexual but having a contempt for men he has conquered this tendency or, he might have developed a desire for the impotent woman or even a corpse.*

His psychical gesture seems to indicate that he is looking for a line of development for maxims of conduct.

He is walking at the very edge of the pavement and moving along the very limits of bourgeois morality. His pen, lead-pencil are found lying in their proper places after his death. He has found the proper limits for his hyper-tense aggressiveness and his reputation and the norm of his sexual commonplaces are enough to prove to himself that he is a man. His reputation gives him ample opportunity for enjoying the illusion of superiority. *He devaluates man in order to make himself a god.*

The higher his position the weaker does his energy become. When his life-line is tending upward this consumption of energy, this advocate's love of hunting decreases. When the hope of a post in the ministry is held out to him he becomes human ; social feelings suddenly develop and burst asunder the heavy coat of mail protecting his attitude from his fellowmen. Eysenhardt passes through a transformation when he feels himself in close proximity to his godlikeness.

How Eysenhardt changed

Is such a change in a man, or let us say, in a neurotic, possible? In the developed neuroses we find as a rule so marked a constancy in the manifestations that we get the impression of an integrated mechanism. A deeper knowledge teaches us however that not even in this phase does the psyche always run the same course. A patient may be just pleasantly excited, or he may be depressed or exuberant, despondent or hopeless or joyful, full of initiative or faint-hearted, in short, all the traits are found in that antithetic order called by Lombroso bipolar, by me polar and herma-phrodite, ambivalent by Bleuler and "double vie", split personality etc. by others. In the stage ante-cedent to the developed neurosis and which is at times described as neurotic but which is generally that of health, such antithetic actions can likewise be observed. In the form of hesitation and doubt, anxiety, shyness, fear of taking a decision and in the trembling experienced when in the presence of anything new, we perceive active and passive traits and impulses, some of which approxi-mate to reality, some to the ego ideal. The developed neurosis shows itself as a safeguard of increased strength

and forces to the front the more fundamental characteristics. *" Ambivalence" proves to be the integrated methods
of attaining the goal.*
Hofrat Eysenhardt was expecting the final consummation of his ambition. We know, however, that such
an advent can never take place satisfactorily because
the guiding goal is *imaginary* and placed too high for
fulfilment. We know that many a neurotic looks
forward to happy events with inward trembling and
hesitation although he is, at the same time, perceptibly
exalted and transported to such an extent by his intensified personality consciousness that he becomes "another
man". The author describes this stage humorously
and allows Eysenhardt to change into a modern man
whose whole external appearance seems heightened.
A modern elegantly trimmed beard takes the place of
the short bristly full-beard. Here too a neurotic trait
is mentioned, the fact that he rather mourns the loss
of one of his bodily possessions. We suspect that
Eysenhardt whose "masculinity" has been curtailed,
is mourning the loss of his manhood. He now becomes
approachable and kindly disposed, for the automatic
raising of his ego-consciousness permits him to waive
part of his "distance". He freely gives advice and
encouraging praise, shows himself more liberal and
casts off some of that intense desire always to prove
someone to be in the wrong. He is playing his old
rôle, is still the same angular person *Steinherr knew him
to be but in a more propitious position.* The accused also
profit by his change, for they are no longer the necessary
sacrifices to his sadistically incited lust. Even his
physiognomy loses its expression of tense desire for
domination. His safe-guarding trait of thriftiness is
softened and even his emotions from our view-point
apparently primary and unalterable elements exhibit
a change of emphasis to the degree at least of making
the formerly pleasurable exercise of his profession now
appear a terrible burden from which he would like to
be freed. *Omnia ex opinione suspensa sunt.*
His life and attitude show the neurotic safeguarding
preparations for the anticipated appointment and *his
memory discloses those reminiscence-residues favourable to
these preparations.* In the midst of it all the old fear of
uncertainty reappears, the fear of taking decisions,

agoraphobia.   As Berger says in another place, Eysenhardt in his sense of incomplete manhood has a presentiment that just as his father had defeated him so now
he would succumb again.

A lower incisor loosens and breaks off while eating.
The symbolical influence of this event interpreted by
Eysenhardt as another sign of inadequacy, the loss of
some bodily possession damaging to his masculine
power, strikes him with all the force of a superstitious
impulse or, whatever it is, that intellectual people conceal in its place.   *The approaching end!*   All is vanity!
The truth overwhelms him almost at the very moment
of his ardently-longed-for triumph, the triumph for
which he had worked throughout life, toward which his
whole life-plan had been directed !   The old uncertainty
holds him in its vice.   What if his intellectual powers,
his main weapons disappear?   So again he takes recourse to his old method, the method to which he was
accustomed.   He wants some proof of his powers, some
certainty, an examination.   *By means of the self-criticism
to which he subjects himself it is within his power either to
lower or raise his prestige.*   What he is most afraid of is
not reality but the semblance of reality, *i.e.* whether he
is to be deprived of his worldly power.   In this condition
of hypochondriac doubt *his construction of fear spurs him
on to take even greater precautions.*   A sensation of
pressure on the heart, slight attacks of anxiety these are
but intensified hallucinatory safeguards and warnings.
The magnificently constructed rôle of the self-complacent
ego has, however, been shaken to its foundations.
When disappointment follows and his triumph, em-
bodied in the post of minister of justice miscarries this
comes upon a man who is already sick, a prey to uncertainty and who has been cut loose from his old
safeguarding constructions.

What will happen in all these instances where the
path to victory has been cut off and the harrowing
feeling of decreasing manhood seeks some way of pulling itself together again?   Attempts and preparations
come to the front to demonstrate that the personality
once possessed has not really suffered and that, on the
contrary, it is now even more firmly fixed.   The motor
habits of Eysenhardt take him more frequently to
Kaertner-strasse and its side-streets than before.   We

may assume that his degenerate sexuality, as in all cases of neurotic climacterics, has not developed from any biological wave but from the desire to redeem his fortune; that, in other words, it is a self-deception whose basis is the intensified will to power, *the intensified neurotic guiding-line.* Berger seems to incline towards this view even when he acquits Eysenhardt of the charge of sensuality, for he makes him feel that his slight lapses are rather to be interpreted as acts of secret despair, *i.e.* what we call *the masculine protest,* when humiliation, the reappearance of an inferiority feeling and the sinking of the sense of personality, are involved.

But there is another respect in which Eysenhardt has undergone a transformation, and this transformation shows us to what an extent the development of a character under the stress and tear of the world, is dependent upon the person's own opinion of himself. It is, in other words, changeable, and can like every *other scheme be exchanged* for another, since the character-picture never represents a purpose in itself but a psychical attitude by means of which the personality ideal is either to be attained in the quickest manner possible or its attainment attempted in some circuitous way, despite the appearance of insurmountable obstacles. Eysenhardt becomes more human and more humane to show that if he wills it he can be these too. " His ego hermetically sealed against contact with any other personality moves more freely ". His conscience awakens. We may justifiably assume that *this awakening is a contrivance of the psyche* for the purpose of raising the ego-feeling when it appears to be in an insecure situation. This and the realization of the mistakes one has committed bring the penitent nearer to God. It presupposes an opponent upon whom the hero's superiority can be proven. *But who is Eysenhardt's opponent?* Whom does Eysenhardt desire to put in the wrong this time, Eysenhardt whose whole life-plan has been to prosecute others for their mistakes? Whom does Eysenhardt, who always possessed complete control over all his expressions and thoughts, now accuse? His thoughts, etc., have now gained ascendancy over him and *he is forced to take his guiding-line literally*, to strengthen the fiction of his god-likeness and adhere to it to the bitter end. *His opponent now is the state*, the ruling regime, the patriarchal and paternal power that punishes and rewards. Eysenhardt's humiliation was a mistake, for the state had possessed no better servant. This servant had, however, an unquenchable ambition to become the judicial ruler of the state, and when he found himself cheated of his fiction and of his assumed right, *he put into operation those mechanisms that, to his mind, were most dangerous* for the state. The transformation of his attitude to one of mildness and soft-heartedness was the strongest attack and the most powerful revolt that he could make against the state. "Mildness is anarchy" he had always preached, and he therefore became mild.

We have here *a change in the guiding-fiction*. Eysenhardt at first wished to act as he had done in the case of his father during his early preparations for life, to rule by subjugating others. When this development was blocked just within reach of the goal, he created still stronger protections and safeguards, and *led a revolt in the form of judicial clemency*.

Hofrat Eysenhardt's mysterious Experience

The letter in which Eysenhardt described his sufferings was not burnt. The author states that he forgot to burn it. Berger is too good a psychologist to stop at this point. Let us therefore continue along the above lines. Eysenhardt selected the arrangement of forgetting in order to incite himself to further revolt and to show the public where loyalty to the state lead.

Remember that Eysenhardt's fiction was to control from the beginning of his career his masculine protest. This consisted *in attaining domination by subjecting himself to the powers of the state*. This fiction of his can be traced very far back, at least as far back as the time when his direct attack against his father failed and he was forced to make a detour. Directness did not remain one of his characteristics. Now we find him defeated again on his main line and at a time when death had already sent him a messenger. What could possibly be expected but that he would abandon his detour and proceed to a direct attack against the state that had so ungratefully repaid his loyal services, that he would reject those maxims and laws that had hitherto bound him both in his interest and in that of the state. All these surgings now partially expressed themselves and *his anarchistic mildness became strengthened.*

Nerve specialists have all had numerous experiences with the revolt engineered by ageing people, their giving up of positions, deserting their families and the world in order, on all sorts of pretexts, *to bring about a change in the form of their guiding-line.*

Eysenhardt at this stage tried to approach the medical profession which he had formerly despised as destructive and anarchistic in character. He regarded an interview with a physician however as a humiliation and therefore wrote down his hypochondriac and anxiety conditions and attempted to exorcise the sick person within himself by speaking of himself as though he were a different person, saving in this way his feeling-personality.

This was at the time when he expected his preferment and when the very upsetting event of the loss of his tooth occurred. Connected with it were trains of thought and emotional consequences which made him feel his capacities, particularly his memory, to be waning.

Here we have the typical "*hesitating attitude*" *of the neurotic* whenever he finds himself in the presence of a new situation, or that a new task is about to confront him. Eysenhardt with his firm grasp on the normal environment that had permitted him all his triumphs, had lost all his elasticity and hardly trusted himself to make the necessary changes for his new position.

Here the poet Berger comes to our rescue and describes the tentative preparations he made, the transformation of his outer person, the brightening of his features, etc. We infer from these fundamental facts and his compulsory execution of them, the existence of *an inward insecurity* demanding compensation. It is the same feeling of insecurity that has driven him out of society and from associating with respectable women. *He feels confident only of dominating prostitutes and criminals.*

The psyche, in particular the neurotic psyche, has a very peculiar method and contrivance at its disposal for meeting insecure situations. *It underestimates its own powers* and insists upon its possession of some inferiority so that it may gain room for expansion. This is the only position that a neurotic really knows well and from which he is able to form an estimate of life. Every prick of envy, of incited craving for domination and aggression will then become more perceptible, caution will mark every step he takes so that he may gain victory. *It is this "hesitating attitude" of caution* that makes neurotics develop misgivings as to their abilities. It is thus not a mere evasion of Eysenhardt if he imagines that his memory has suffered, for it represents, on the contrary, his strongest means of protection, the best method of warning himself, of re-doubling his attention, mobilizing his forces so that he may attain his guiding-goal and personality-ideal or, at least, spare his own feelings if he cannot other-wise succeed by some pretence of illness.

Now what rôle does the lost tooth play in this cŏn-nection? It is impossible to over-estimate Eysenhardt's evaluation of even the smallest parts of his body. Because of his feeling of inadequacy the neurotic can stand no loss of any kind. Nor should we exclude the well-known symbolical significance of the loss of a tooth. Its loss has at all times been associated with thoughts of death, old age and pregnancy. In dreams, phantasies and poems we find the tooth standing for something growing, some after-growth, as an expres-sion of masculine power, and its loss is consequently the symbol of emasculation. The emotional idea that the novelist wishes to convey is probably identical. Eysenhardt takes the loss of his tooth as a sign of the decrease of his creative powers. Did he have to interpret it in this fashion? Remember that Cæsar when falling, on his landing in Egypt exclaimed, "Africa, I seize you by the hand!" Why did Eysen-hardt set so high a value on this event and why did he not interpret it in another way? The answer is simple enough—*because this evaluation was of help to him*. He found himself, according to our view, in a hesi-tating attitude demanding caution and just before a decision and change in his situation. *This tooth fell out at a most opportune moment*, or to put it in a different way, he utilized this event in order to increase the strength of his safeguards.

His logical faculties then came under the sway of his end-purpose.

Then came his humiliation. His expectation of obtaining *a post in the ministry* was not fulfilled. In consequence of this set-back a series of hallucinations appeared every night, generally in the form of figures of men, occasionally of women, and he was able to recognize from certain details that they were all people he had sentenced. These hallucinations interfered with his sleep and filled him with fear. I cannot here enter into the discussion of these details brilliantly described by Berger. They seem to have the purpose of demonstrating the need for the establishment of some illness and *the danger to the existence of the state of his penitence.*

My observations of psychotics and neurotics lead me to believe that the latter resort to hallucinatory images when they are about to develop safeguards of particular clarity and penetration.

As a matter of fact Eysenhardt's hallucinations always called up his feeling of inferiority. For instance he allows others to demonstrate their superiority, to accuse him on account of his severity, to suggest to him that he also is a criminal just as Marcus Freund had actually called out to him during the latter's trial. The figure of this man in his series of hallucinations has the same significance and shows even more definitely the vulnerable part of Eysenhardt's psyche, that part to which attention has already been drawn. Eysenhardt like Marcus Freund *is afraid of woman* and finds pleasure only in prostitutes as Freund had in children. The analysis of perversions found among neurotics shows the succession of events to be as follows : fear of woman, at best excepting prostitutes, followed by sex gratification only through children. Such a person may as a matter of fact proceed along this line as far as necrophily or homo-sexuality. The worthless fickle woman is the ideal of most neurotics and their policy will always be to depreciate a woman until they have rendered her worthless.

It is along such a line that Eysenhardt obtained the clearest insight into his own character, because in his feeling of inadequacy which events had recently intensified we find him craving for increased indulgences so that he may begin to develop his masculine protest. Has he any presentiment that this path leads to the craving for the child ? He protects himself at any rate by developing warning hallucinations and terrifying images. *He has his hallucinations just as others have a feeling for society or a religion*, in order to protect himself by means of an aggressiveness which defeat has called forth.

Two other conditions favouring hallucinations co-operating with each other are found. *His illness* and the hallucinations—the accompanying anxiety condition as well as his doubts as to his abilities, demonstrate him to be ill—destroy *a wonderful instrument* forged for the use of the state. *In accusing himself he is accusing the state*, the administration of the law, public safety of which he had been one of the guardians, and by his penitence he is shaking to its very foundations the concept of justice he had held. He is delivering body blows at his opponent now, his real opponent, the state, the ruling classes—all of whom have contributed to his defeat.

The psychic situation portrayed so concisely by his hallucinations aid us in what follows. In a moment of deep humiliation he conquers his desires for revenge by erecting terror-inspiring spectres which are to show him what would happen if he proceeded on his normal course. The meaning of his aggressiveness is a neurotic and hostile preparation directed against his sleeping and unsuspecting master, whom he is threatening in much the same way in which he once threatened his father. His neurotic perspective, in its search for security, sought and found in Marcus Freund a threatening reminiscence. And so Eysenhardt becomes again the victor.

When he accepted the presidency of the espionage case upon whose proper conduct the welfare of the state might depend, he felt that he had returned as conqueror. He made his preparations as on former occasions. "He did not think of Marcus Freund any more", because he did not need him any longer. His protesting sexual tension had become allayed.

Against "ladies" he was also able to protect himself, for here his old construction of shyness when in their presence still proved efficacious. But he fell a victim to a child. "Daimonic" femininity conquered him, as from childhood he had had a foreboding it would. This was however *from the very beginning a construction of his own making*. He now had but one

alternative left if he wished to evade the compelling
power of the triumphant woman—death.   He proceeded
along this path firmly and thus fulfilled two of the above
enumerated conditions :—he deprived the state of a loyal
servant whom it could ill afford to spare, and left
behind him among the mass of people a shattered faith
in the course of justice.   The first of the reasons for his
hallucinations, namely that he should shrink back before
the idea of violating a child, had become meaningless.
So once again had he aimed at the head of his father,
the father who had punished him for his craving for
love, but this time it was himself he had to strike if he
wished to hit the real enemy.

XXIII

Dostoevsky

(Lecture delivered in the Tonhalle of Zurich, 1918)

BELOW the earth in the mines of Siberia, Dimitrji Karamasov expects to sing his song about eternal harmony. The guilty and yet innocent patricide takes up the cross and finds his salvation in the all-forgiving mutual harmony.

"For fifteen years I was an idiot", says Prince Mischkin in his amiable smiling manner, the man who could interpret every twist in a hand-writing, who gave utterance to his ulterior thoughts without the slightest embarrassment and who immediately recognized those of others. We have a greater contrast here than can well be imagined.

"Am I Napoleon or am I a louse?" Roskolnikov ponders in his bed for more than a month in order *to cross the line* set by his former life, his community-feeling and his experiences. Here again we have the great contrast, the contrast in which we ourselves participate and which we ourselves feel.

It is the same with his other heroes and is the same in his own life. "Like a hot-head" the youth Dostoevsky flew about under his parental roof and if we read his letters to his father and his friend we will find an extraordinary amount of humility, submissiveness and acceptance of his often tragic fate. Hunger, torment, misery, of these he was to taste frequently enough in his life. He passed along life like a pilgrim. The young hot-head took the cross upon himself like the wise Sossina, like the all-knowing pilgrim in "Youth" and he walked step by step, gathering together all experiences, embracing all humanity in one broad embrace, for the sake of obtaining knowledge, of touching life in all its phases, to seek truth, to seek *the new teaching*.

Anyone who holds within his breast such contrasts, who is compelled to bridge such contrasts, must indeed drink deeply if he desires to gain any repose. For he will be spared no trouble, none of the sufferings of life ; he will not be able to pass even the most insignificant bit of life without trying to see how it fits into his formula. His whole nature impels him onward toward an *integrated* interpretation of life so that in his eternal oscillations when in this state of restlessness he may find security and rest.

To gain repose he would have to be able to arrive at *truth*. But the road to truth is beset with thorns, demands great exertions, great perseverance, a tremendous training of mind and soul. Is it strange therefore that this restless seeker after nature came far nearer to true life, to the logic of co-operation than others who could far more easily have taken an attitude toward life?

He had been brought up in needy circumstances and when he died all Russia in spirit followed his cortege. He who enjoyed working, who was full of life, who always had a word of encouragement for himself, his friends, was more incapable of work than other people, for he was afflicted with that frightful disease, epilepsy, which often prevented him from making any progress for days and weeks. The " criminal " to whose legs chains had been bound for four years in Tobolsk and who for four years was compelled to serve as a convict in a Siberian infantry regiment, this noble innocent sufferer leaves his prison with the following words and feelings in his heart :—" My punishment was just for I had evil intentions in my heart against the government. But it is too bad that I must now suffer for theories, and for a cause that is no longer mine ".

The contrasts in the life of his country were of course numerous. When Dostoevsky appeared before the public, Russia was in a ferment and the question of the freeing of the serfs was uppermost in everyone's mind. Dostoevsky was always impelled toward the " poor and lowly ", toward children, toward sufferers. His friends told many a tale of the ease with which he made friends with beggars who came to visit his friends as patients, how he would draw them to his room, entertain and try to understand them. When in prison,

his greatest misery was caused by the fact that the
other convicts regarded him as a nobleman and withdrew
from him. His persistent longing was to understand
and analyse the meaning of prison life, of its inner laws,
to gain a knowledge of those boundaries within which
an understanding and friendship with the others was
possible. Like many great men, he utilized his banishment for the purpose of developing a sensitiveness even
under petty, oppressive circumstances, to practise his
penetrative vision in order to attain to knowledge of
the inter-connections of life and then to call a halt and
unite in one synthesis all the antitheses that threatened
to shake him to his foundations and confound him.

Amidst the uncertainties of his psychic contradictions the goal of his striving was the discovery of some
valid truth. He himself was alternately rebel and
obedient slave, was drawn to abysses from which he
shrank back frightened. To obtain truth he made
error his guide. His principle had been for a long
time, even before he gave it expression, *to approach
truth through falsehood*, for we never can be certain of
possessing truth and have to be prepared to resort to
infinitesimal lies. Thus he grew up to be the enemy
of " Western " culture, whose essential traits appeared
to him to be *a striving to arrive at falsehood through
truth*. He could find truth only by uniting the antitheses struggling within him, the contrasts that always
expressed themselves in his creation and threatened to
destroy him and his heroes. In this spirit did he accept
an invitation for the rôle of poet and prophet and he
proceeded to establish limits for his *self-love*. *The limits
of power intoxication* he found set *by the love of one's
neighbour*. What had originally spurred him on was a
clear-cut striving for power, for domination and even
in the attempt to include all life in one formula there is
manifest a great deal of this impulse towards superiority.
In all the deeds of his heroes we find this up-stroke
impelling them to raise themselves above others, to
accomplish Napoleonic tasks, to approach to the very
brink of the abyss, even to suspend themselves over it,
running the danger of falling into its depths and being
shattered. He says of himself: " I am reprehensibly
ambitious ". However, he succeeded in making his
ambition of some use to the community. He proceeded

similarly with his heroes; *he permitted them all to madly transcend the limits that he had discovered from a realization of the logical demands of communal co-operation. He drove them all, by inciting their ambition, vanity, self-love, on to the uttermost confines of life and then set the chorus of furies upon their path and drove them back again to the boundaries* imposed by human nature where he allowed them to sing hymns in harmony. There is no *image* so often occurring in his work as that of a "*boundary*" occasionally also the picture of a wall. He says of himself, "I have a mad love of penetrating to the limits of the real, there where the phantastic begins". His attacks he describes as making him feel as though an intoxication of joy enticed him to the furthermost limits of the sensation of living, where he felt himself near God, so near indeed, that only one step would have sufficed to cut him off from life. This picture recurs again and again in all his heroes and has a profound significance. Let us listen to his new messianic teaching—The great *synthesis* of uniting *heroic life with love of neighbour* has succeeded. It is at this boundary line that the destiny of his heroes, their fate seemed to be consummated. To that limit he too was induced to go. There, he had a presentiment, he would find the richest fulfilment of human worth in the form of fellow-love and so he drew this boundary line with the greatest precision, with a precision that few had ever succeeded in doing before his time. This goal became of particular significance for his creative faculty and his ethical stand-point.

Again and again he and his heroes were tempted to advance to the uttermost limits of experience, where groping and hesitating he brings about their amalgamation with humanity, in deepest humility before God, Czar and Russia. For this feeling that held him in a vice and which might be called the limit-feeling, one which caused him to call a halt, one which had become transformed into a safeguarding feeling of guilt—as his friends often spoke of it—he knew no cause. Strangely enough he brought it into relation with his epileptic attacks. The hand of God appeared whenever man in over-weening conceit wished to transcend the limits of his *community-feeling* and warning voices were heard, recommending introspection.

Roskolnikov, who bravely pursuing his thoughts of murder, who on the impulsive feeling that everything is permitted chosen natures, was already thinking of the nature of the weapon to be used, lies in bed for months before crossing the line. And finally when with his club concealed under his coat, he runs up the steps to commit the murder, *he finds that he has heart-palpitations.* In this heart-palpitation we recognize the voice of life, and in it Dostoevsky's sensitive feeling for the limits of life are expressed.

A number of his creations picture, not an isolated hero overstepping the limits of neighbourly love, but, on the contrary, a man lifting himself up out of insignificance and dying nobly and heroically. I have already mentioned the novelist's love of the small, the insignificant. In such cases the men of lowly origin, the ordinary man, the prostitute, the child, become the heroes. They all suddenly begin to assume tremendous size until they come to the boundary line of the all-embracing human heroism to which Dostoevsky wishes to conduct them.

Throughout his whole youth the concept of the *permissible and unpermissible,* of the boundary line, had been brought clearly home to him. In his early manhood the situation remained the same. He was handicapped by his illness and his spirit was very early affected by his harrowing experience when about to be executed, and by his banishment. In childhood, his father, apparently a rather strict and pedantic man, appears to have tried to cope with the boy's stubbornness, his unbroken fiery spirit, and apparently he drove him too forcibly toward the boundary line.

A short fragment entitled "St Petersburg Dreams" dates from early life and we should for that reason expect a definite line of action to be manifest. If anything may be inferred logically from the development of an artist's soul it must refer to lines of connection leading from his earlier work, his sketches and plans, to the later forms of his creative activity. But we must remember first and foremost, that the orbit of artistic creation passes outside the battle of life. We may consequently assume that every artist will show a turning-off, a halt, a retreat, as soon as the normal expectations of society confront him. The artist who out of nothing, or let us say, out of an anxious attitude toward the facts of life, creates a world and who, instead of an answer in terms of practical life, gives us a puzzling artistic creation, such a man is averted from life, and its demands. "Well, but I am a mystic and dreamer!" Dostoevsky tells us.

We obtain some notion of Dostoevsky's method of attack as soon as we discover exactly *at what point of man's activity he halts*. That, he indicates clearly enough in the above sketch. "As I approached the Neva, I stopped for a moment to cast a glance up the river into the misty cold and indistinct distance where the last traces of the purple dusk disappeared". Then he hurried home and like a normal man dreamed of Schiller's heroines. "The real Amalia, however, I had never noticed; she lived in my vicinity". . . Intoxicated with love, he preferred to suffer and found this suffering sweeter than all the pleasures of life. "Had I married Amalia I would certainly have been unhappy". Is it not the simplest thing in the world? One is a poet, indulges in dreams at the proper distance from the turmoil of life, stops for a moment to find the sweetness of imagined love unsurpassable, and realizes "that reality destroys even ideal constructions. Do I not wish to travel to the moon!" That means, however, that he wishes to remain alone and to love nothing earthly!

Thus the poet's ramparts became a protest against reality and its demands. This is different from what we find in *The Idiot* or in the case of the sick man who had "neither protest nor voice". Dostoevsky did not know that his endurance of misery would one day be his distinction. When by annoyance and reproach he was forced out of his orbit, he found the normal man within himself, the destroyer and revolutionary Garibaldi. In discovering this he discovered what no one had understood until then, that humility and submissiveness do not signify final acts but are revolts indicating the "distance" that is to be overcome. Tolstoi also understood this secret and preached it frequently enough to deaf ears.

A real secret may be published in the newspaper and yet no one will know anything about it. No one knew, for instance, on whom Harpagon Solowjow wished to revenge himself by starving himself and dying in misery while concealed among his dirty papers was hidden a fortune of 170,000 roubles. How he must have enjoyed himself inwardly when he shut himself off sadly and helplessly from his cat, his cook, and his housekeeper, and remained in debt to everyone! He held them all in the palm of his hand, forced them all to beg, all those who only recognized money as a power and prayed to it. True enough this resulted in his developing a peculiar obligation, and methodically doing violence to life. He himself had to starve and perish in order to carry out his method of attack. "He is elevated above all desires". Must a person necessarily be crazy to do this? Well, Solowjow is willing to make this sacrifice if necessary. For then he could without any responsibility show his contempt for mankind and its conceited fortune-chasers, harass everyone who comes near him. He has everything that would enable him to enter the best of society and yet, he halts for a moment, throws his magic wand into the dust-bin and feels great and elevated above mankind.

The strongest point in Dostoevsky's life is that all his magnificent creations were to arise in the following way namely, that the act was to be regarded as futile, pernicious and criminal and *that salvation was to lie in submission as long as submission contained within itself the secret enjoyment of superiority over others.*

All biographers of Dostoevsky have busied themselves markedly with explaining one of his earliest *childhood reminiscences*, that he himself mentions in his *The House of the Dead.* For the better understanding of this reminiscence let me give something of the mood in which it arose.

At a time when he had almost despaired of making any *connections* with his fellow-prisoners he had resignedly thrown himself upon his bed and mused on his childhood, on his whole development and life-experience. Suddenly his attention becomes fixed upon the following reminiscence : One day, wandering too far from his father's estate and cutting across the fields, he suddenly stopped, frightened at the voice of someone calling, "The wolf is coming!" He hurried back to the shelter of his father's house and there he saw in the field *a peasant* and to him he ran for protection. Weeping and frightened he held on to the peasant's arm and told him how he had been frightened. The peasant made the sign of *the cross* with his fingers over the boy, consoled him and promised that he would not let the wolf devour him. This reminiscence is generally interpreted as if it characterized Dostoevsky's bond with the peasantry and the religion of the peasantry. *However, the important thing here is the wolf, the wolf that drives him back to man.* This experience persisted in him as the symbolical expression of his whole striving, because it lay in the direction-line of his activities. What made him tremble at the idea of the isolated hero is comparable to the wolf in the experience. The wolf drove him back to the poor and the lowly and there, in the sign of the cross, he tried to make his connections. There he wished to be of help. This is what he means when he says, " My whole life belongs to my people and all my thoughts to humanity ".

Even though we emphasize the fact that Dostoevsky was a Russian and an opponent of modern culture, that the Pan-Slavic ideal had taken firm root in him, this need not be in contradiction with his spirit, the spirit that wished to search truth through error.

In one of his greatest messages, in his speech *In memory of Pushkin*, he attempted nevertheless to establish a connection between Western Europe and the Russophiles. The effect that very night was glorious. Adherents of both parties rushed to him, embraced him, expressed themselves in accord with his standpoint. But this unanimity did not last long. Men had not as yet thoroughly awakened from their slumber.

While Dostoevsky was trying with all his intensity to put into effect and carry to the masses the longing of his heart, the consummation of an all-embracing humanity—a task for which he had been destined—he also formed for himself a concrete symbol of this fellow-love. This would naturally suggest to one who was attempting to save himself and others, the idea of a saviour, *a Russian Christ,* who had turned aside from the merely human, from worldly power. His confession of faith was simple, " For me Christ is the most beautiful and the most exalted person in the history of the world ". In this passage Dostoevsky discloses with incisive

sharpness his guiding-goal.   It was thus he had
described his attacks of epilepsy where in his feeling of
rapture he had ascended, had attained eternal harmony,
felt himself in the proximity of God.   His goal was to
be with Christ always, bear His wounds, fulfil His task.
He attacked isolated heroism, that heroism which he had
experienced personally perhaps more keenly than anyone
before him, recognized it as a diseased conceit, as self-
love in contrast to that feeling of a common bond which
to him was inherent in a love of one's fellowmen and in
the logical demands of society.   "Bend your knee, proud
man!"   To those who had given up, who hurt in their
self-esteem were striving for peace, he cried : " Work,
sluggards ! "   People who referred him to human nature,
to its apparently external laws, in order to refute him
he answered by saying, " The bees and the ants know
their formula, it is only man who does not know his ! "
We can add the following to the inferences that flow
from Dostoevsky's striving : *Man must look for his
formula and he will find it in a willingness to help others, in
a capacity for sacrificing himself for his people.*

Thus he became a solver of riddles and a God-seeker.
He felt his god more intensely than most other semi-
sleepers and dreamers.   "I am no psychologist", he
once said : "I am a realist".   And here he strikes at
the point separating him most sharply from all artists
of modern times and from all psychologists.   He was in
intimate connection with the community-feeling, with
the very bases of society, the one true reality we do
not completely know but would like to understand.
And that is why he could call himself a realist.

Let us now look into the reasons for the tremendous
effect exerted upon us by Dostoevsky's personages.
The main reasons are to be sought *in their integrated
unity*.   No matter at what point you take and examine one
of his heroes you will always find him with the complete
paraphernalia of life and ideals.   To find analogies we
would have to go to the realm of music where the
same holds true, for a melody discloses in the course
of its harmonic development all the currents and movements of the whole piece again and again.   So also
for Dostoevsky's figures.   Roskolnikov is the same when
lying in his bed and pondering over the murder he is
to commit, as when he ascends the steps with his heart

palpitating ; he is the same when dragging the drunkard from under the wheels of the wagon giving his last penny for the man's starving family. This it is which creates singleness of purpose in these characters and is at the bottom of the influence they exercise upon us. Unconsciously we carry away in the person of every one of his heroes a firmly fused plastic figure as though it had been cast in some imperishable medium, figures similar to those in the Bible, of Homer, of the Greek tragedies where we have but to mention the names in order to bring before our soul the whole of their influence.

There is another difficulty in understanding the effect Dostoevsky produces, but fortunately the conditions necessary for solving it are at hand. The difficulty consists in *our realization of the double axis on which every one of these figures revolves, each axis marvellously fixed to a definite point.* Every hero moves securely in a space bounded on one side by isolated heroism where the hero becomes a wolf and, on the other, by the sharply drawn line of love of fellow-men. This double axis gives each of his characters so secure a hold and so fixed a view-point that they remain firmly imprinted upon our memory and feeling.

One word more about Dostoevsky as a moralist. He was forced by circumstances, the antithesis in his own nature which he had to negate, the tremendous contrasts in his environment which he had to bridge, to look for formulas that would both embrace and help his deeply-felt longing for an active expression of love of man. And so he reached that formula that is to be placed far above the categorical imperative of Kant— *"That every person participates in the guilt of his fellow-man."* We know to-day more than ever before how deep this formula goes and how intimately it is bound up with the truest realities of life. We may deny this formula but it will always reassert itself and give us the lie. But this formula means far more than just an idea of love of fellow, which is indeed frequently misunderstood, arrived at through vanity or just a form of the categorical imperative that retains its value even in the isolation of personal ambition. If I participate in the guilt of my neighbour and in the guilt of everyone, then I have an eternal obligation impelling me to

T

assume this responsibility and commanding me to pay the price.

Thus he remains both as artist and moralist a great and unapproachable figure.

His achievements as a psychologist have not yet been exhausted. We venture to say that his psychological seer-vision penetrated deeper than the science of psychology because he was better acquainted with nature and psychology has developed conceptualistically. Anyone who like Dostoevsky has tried to ponder *upon the significance of laughter*, upon the possibility of learning to recognize a man better from his laughter than from his life-attitude, anyone who went so far that he came upon the idea of *the accidental family*, where every member lives for himself, isolated from the other, and implanting in their children the tendency for still greater isolation, greater self-love, that man has seen more than can be expected or demanded from any psychologist. Anyone who remembers how Dostoevsky in *A Raw Youth* lets a boy under his bedcover give expression to his phantasies by ideas of *power* will have realized the truth and sensitiveness of his description of *the origin of mental ailments* in life as serving the purpose of revolt; anyone who has felt to what a degree Dostoevsky has recognized *the tendency to despotism* implanted in the human soul, he will admit that Dostoevsky must be regarded as our teacher even to-day, as the teacher Nietzsche hailed him to be. His understanding and his discussion of the dream have not been superseded even to-day and his idea that no one acts or thinks without a goal or a final climax, coincides with the most modern results of students of the psyche.

Dostoevsky has thus become a great and endeared master in a distinct number of fields. His realistic portraiture of life explains why his work comes upon us like a flash opening the eye of the sleeper. The sleeper rubs his eyes, turns around and knows nothing of what has happened. Dostoevsky slept little and woke up many times. His creations, his ethic and his art take us very far in an understanding of human co-operation.

XXIV

New View-points on War Neuroses

(January 1908)

THE new literature on war neuroses has repeatedly and persistently insisted upon the small degree in which our present neurological attitude differs from that which prevailed before the war. We have the same material, neurologists tell us, the same etiology, the same course of the illness and the same difficulties. It is only in connection with therapy that fundamental changes have occurred and these have resulted from conditions imposed by the war and the military situation.

We ought however to emphasize one new and important change and one that is likely to increase the difficulties of present-day neurological investigation. The treatment of neurosis among the civil population in times of peace had as its unexpressed but self-evident object the patient's cure or at least freeing him of his symptoms so that he might be able to find himself again and pursue a course of life dictated by himself. Military neurology had as its object naturally enough not the desire to cure a man for his own sake but for the sake and the advantage of the army and the "state." Medical ideas of the purpose to be served and purely medical considerations were thus mixed up with what ought always to be an objective science and therapy. However necessary and desirable such purely medical considerations may be they clearly increase the difficulties for a proper understanding of the problems since the picture of the disease to be investigated would then have to be inordinately stressed on one side or the other. Our problem thus narrows down to the *manner in which a neurotic behaves in a situation imposed upon him from without.*

There is enough pre-war material at hand for enabling

us to obtain some insight into the peculiar position this question occupies. Practically every physician knows the results of the variously graded suggestion-therapy as applied to single disturbing and insistent symptoms. Unfortunately the belief was frequently indulged in, that a permanent cure had been effected, a belief that oral information and letters seemed to corroborate even when the patient was at that very moment undergoing treatment either for old or for some new manifestations of his trouble.

Let me remind you of the results brought to the fore-ground in the treatment of symptoms where the object was not so much curing the patient as enabling him to perform some set task. A law student, for example, just before his examinations complained of insomnia, tiredness, forgetfulness and head-aches. His examination was to take place within eight days. Let me give you all the steps in the cure of his case by no means an infrequent one. Undoubtedly instances do exist where either through the doctor's suggestions or by some other therapeutic procedure a student is successfully helped over an examination. (For example, by suggestions to remain awake, hypnosis, applications of cold water, electric treatment, medicines). In the case of a neurotic the words of the physician or indeed of any person are quite enough to improve the patient's condition.[1] Everyone will be in agreement with me in considering such cases, no matter what the nature of their symptoms, as slight and lying on the border-line of the normal. The foregoing treatments were of course, not always successful. Some students took their examinations and found themselves utterly unable to concentrate their attention. In a large number of instances the symptoms became exaggerated and they then used their sufferings as an excuse for changing their profession. Occasionally a severe neurosis developed or suicide took place. Quite a number of those whose condition became aggravated regarded the treatments they had undergone as responsible and were generally corroborated in this supposition by the next doctor they visited. I remember a case where a

---

[1] Visiting a physician means to half of the "neurotics" a decision to improve to give up a symptom that has become unnecessary. All the tendencies found in modern neurology are founded on these 50 per cent. cures.

man cured his wife's fear of being driven fast by spurring
on the horses to even greater speed.

No one would claim that the above cases were cured.
Barring a few people not even the war neurologists
ever believed that they had done more than rid the
patient of his symptoms and they always preferred after
treatment to keep these men out of the front ranks. In
contrast to the treatment given in peace times where
the physician always has some purpose and attempts
with the patient's co-operation to carry it out, the war-
treatment had for its immediate object making a person
fit for active military duty although the nature of this
service could be gradually reduced and made lighter.
The neurotic was thus even if kept behind the front or
in the very rear continually confronted by new and vital
decisions arising from the success of the treatment. The
authorities are quite right in emphasizing the importance
of the " atmosphere " in the infirmary. This atmosphere
is however by no means merely the result of the attitude
adopted toward the inferences drawn from the cures but
is made up of hundreds of details among which are
included, to a smaller or greater degree, some assumptions of a more or less justified nature about the subsequent question of utility and the problems of the future.

The question of the granting of a pension must be
included here although we do not wish to imply that
the annual grant of money ever appeared to the neurotic
as a goal worth striving for. This was not even true
for the patient who became hysterical about the possibility of accidents befalling him. The pension has,
however, for the war neurotic a value like that ascribed
to a war-medal. It is an official document and a
certificate of illness to be shown the patient's relatives. It
can also be used to protect himself from further attempts
to drag him back to military service. Every neurologist
must have been struck by the very critical tone employed
by the pensioned invalid whenever he is being re-
examined and by his insistence that his papers should
be perused. The " imaginary pension " is what most
impresses the neurotic, even when he seems to be obeying conscious logical interpretations like fear, danger,
home-sickness and personal gain.

Every move of the physician is, as in peace time,
answered by a contrary effort of the patient. I always

examined neurotics away from their home and their relatives. As long as this reaction can be regarded as a purely neurotic one and as long as it persists, both the absence or the occasional presence of relatives, their distance or their nearness, will affect him in the same way. Every irrational bias on this question renders the simplification and at the same time the process of amelioration more difficult. Demands made by private nursing-homes can for example be definitely made dependent upon the nature of the betterment produced.

It is always possible to prove that the "lability" of the neurotic symptoms arises from the neurotic's position and we may claim that it is *a position-illness*. It is for that reason that it is so vital for the neurologist to possess a complete understanding of each individual attitude and every aspect of the patient's language, a knowledge which it is at times difficult to obtain.

Forming one part of the neurotic's "*position*" is the nature of the treatment used. The problem becomes insoluble if the sick man is treated by more than one physician. Small neurological nursing homes are for that reason to be recommended. Records of cures obtained there would be of service and methods of treatment could then be evaluated according to their success. Only information about cures should be accepted when given by the physicians who had actually treated the patients.

Only those methods of treatment can be taken into consideration as part of a true *psycho-therapy* that have succeeded in unmasking the patient's psyche. All the "psycho-therapeutic" measures used in present day nervous treatments must therefore be excluded from this definition and regarded only of value as general maxims to be applied. In war-time whatever success they possess is derived entirely from the use of authority and the bestowal of a "minimum of comfort." In the first method of treatment hypnosis, waking suggestion, sham neurosis and the "psycho-therapeutic" preparation before the actual cure, ought also to be included. Heroic methods often take the form of such painful procedures as the water-bed, frightening the patient, depriving him of certain objects and the conscious aggravation of his condition. At best the Frank method recommended by Sauer is but a make-shift for it tells us too little of the psychic make-up of the patient, puts him too much in the power of the physician and seems to be operating with a kind of "counter-shock." The success these methods can be shown to have had in war-times and occasionally during peace, is based upon the neurotic disinclination for treatment—itself a neurotic symptom.. Followers of Freud apply this method to officers and the Kaufmann method to the troops with approximately the same results.

The greater insistence upon action in the methods adopted to-day is quite noticeable among all the practitioners. Bringing the patient into more favourable surroundings, calming him and waiting are no longer regarded as of any importance. The fundamental point in present-day war neurology is the attempt to destroy the neurotic's obstinacy by calling forth counter traits of the individual. I mean the examination and the disclosure of the neurotic obstinacy. Such is the case in that therapy which externally impresses one as milder but which is in reality more drastic and fundamental and which apparently promises a quicker and more durable success in those cases where neurotics are employing their war experiences as subterfuges. This method likewise cannot entirely prevent the patient's psychical "position" from becoming aggravated and it suffers unfortunately from the taint of being after all but a sham procedure.

The question as to whether neuroses are acquired or inherited has not been entirely neglected but the educational factor, the influence of environment and children's imitation of their neurotic parents have become of more importance than before. The frequency or the regularity of a neurotic pre-history is to-day always insisted upon. The parent's position in life and society as understood by individual psychology is from a prognostic point of view held to be decisive. The individual-psychological penetration into the psychic picture presented by a patient, the proper kind of anamnesis and a better understanding of the patient's view-point toward life than has hitherto been obtained is bound to give us the safest guide as to the extent of the aggravation absent in no neurosis and will also aid us in unmasking all shams.

A view fairly dominant today is that which insists that the symptom preferably selects a type of disease from which the patient has formerly suffered and locates it in the same place. That is simply insisting that it develops in connection with an organ of inferiority, or that the symptom represents a permanent fixation of such normal manifestations of an affect as trembling, nausea-fixation, speechlessness, etc. Very few attempts have been made to study the cause of this fixation. One of the favourite assumptions is that the tendency toward fixation is a neurotic trait like the lability of the symptom. We might assume from the "position" of the patient that the real explanation is that the neurotic fixates a symptom *by identifying himself* with it if it suits his purposes and rejecting it if it does not. Similar things are found among normal people under normal conditions.

I wish now to comment upon a number of statements, observations and suggestions made within the last two years in various publications. Schanz (1) regards the starting point of ague to lie in the deficiency of a vertebral segment which Blencke (2) insists actually exists and which manifests itself, if at all, only indirectly in ague. "Neurasthenic" pains can be more frequently attributed to this deficiency. We can often satisfy ourselves of the existence of a naevus either at the place where the pain is felt or in one of its segments. This finding, together with a minimal degree of scoliosis or kyphoscoliosis generally present simultaneously, protect the diagnosis against the suspicion of simulation being present. Andernach was always successful when using verbal suggestion followed by the application of the Faraday brush. He insisted likewise on atmosphere favourable to suggestions. Rottmann, followed by Josef and Mann, tried to conquer the patient's psyche by a sham operation during narcosis and imposing bandages afterwards. Kalmus and E. Meyer favour the Kaufmann method which has *recently become milder*. It now consists of a preparation in the form of verbal suggestion followed a few days later by faradization but with *electrical currents of medium strength* and interrupted by military gymnastics. E. Meyer wishes to exclude from this treatment psychopathic patients of the neurasthenic type, for example, all those who have major attacks of hysteria or general psychical manifestations, in other words severe cases. Incidentally let

me add that the physician is of more importance than
the nature of the treatment. Simulation should not be
assumed *too hastily*. As we are always bound to find
irritations of the psychopathic constitution *faradization*
is to be rejected.

Liebermeister (3) seems to have some important
suggestions. As his treatment is not allowed to be
practised outside of Germany I can only refer to remarks
taken from reviews of his work. I infer from these that
he insists that the practitioner should either pledge
himself to bring about a cure or not accept payment.
Adler (4) has come to the same conclusion. He stresses
in addition the importance of the individual-psychological method and an educational therapeutics by
means of which the neurotic fundamentals of character
persisting since childhood, can be shown to be defective
or erroneous. If we disregard all schematic interpretations we shall find that the neurotic instinctively protects
himself against the general demands of life by resorting
to a subjective feeling of weakness. By self-identification with a danger he attempts *to protect himself* against
a real danger. The neurosis thus becomes a means of
evasion. The prognosis will be more favourable if
there are indications of an earlier active cooperation in
the patient's previous history, of progress in school,
friendship, love affairs, marriage at a proper age,
children, occupation, etc. The neurotic always betrays
himself by his tendency to adhere to the "protecting"
small family-circle. Both the symptoms and their
fixation are dominated by the "safeguarded future
goal." It is quite easy to distinguish between simulation and true neurosis. The above statements taken
from a lecture directed against the use of high-voltage
currents terminated with the warning that "all methods
of treatment were to be avoided that hurt people's
dignity." Lewandowsky (5) says very much the same:
"Sick people develop a neurosis in order to secure
safety. Among some of them an inherited inability to
subordinate one's self, an unwillingness toward adaptation plays a prominent rôle in the development of the
desire to remain at home . . . The real cause of the
illness is not to be found, however, in their past history
or in a traumatic condition of any kind but in the future,
in those things that the patient no longer cares to

endure . . . The illness allows him to gain his wish to run away from danger." Lewandowsky also stresses the danger of bringing many neurotics together in one place on account of the possibility of infection. He considers the treatment more difficult when the patient is in his own home, because that is where after all he most wishes to be. He does not however indicate what means against the desire to remain at home are to be adopted. The writer quite correctly points out how one cure brings others in its wake. I too remember a number of clear-cut cures accomplished by a nurse speaking to patients of other patients who had been cured. Lewandowsky possibly exaggerates the importance of military rank upon the success of the treatment. His treatment consists in attempts to aggravate the situation, supplemented by suggestion, by faradization, although different from that used by Kaufmann, and by hypnosis. He rejects the employment of either sham-operations or sham-narcosis. Meyer (6) regards every method as good as long as the physician believes in it and applies it fearlessly. The important thing is to convince the neurotic that he can be of use in his former occupation. Raether (7) describes an application of the Kaufmann method consisting of a kind of psychotherapeutic introductory treatment followed during the same visit by an application of the faradic current. Subsequent treatments should follow. The results showed that 97 per cent. of the people were cured and rendered capable of undertaking civil occupations. L. Mann (8) points out that as early as 1911 he had already used verbal suggestions and subsequent applications of the faradic current.

From Naegeli's (9) work, *Unfalls-und Begehrungsneurosen*, I would like to call attention to the fact that cures took place and working capacity was restored as soon as the nature of the vitality of the individual was discovered. He strongly opposes Oppenheim and denies as most people did then, the existence of " accident neurosis."

Troemner (10) shows the existence of a pseudo-clerodermatic form of traumatic neurosis (Oppenheim) which he interprets as the hysterical paresis accompanied by tropho-neuroses in consequence of an injury to the back of the hand due to the wearing of a bandage for two months. The same author describes one of the manifestations of "bilateral monæsthesia" in which two widely separate points of a compass applied at the same time were felt as one. He regards this as a utilizable demonstration for the existence of an hysterical restriction of attention. Leusser (11) comments on a case of tachycardiac paroxysm extending over four generations. Heinze (12) describes the success obtained by the hypnotic treatment of hysterical war-manifestations. He obtained 86 per cent. cures and was even successful in cases of stimulated hypnosis. None of these patients regained complete working capacity and in spite of the curing of their symptoms only a small number could be put to military work. He regards neurotic war diseases as transient reactions developing out of psychopathic inferiority. Minkowski (13) calls to mind a case of Israel's thirty years ago, when the latter performed a sham operation upon a patient and where the success lasted until such time as the patient discovered the truth. Bumke emphasizes the tremendous complication of psychic situation pictures. He claims the same to hold true for hypnosis. Some of the patients are refractory, others use hypnosis to protect the line of retreat, while still others are so over-joyed at the cure that we hardly have the right to assume that a "wish idea" existed. Bumke's experience led him to the conclusion that no pension be granted or that the possibility of the patient's being able to work denied. All physicians should definitely oppose all sham operations and other treatments suggested, because the personnel must be properly educated first of all not to employ either compulsion, punishment or deception. Kraus (14) seems to have missed the whole nature of neurosis, in which the symptom is of course only a means, if he claims that neurasthenia is not the sole concern of neurology. His argument is apparently based upon the fact that he regards constitutional causes and organ inferiority as necessitating neurosis but not as bringing one to it.

Mohr (15) finds the essence of depressions to consist in a conflict of the feeling of duty with the desire to evade unpleasantness as found developed among many conscientious and scrupulous people. (We might if we so desired say something about " unsocial conscientiousness "). A cure can only be secured through psychical influences. The following conditions are necessary to the treatment: small nursing homes for about twenty to thirty patients and one physician; separation from home; exclusion of other treatments and the application of psycho-therapy leading the patients to dominate their symptoms. Weichbrodt (16) points out the fact that the disease often makes its appearance long after the trauma. Occasionally it arises through reappearance of the trauma or, in the case of soldiers who have not yet been at the front, at the prospect of such a reawakening. With regard to the question before the soldier, namely, shall he go home or be sent to the rear? the author refuses to give a direct answer. He thinks that the Rothmann method merely fixes the patient's thoughts upon his disease. Narcosis he suggests might also be abandoned. The Kaufmann method he would retain. In the use of hypnosis he regards the authority of Nonne as of the greatest importance. Nonne's method consisted of a bath of twenty-four hours' duration that might at times be extended to forty hours. An intensification of its effect occurs if the bath takes place *in a closed and noisy place.* The success does not extend to hysteria, but only affects the neurotic disturbances. Permission to go out or the granting of a furlough is to be denied. Few of the patients invalided in this fashion can be used for war service but they are all capable of following their own occupations. He is not in favour of pensions. The treatment is not suitable for officers. Alt (17) only believes in "hinterlands neurosis." According to his view 75 per cent. of his patients can be used for barrack duties. Quensel (18) regards the war neurosis as a combination of a real disease and a reaction against circumstances. Jolly (19) regards 1 to 3 per cent. of the war neurotics as capable of field duty and lays particular stress upon the therapeutic value of work. Hypnosis did not appear to be of great value but he praises the electro-psychic treatment. He recommends weak applications of currents supplemented by exercise. "What is to be taken into consideration is not how the men receive their discharge but what happens to them afterwards." His inquiries showed the following results: of 41 hysterical patients 30 were unfit; 3 in active service, 5 B 1 and 3 C 3. Of 23 neurasthenics, 1 was in active service, 15 B 1 ; 3 C 3 and 4 unfit. Of 14 cases suffering from slight disturbances, 5 were in active service and 9 g.d.f. In one third of the hysterical cases the intelligence of the patients ranged from slight feeble-mindedness to imbecility. This author makes an exceedingly important remark without following it up. He found a very large number of *unskilled workers* among his examples. The enormous amount of data gathered by the Cracow Nervenzentrale gives the same result. A fact of considerable significance can be gleaned from this Cracow material ; for example, clear-cut and easily discernible instances of war neurosis are relatively rare among officers. This seems to indicate *that only wavering natures and those exhibiting timidity when faced by their social obligations, become afflicted with neurosis.* Kehrer (20) definitely gives up all hope of being able to restore any perceptible number of war neurotics to active military service, but urges practitioners to do their best to turn them into people who might be useful workers behind the front. His method is based on the idea of *aggravating the patient's condition* in every way including therein the restriction of nourishment, milk diet and "forcible or compulsory exercise." He criticizes the misuse of the faradic current by non-medical practitioners and expresses his disappointment with a psycho-therapeutic that tries to explain the symptoms without however further entering into the question. He also lays great stress upon the atmosphere being of such a kind that everyone would be willing to say that he would not leave unless cured. He wants to place the military authorities in control.

Sauer (21) together with Frank accepts the early view of Breuer-Freud according to which the neurosis is a kind of compressed affect. He rejects Freud's later view of the sexual origin of war neurosis. He attempts to diminish the "tension of the affect" by having the affect revive in the hypnosis. He mentioned cures that were subsequently corroborated by letters received from the field. Wexberg years ago justifiably insisted in regard to these and similar theories, that anyone who is changed by an experience or trauma does not become ill on account of it but is already ill. We must further take into consideration the fact that little is learnt of the patient's nature by this treatment, so that it might be

contended that it is not dictated by any knowledge of
the causes and that any aggravation of the situation is
due to an unscientific method. It is quite natural to
assume that the patient discloses more about his psychic
life and goal in these therapeutic treatments than the
physician notices and that while in this position he is
in reality beginning to abandon his symptoms. That
does not mean that the practical utility of the method
is thereby denied. The fact should also be mentioned
that this writer prefers hospitals to be situated in the
patient's native place. Jalowicz (22) emphasizes the
rarity with which neuroses arise on the field of battle.
Of twenty-five cases he found only two where the
individuals had not been under treatment before. He
calls attention to the existence of a "battle tonus"
in the front ranks hostile to the development of a
neurosis and shows the misuse of the traumatic "shock
due to entombment." He insists that he never found a
neurosis following a real "entombment." He also
insists as against Oppenheim on the possibility of a
transition from simulation to true neurosis, and warns
against sending the man home too quickly. However
his opposition to Oppenheim is only an apparent one
for Jalowicz like the former is not really thinking of the
origin of the neurosis in those cases which begin as
simulations but of the neurotic symptoms themselves.
The "symptom susceptibility" does in truth require
for its full development *a number of preparations* and
arrangements of which some, as practice during peace
time shows, fall into the category of simulations and
aggravations. These latter occur in the "latent period"
and can be best studied and predicted in dreams.

Sommer (23) cured functional deafness among soldiers
by an experimental psychological method. While the
patient is sitting in front of an apparatus for the analysis
of finger movements a bell is suddenly sounded behind
him. A movement of the forearm follows proving that
he has heard the tone. Practically all of his cases also
suffered from a physical injury such as rupture of the
ear-drum. Sommer finds the essence of the neurosis to
lie in a "pathological compulsion towards the suppression of reflexes". This can hardly be taken to be
more than a round-about manner of describing the facts.
Nissl v. Meyendorf in his discussion of the above claims

that in these cases of deaf soldiers the probability is that they could really hear. The therapeutic effect of Sommer's method is perhaps to be regarded as similar to that obtained by dismissing new cases after thorough examination with the statement that "no such disease exists." Imhofer (24) points out the difficulty of unmasking individuals who are simulating deafness and that a great deal of time, continuous observation and, in some instances, a particularly ingenious physician, are needed. The whole organic make-up and previous history of the patient is important. The anæsthesia of the ear-drum is unimportant. The results obtained from the organ in a static condition are however significant. The psychology of people actually deaf is also to be used. Idiocy is also to be reckoned with.

Erich Stern (25) finds the pathogenesis of psychoneurosis to consist "in a lability of the psycho-neurotic individual factors out of which there then develops a labile equilibrium of the entire psyche."

Struempel (26) distinguishes between two groups of functional nerve diseases; first those diseases that have nothing at all to do with consciousness and second those that are connected with a changed condition of consciousness. Among the first he includes epilepsy, chorea, eclampsia, myasthenia, tetany, real neuralgia and migraine. These he calls somatic functional neuroses. He finds it difficult to place tick, tremour, myoclonia and vasomotor secretory traumatic neuroses. Manifestations connected with the loss of functions such as degenerative reactions, reflex rigidity of the pupils, absence of reflexes and their pathological intensification with increased reflexogenous zones, all suggest the above being really organic diseases. In favour however of their being psychogenic in origin are the irritability symptoms, the characteristic anaesthesia and hemi-anaesthesia and the possibility of evoking attacks by suggestion. It is possible that this division is too finely drawn in some respects, for example, in the importance assigned to reflex intensification and the extension of the reflexogenous zone, a condition which is frequently found in psychogenic war neuroses especially where an *unconsciously acquired spasm* is noticed. This fact has been remarked by practically every observer.

Rothe (27) recommends the practice of stoicism as a method of combating stuttering. Considering the frequent failure of most treatments this is indeed an interesting view. Rothe quite rightly attempts to obtain a psychic transformation of the whole man in the conviction that "stuttering for the stoic is a test imposed by fate and the man must then prove himself worthy by developing calmness," for otherwise the basis of the evil remains unknown and if, at best, it does disappear this takes place without the physician getting any knowledge of it.

Stertz (28) lays stress on the normal affect-radiations and their hysterical symptoms. The former are to be regarded as physical and not psychical. The hysterical types of reaction are independent of the synchronous organic changes and are the outgrowth of a definite kind of predisposition. Like Charcot and Breuer, he finds another cause for the outbreak of the disease in the "hypnoidal condition". The tendency toward "fixation" is perhaps a general principle of psycho-pathological predisposition. Hysterical complexes may exist without desires, wish concepts, expectations and fears. If however these do exist, as in the case of pension- and war-hysteria, they constitute a never-failing source of energy for the feeding of the disease. The apparent objection as to whether "lability" of the symptoms and their fixation represent a general pre-disposition and when the one or the other is operative Stertz does not consider at all. Nor does he mention the means by which he has succeeded in excluding the definitely-given goal of hysterics. On the other hand his conception of the pension- and war-hysteria approxi-mates to that of the "actual position". Zangger (29) argues from the view-point of a person who believes in neuroses being cured by improving the character of the patient and by a sharpening of his intellect. Dubois (30) rightly, although without any weighty reasons, attacks the concept of "conversion" of the Freudian School. He feels "all observable nervous disturbances to be ordinary emotional physiological manifestations of an emotional situation differing from the normal only in their intensity and fixation". This is correct to the extent that we never actually perceive hyper-physio-logical manifestations. The concept of "conversion" presupposes, even in its most minimal significance, the conservation of psychic energy and owes its existence to the fact that the physician designates every reaction deviating from his own as a conversion. Overlooking the existence of individual and utilitarian reactions Schuster (31) comes to the conclusion that in cases where the function is pathologically changed either permanently or transiently, the anatomical substratum has in some fashion deviated from the normal.

Nonne (32) in his suggestion method is only concerned with freeing the patient of his symptoms. His method is applicable to officers also. The capacity for revision is great. He rarely is able to restore his patient to full capacity for field service. The main value of his treatment consists in its success in obtaining an a.v. and obviating the necessity of granting pensions. In 42 new cases 26 were able to do full work, 16 were still suffering but could perform light duties and 2 had relapses. The original Kaufmann method has here been transformed into a *persuasion method* helped along by faradic stimulation.

Strasser (33):—"Every thing that can creatively develop from the imaginative faculty of man can be utilized in the symptom complex of a functional emotional or neurotic disease. Every psychic activity is to be understood as in the main an anticipatory preparation for the future. *The final orientation* of the psychic event which people like to ascribe only to the 'pension hysteria', can be shown to exist in every neurosis. The belief that something has been created can express itself functionally in exactly the same manner as the creation itself. 'Trauma' has the ability to push aside personal responsibility. Numerous tracts lead from the healthy condition to that of neurotic disease and practically every individual preserves in some form, either a memento or some *protective mechanism* of this development. From the individual-psychological viewpoint we must recognize behind every neurosis the existence of a weakling whose incapacity for adapting himself to the ideas of the majority calls forth an *aggressive attitude* taking on a neurotic form. The proper therapy must solve the fundamental conflict between the duty to the community and to the individual."

War neurosis has accelerated the discussion of the

U

fundamental questions in the psychology of neuroses. The further study of the data and the numerous writings on the subject will probably lead to integrated viewpoints approximating to ours.

LITERATURE

1. SCHANZ, *M. m. W.*, 1916, H. 12.
2. BLENCKE, *Ibid.*, H. 32.
3. LIEBERMEISTER, *Ueber die Behandlung von Kriegsneurosen* (Halle 1917).
4. ADLER, *Lecture delivered before the meeting of Army Physicians at Cracow*, Nov. 1916.
5. LEWANDOWSKY, *M. m. W.*, 1913, H. 30 : *Feldärztliche Beilage.*
6. MEYER, *Ther. Mh.*, June 1917.
7. RAETHER, *Arch. f. Psych.*, 1917, vol. 57.
8. L. MANN, *D. m. W.*, 1917, No. 29.
9. NAEGELI, *Unfall- und Begehrungsneurosen* (Stuttgart 1917).
10. TROEMNER, *Aerztlicher Verein in Hamburg*, May 22, 1917.
11. LEUSSER, *M. m. W.*, 1917, n. 23.
12. HEINZE, *Med. Sektion d. Schles. Ges. f. vaterl. Kultur zu Breslau*, March 9, 1917.
13. MINKOWSKI, *Ibid.*
14. KRAUS, *Kriegsärztliche Abende.*
15. MOHR, *M. Kl.*, 1915.
16. WEICHBRODT, *Arch. f. Psych.* vol. 57, H. 2.
17. ALT, *Ibid.*
18. QUENSEL, *Zwanzigster Vers. mittledeutscher Psychiater u. Neurologen in Dresden*, Jan. 6, 1917.
19. JOLLY, *Ibid.*
20. KEHRER, *Zschr. f. d. ges. Neur.* vol. 36 H., 1 and 2.
21. SAUER, *Ibid.*
22. JALOWICZ, *Ibid.*
23. SOMMER, *Zwanzigster Vers. mitteldeutscher Psychiater u. Neurologen in Dresden*, Jan. 6, 1917.
24. IMHOFER, *W. kl. W.*, 1917, no. 23.
25. ERICH STERN, *Sommers Kl. f. psych. u. nerv. Kr.*, 1917, vol. 10, H.1.
26. STRUEMPELL, *M. Kl.*, 1916, vol. 36.
27. ROTHE, *Zschr. f. ges. Neur.* 1917, vol. 36.
28. STERTZ, *Ostdeutscher Verein f. Psychiatrie*, Dec. 1916.
29. ZANGGER, *Neurol. Ges.*, Berne 1916.
30. DUBOIS, *Ibid.*
31. SCHUSTER, *Neurol Zbl.*, 1916, H. 12.
32. NONNE, *Wandervers. d. süddeutschen Neurol. u. Psych. in Baden-Baden*, June 1917.
33. STRASSER, *Schweizer Korr.*, Bl. 1917, no. 9.

XXV

Myelodysplasia (Organ Inferiority)

In my *Studie über Minderwertigkeit von Organen* I was able
to show in connection with the study of the urinary
apparatus that all pathological changes whether functional or morphological are associated with an hereditary
inferiority of the organ and the nerve superstructures.
This inferiority frequently remains latent and the result-
ing deficiency is compensated for in some way. Very
often the inferiority discloses itself at one point of the
organism and dominates the whole picture of the
disease.

I pointed out there that the most definite manifestations were the inheritance of the disease and its
occurrence in families ; childlessness ; signs of degeneration ; and anomalies of the reflexes. In conclusion
starting from one of the signs of inferiority, *enuresis*, I
was able to show that others were connected with it.
In my statistics, consisting at that time of fifty cases
but which since then have been considerably augmented,
I succeeded in proving the unified and exclusive nature
of the symptoms of organ inferiority.

An important part was there shown to be played
by the *segment inferiority* which in cases of enuresis is
expressed in the inherited anomalies of the lower
extremities and in the arrangement of the naevi, neuro-
fibromata and angiomata found in the affected area.

What I was most concerned with was to substitute
for the concept of "disposition", a hypoplastic and
dysplastic predisposition of organs and their nerve
superstructures so as to strengthen our case by a
clinical demonstration of the inferiority symptoms
mentioned above.

Since my work covered the anomalies and the
diseases of the whole organism my conclusions, summed
up in my theory of organ inferiority and which I tried

to prove held for the whole organic system should on account of their fundamental importance, be given a more prominent place. It was possible to show repeatedly that the organ inferiority developed genetically *affecting the whole organ and its nerve superstructure* yet manifesting itself only in certain places. I refer to pages 7, 10, 22, 25, 30, 31, 47, 53, 57, and 61 of my book where I said : "We must insist that the already described synchronous occurrence of multiple organ inferiority extends to individual parts and to the nerve tracts of the central nervous system, that frequently the efficiency of an organ corresponds proportionally to the efficiency given by nature to those particular nerve tracts that are connected with its associated organ, from which it receives stimulation and to which it carries impulses."—Adler, *loc. cit.* Cf. also the appendix, page 75 (On the inferiority of the Urinary Apparatus, the history of individuals afflicted with enuresis, their family-tree etc.) : I said : "I must here confine myself to showing how the focusing of the inferiority manifestations by means of enuresis comes about and to prove by specific cases the synchronous inferiority of the central nervous system and the sexual apparatus." On p. 78 of the same book I state that "an originally inferior psychomotor superstructure is found associated with that organ which inadequately responds to its environment, namely the bladder. . . ." The foregoing quotations as well as the whole aim of my book was to prove that inferiority might manifest itself morphologically and functionally (cf. pages 5-17 of my book) at certain definite places in the organism and its "nervous superstructure."

Alfred Fuchs propounds the following view in his study of *Myelodysplasie* (*Wiener Med. Wochenschr.*, 37, 38, 1919) :—"There is a possibility that the picture shown by a few perhaps even by many diseases which seemed up to the present to imply a functional neurosis will turn out to be due to a neurosis that can be traced back *to a congenital hypoplasia or dysplasia* of the lower sections of the spinal cord." His work which called attention, in the main to interrelations already described by me from the study of which the same conclusions were drawn as those I had reached from an examination of the very extensive body of facts in my possession, induced Fuchs to postulate six groupings of the factors belonging to the symptom-complex of myelodysplasia :

1. Sphincter debility particularly enuresis nocturna in adults.

2. Syndactyly. In discussing it Fuchs mentions some additional symptoms such as congenital pigmentation arranged in mechanical order extending from the sixth dorsal vertebra to the middle of the os sacrum ; hypertrichosis lumbalis and pes planus.

3. Disturbances of sensibility.

4. Defects in the lower portion of the spinal column and the os sacrum ; rudimentary development of a spina bifida occulta and presumably the presence of supernumerary sacral vertebrae and changes in shape of the lower lumbar vertebrae, etc.

5. Anomalies of the reflexes.

6. Deformities of the bone structure of the foot and trophic and vaso-motor disturbances of the toes.

The first symptom I have discussed together with a number of other childhood defects in my previously mentioned book, where a whole section is devoted to them (II. Anamnestic References). There I regarded these defects as *significant indications belonging to inferior organic systems* and came to the conclusion "that hereditary defects of children, their existence in the parents, their brothers and sisters and subsequently their own children, must be looked upon as *suspicious suggestions of inferiority in the organ connected with the particular defect.*" Since Fuchs regards as of equal value both the enuresis of *adults* and of children I am saved the trouble of proving the similarity of our views on this point. That my conclusions go further need not be considered. But as an example take my suggestion that other parts of the system and not merely the associated nerve tracts may be the indication and the result of inferiority. In a study of nephrolithiasis (*Wiener Klinische Wochenscrift,* no. 49, XX.) I was able to show its connection with enuresis and thus justify that statement in my book where I claimed that a large proportion of the diseases of the urinary apparatus were connected with an hereditary inferiority of the organism which then expressed itself in the form of enuresis. Other signs of inferiority are also present such as *anomalies of the lumbar vertebrae* subsequently proved by *Jehle* and other scientists to hold for "lordotic albuminuria", a disease in which anamnesitic enuresis always plays an important part. My suggested connection of enuresis and other indications of inferiority of the same type with tabes, I was subsequently able to confirm in other cases. I had previously pointed out the similar observations made by H. Schlesinger (a combination of nephrolithiasis with syringomyelia and tabes) and by Israel (dystopia of the kidneys, and hydrocephalus).

The question that I would now like to ask is whether *myelodysplasia* really constitutes "*an etiological element of importance*," as Fuchs believes and whether enuresis can actually be traced back "*in all probability to a congenital hypoplasia or dysplasia* of the lower sections of the spinal cord"; or whether on the other hand as I first emphasized it cannot be shown to belong to a *defective embryonic functioning of a urinary apparatus and nerve superstructure inferior as a whole.* As this question contains the only *fundamental deviation* from my views I feel constrained to enter upon it briefly although the main points can be found in my earlier articles. In favour of the independence of the therapeutic effects obtained through psychic influences is to be mentioned [1] first the actual success obtained by its employment, a fact that Fuchs also mentions. Equally corroborative is the fact that despite marked uniformity the course of the disease is variable that very often transitions occur into pollakiuria, dysuria, a greater retentive capacity caused by *over-compensation* (cf. my *Studie*), and finally anomalies in the bladder-discharge. The appearance of all these manifestations, one following the other, are due to psychic causes. For the facts to fit into Fuchs' theory it would be necessary to regard the clear-cut picture presented by an illness as common as enuresis as due to some anomaly of the spinal marrow which would always produce the same effect, an assumption disproven by the one circumstance that enuresis is not even invariably found in hydromyelia. That it could be invariably caused by the manifold and abortive anomalies that I and Fuchs subsequently assumed, is consequently an unwarranted hypothesis. More

---

[1] Paul Federn was able to observe, in a large number of cases, how enuresis was arrested by a change of environment.

justifiable is the view flowing from the doctrine of inferiority according to which enuresis indicates a functional arrest at an early stage of development and an inferiority of the organic system. Other morphological signs of inferiority both in the organ itself and in the afferent and efferent nerve tracts and the central nervous superstructure may likewise be found to be associated with it.

Every one of these additional anomalies *can, under suitable conditions, themselves become active causes* and create symptoms but cannot call into existence *an enuretic complex.* " *The organic nerve diseases* are however according to our premises only special instances where a localized inferiority has led to inflammatory or degenerative changes." (Cf. *Studie*, p. 69.)

With regard to the second point *syndactylism* I, like Fuchs, see in it only the bringing into prominence of one of the many peripheral *degenerative signs* from which the inferiority of the lower extremities is to be inferred. Its connection with the inferiority of the urinary system (as well as with the sexual and excretory systems), I have stressed in my *Studie*, etc., where I explained it as due to the participation of adjacent segments. In chapter three of my *Studie* I took the attitude that the peripheral degenerative stigmata like the defects of children, indicate inferiority of the organ and the superstructure with which it is connected. "If any trace of this embryonic arrest (in the organic system) extends to the body extremities and is there detected by the scientist, it takes the form of well-known degenerative stigmata." It is Fuchs' merit to have discovered what according to him is one of the most frequent signs of degeneration. Though we are justified in speaking in this case of a co-ordination as I mentioned in connection with Fuchs' first point, we have no right nevertheless to speak of "coincidence" as Fuchs does in his summary or to regard syndactylism as a "symptom" of myelodysplasia. If however it really is coincidence then Fuchs' view that degenerative indications and stigmata are to be interpreted as peripheral signs of inferiority of the organ to which these signs belong is in accord with my own, the latter being then indeed strengthened by this discovery of the rôle of syndactylism.

The appearance of degenerative signs in the lower extremities together with enuresis, I myself pointed out and I shall return to the subject briefly again.

In my *Studie* a prominent position is assigned to a view emphasizing the *importance of the naevus* and other anomalies of the blood vessels as signs of inferiority of *the organs connected with them segmentally* (cf. p. 40 of my *Studie*).

According to this *naevus theory*, a number of external stigmata such as naevi, angiomata, teleangiectasies and neurofibromata exhibit "connections" with the segments of the respective internal organs so that their presence indicates an inferiority of the segment ("a segmental deficiency"). This is not to be taken in Fuchs' sense as signifying that the naevus is dependent upon anomalies of the spinal marrow but as indicating a peripheral co-ordinated inferiority symptom.

That these stigmata are frequently found within the area of inferior or diseased organs, occasionally longitudinally displaced, I was able to observe in a considerable number of cases. I was also able to confirm my belief that these connections hold true in the case of inferiority of the urinary apparatus. Following me Robert Frank[1] called attention to the signs of *pulmonary tuberculosis* found in these cases but interpreted them differently. Josef Uhrbach[2] mentions the "naevus theory" in his study of tabic bone and articulation diseases and accepting my interpretation, infers the existence of a predisposition to tabic arthropathia due to the presence of inferiority signs (naevi on the back and the belly, genua vara and vein ectasia). Sigmund Steiner has been re-examining my conclusions on the basis of his very extensive material and has corroborated my statement that for the majority of the anomalies of the spinal column a naevus can be shown to exist, a fact that certainly speaks in favour of an inherited inferiority of the spinal column in cases of curvature.

In my book I also recognized and mentioned other signs of inferiority of the enuretic complex such as *anomalies of the spinal column, pes planus, lordosis hypertrichosis and suggestions of spina bifida.* The frequency of the enlarged hiatus sacralis and its demonstration by

[1] *Münchener Med. Wochenschrift*, 1908.
[2] *Wiener Klin. Rundschau*, nos. 31 and 32, 1919.

Roentgen rays I regard as a valuable contribution to our knowledge of inferiority signs. In this case neither can the coincidence be denied nor the independence be rejected. It would be just as correct to call myelodysplasia a symptom of the naevus as the reverse.

I have barely touched on the third point, *the disturbances of sensibility* in organ inferiority. A reference was made to the connection with the zones of Head and an attempt made to connect meralgia paraesthetica with the inferiority of the urinary apparatus (Pals' earlier discovery of the coincidence of the meralgia paraesthetica made it possible for us to draw this disease definitely into our discussion). This is all the information that I can at present furnish on this point. The description of a "feeling of dullness" in the lower extremities, a condition that according to Fuchs is to be brought into close relation with the enuretic complex certainly constitutes a notable extension to our knowledge in this thorny field. To interpret this as an "*organic spinal symptom*" merely reflects the author's stand-point. This dullness may just as well be an expression of cerebral as of peripheral inferiority and represents either a qualitative, or on the analogy of bone and skin anomalies, a morphological variety. The results obtained from such sensibility tests will always depend as much upon the training of the brain and the course of the childhood defect as upon enuresis. The final decision always rests upon the compensation made by the brain, and it is always justifiable to assume that brain inferiority is at the basis of all inferiority manifestations and consequently of any co-ordinated enuresis. In the discussion of the inferiority of the sense organs given in my book I showed that the inferiority symptoms are disclosed in the absence of partial perceptions, by "dissociated sensation stoppages" as well as often by an intensified capacity for perception. The latter is to be interpreted as a compensation tendency from which occasionally hyper-compensation arises and at times artistic abilities take their origin.[1] These explanations render any direct dependence upon myelodysplasia of

---

[1] Colour-blind individuals may be taken as examples, for some of them, "the Daltonists," are prominent painters. This perceptive symptom, colour-blindness, is based upon peripheral inferiority. Similar *peripheral stigmata* can be shown to exist in the other sense organs.

even the sensibility disturbances doubtful for the majority of cases and justify the attempt to include this "symptom" as co-ordinate with the others. It should be placed on a level with toxic, neurotic and the extensive hyper-aesthesia symptoms found in moral insanity.

Point 4 *the persistence of an opening in the canalis sacralis* etc.—I called them suggestions of spina bifida in my *Studie*—really represent the cardinal point of Fuchs' presentations. According to my theory they fall in the category of signs of segmental inferiority and retain their individual justification and are independent of the inferiority of the spinal marrow. Anomalies and personal carriage associated with the lumbar vertebrae are frequently met with and are, at times, found connected with diseases of the kidneys such as nephrolithiasis. We would have to go as far back as Gall in the history of medicine if we wished to be really fair in the question of the origin of the concept of the coincidence of the frame-work of the spinal column with the efficiency of the spinal marrow. Fuchs' observation about the frequency of hiatus anomalies thus constitutes an increase in the number of inferiority signs even if not in his sense.

With regard to the fifth point let me refer to the fourth chapter in my *Studie* (*Reflex Anomalies as Indications of Inferiority*), where I came to the conclusion (page 44) that the absence of certain manifestations in the case of an inferior system of organs, represents "motor insufficiency, deficient production of the respective gland secretions and *above all a more deficient development or, even an absence, of reflex actions of all kinds. They may however also mean just the opposite,* namely motor hyper-activity, hyper-secretion and *intensification of the reflexes.*"[1] Let me again at this point call attention to the question of a defective reflex mechanism with an inferior organ and childhood defects, such as enuresis, blinking, stuttering, vomiting, etc. Connected with enuresis we find sphincter cramp, "an additional sphincter reflex" (defective reflex) and the not uncommon Freudian adductor phenomenon that represents a partial myotonia. The non-appearance of the inherited reflex mechanism is dependent upon the extension of the peripheral tracts, those of the spinal marrow and of

---

[1] This passage is not italicized in the text.

the brain. Toxic influences (of the thyroid gland and the epithelial cells) as accessories of manifold inferiority can no more be summarily dismissed than can the symmetrical or unsymmetrical compensation of the spinal marrow and brain. Morphological changes may consequently be looked upon as originally co-ordinated stigmata capable under certain circumstances of giving rise to "symptoms". Apart from this *an embryonic character* is predominant in the reflex anomalies, as I have tried to show in the case of changes in the palatal reflexes connected with organ inferiority.

With regard to the sixth point, *the inferiority signs in the lower extremities*, in addition to what I have already stated let me mention *disproportionate size of the legs*. The deformities that Fuchs mentions—pes planus, varus valgus, are no more to be brought into relation with the "spinal marrow symptoms" than are the above-mentioned inferiorities.

The remarks made in my *Studie* in connection with the summary of the traits of the enuretic-complex I would like to quote briefly not only to show their identity with Fuchs' conclusion but also to indicate their divergences (p. 76):

"The segmental inferiority found among people afflicted with enuresis must be greatly stressed. I should not so much emphasize the skin anomalies frequently found in the form of naevi or neuro-fibromata above the kidneys, in the bladder area or in the groin, but the inferiority that affects the whole dorsal side of the rump expressing itself as a primary weakness of urine, stool and semen discharge, that frequently can be overcome and hyper-compensated, and clearly is connected with an inferiority of the spinal marrow in the region of the lumbar vertebrae. Frequently the lower extremities are embraced in this inferiority. This question is of importance for tabes, ischias, stool incontinence and in the history of enuretic families. The spinal column participates therein with the suggestion of spina bifida or deformity, the lower extremities by developing deformities such as unequal length of the legs or diseases of the joints."

Incidentally Fuchs disposes of the "neurotic" theory of neurosis. I myself had passed through the same stage before and believed firmly in the organic basis of enuresis and other defects of childhood. My findings however led me further and impelled me to take into consideration likewise *the synchronous inferiority of the brain.* The childhood defects thus were shown to be " signals indicating the as yet unsuccessful conquest of the inferiority of the peripheral nerves and the central nervous system." In pursuance of this thought and following up my discoveries among neurotics I came to the conclusion that "all manifestations of neuroses and psycho-neuroses are to be traced back to organ inferiority, to the degree and the nature of the central compensation that has not yet become successful and to the appearance of compensation disturbances." Thus I came to the conclusion that enuresis was due, in every case, to an inferiority of the organ and its nerve super-structure and that the compensation developing induces in the inferior brain a "condition of high psychic tension out of which there springs the predisposition of neurosis."[1] That these conclusions have met with some acceptance is, among other things, shown in the very readable work of Otto Gross[2] who starting from a more limited view-point and following up the work of *Anton* comes to the conclusion "that in the psychopathic constitution is to be found the direct expression of a disturbance in compensatory regulations, that indeed there may even be a lack of relation between the compensatory appropriation of the whole brain and its capacity to perform compensatory super-activity."

I would like again to emphasize the fact that the neurotic symptoms preferably attack the area of the inferior organ and its psychic super-structure,[3] that they revive childhood defects or are involved in the assumption shared also so far as I can see by the psychoanalytic school. The insistence that enuresis is to be included entirely among neuroses, a view combated by me, is in the main an achievement of the Breslau school. It certainly cannot be claimed that this school "belongs to a certain speculative tendency."[4]

[1] Cf. also Adler, *Die Disposition zur Neurose* in *Heilen und Bilden.*
[2] *Ueber Psychopathische Minderwerthigkeiten* (Braumüller, Vienna).
[3] Cf. Adler, *Der Aggressionstriel im Leben und in der Neurose,* in *Heilen und Bilden.*
[4] Since then a number of scientists, notably J. Zappert (*Wien. Klin. Wochenschr.,* 1920, No. 22), have supported my interpretation against that of Fuchs who disagrees on a few details.

XXVI

Individual-psychological Education

(Lecture delivered before the Zürich Association of Physicians, 1918)

THE tremendous importance of a thorough, complete understanding of educational questions and the necessity for every physician mastering them up to a certain point, is particularly clear when looked at from the standpoint of the nerve-specialist's treatment. We demand justifiably that the doctor in particular, have a knowledge of men, and we know that such a vital question as the relations between physician and patient, always break down if the physician is either lacking in knowledge of men or in methods of education. It was this attitude and interpretation of his rôle that made Virchow say : " Physicians will eventually become the educators of humanity."

A question that has become acute in our day and which is bound to become even more acute in a short time, is that relating to the relative spheres of physician and educator. It is quite essential to reach some unanimity in regard to the whole range of problems involved and to obtain a bird's-eye view of them. Both sides overlap but co-operative work is entirely absent.

If we but ask what purpose education serves, all the main points involved will certainly fall within the domain of the physician. The education of children so that they may become individuals actuated by ethical principles, the utilization of their virtues for the good of the community, are regarded by every physician as the self-evident presupposition of life. It may justifiably be demanded that all his actions, measures and moves be in conformity with this object. The immediate direction of the education will always be in the hands of the educator, of the teachers and parents, but we may assume that they will acquaint themselves with those questions and difficulties that only the physician can really plumb to their depths, because he must unearth them from out the pathological interrelations of the psychic life. I wish in particular to emphasize the fact that it is impossible to cover in a short time a field of such tremendous extent and that until a unified conception can be reached, it is only possible to touch briefly on certain questions whose more extensive discussion will be the concern of the following future generations. Nevertheless it is important to become acquainted with those view-points that individual-psychology insists are of fundamental significance and whose misunderstanding, it is claimed, will be visited upon the children in the course of their development.

What brings the physician into the closest contact with educational questions is the relationship between psychic health and bodily health, although not however, in that general sense so often spoken of, namely a sane mind in a sane body, a rather unwarranted conception. We all have ample opportunity of seeing physically healthy children and adults whose psychic condition is by no means healthy. It is difficult, if not impossible, for a child with a weak constitution to attain to that harmony expected of physically normal children. Let us take the case of a child born with a poor digestive system. From the very first days he will be cared for most carefully and solicitously. Such children will consequently grow up in a markedly affectionate atmosphere; they will find themselves always protected, their actions directed and circumscribed by a large number of commands and prohibitions. The importance of food will be markedly exaggerated so that they will learn to prize and even over-value the question of nourishment and digestion. It is the children with digestive troubles who form the main contingent of those who put difficulties in the way of their education, a fact with which the older physicians were already acquainted. It has been claimed that such children must become nervous. Whether such a definite compulsion exists is doubtful. It is however true that the "inimical" character of life weighs more heavily upon the souls of children who suffer and invests them with an unfriendly *pessimistic attitude* toward the world. Sensible of their deprivation they demand stronger guarantees for their importance, become egotistic and easily lose their contact with their fellowmen, because the discovery of their ego has rendered the discovery of their environment a somewhat antagonistic element.

The child is beset with a tremendous *temptation* by its relation to the environment, its attitude toward school, to the frequently intensified discomforts entailed by the weakness of the stomach and intestinal tracts *to obtain compensatory advantages* that can be derived from proving himself ill. He will, for example, develop an extraordinary tendency to being spoiled ; from earliest childhood accustom himself to having others clear away all difficulties for him ; it will be more difficult for him to become self-reliant and he will invariably *refuse to make increased efforts* in all the dangerous situations of life. His courage and his self-confidence will be shaken almost to their foundations. Such an attitude persists to old age and it is not easy to change a child who for ten, fifteen or twenty years had been a weakling, pampered by everyone, into the courageous man full of initiative, enterprise and self-confidence, demanded by our times.

The harm inflicted upon the community is of course, much greater than the above standpoint lets us see, for we must take into consideration not merely children with stomach and intestinal weaknesses but all those born with inferior organs, those whose sense-organs are deficient and who, in consequence, find the approaches to life rendered more inaccessible. We frequently find such difficulties mentioned in biographies or by patients. In such cases the physician will have to concern himself not merely with the psychic educational question—but will endeavour with all his powers, to apply some remedy or treatment for correcting defects so that the child may, at an early stage, be prevented from falling back upon his weakness. We will do this all the more energetically if we ourselves realize that we are here not dealing with any permanent deficiences or with smaller or greater difficulties, and that the important point to bear in mind is that an original organic weakness, *when subsequently corrected*, may yet

live on in *a permanent feeling of weakness* and make an individual unfit for life.   These conditions become of extraordinary complexity because the children themselves,
to an unusual degree, strive to make some compensations and corrections.   Only a few succeed in making
any good compensations and most of them attempt,
in some fashion or other, to equalize the differences that
exist (between them and healthy children), to make
up for their deficiencies either by having recourse to
cultural methods or by intensifying both their initiative
and their mental powers.

In all these cases we shall find noticeable traits of
character causing disturbances such as, for example,
psychic sensitiveness always leading to a conflict.   We
must remember that we are here dealing with manifestations of daily life which we cannot pass over lightly for
otherwise both body and soul would be injured.

It is difficult to stress adequately enough how great
is the distress and tension reigning in the child's soul.
It is an easy matter to understand the mental habits of
men who have become useless if we suppose that their
uselessness is a persistence of something they have
brought with them from the nursery.   *Disease and the
idea of disease* means much more to the child than we
generally imagine.   Anyone who wishes to survey the
child's psyche from this angle, will soon discover that
to a child these are important experiences, and that
illness in almost all cases appears not as an increase
of difficulties but as their alleviation, that it is even
prized as a means for obtaining tenderness, power and
certain advantages at home or in the school.

There are a large number of children who always
have the idea that they are ill, who always feel weak.
In all these cases where a persistence of the symptoms
cannot be explained by any medical findings, it proves
that *the children are making use of this feeling of illness* in
order to gain prominence, to do justice to their desire
for domination and importance in their own family.
For example, in cases where long after the whooping-
cough has passed, children still adhere laboriously to a
similar cough.   We find that they invariably succeed in
frightening their families by these attacks.   This would,
for instance, be a case where it would be essential for
the physician in his pedagogical capacity to intervene.

On the other hand there are also parents and educators who take the opposite view-point, treating their children with severity, even with brutality, or wish, at least, to give the children the impression of being so severe.

Life is so diverse that it compensates for the errors of the educator. Nevertheless, a man whose childhood has been spent in a loveless atmosphere shows, even in old age, indications of this bringing-up. He will always suspect that people desire to be unkind to him and he will shut himself off from others, lose touch with them. Frequently such people appeal to their loveless childhood, as if that exercised some compelling force. Naturally enough a child does not necessarily develop mistrust because parents have been severe, to be as cold to others as they have been to him, or to distrust his own powers for that reason. It is, however, in such soil that neuroses and psychoses are prone to develop. It is always possible to disclose in such, a child's environment, *some disturbing individual* who, either through lack of understanding or evil intention, poisons the child's soul. Hardly any person except the physician is able in such cases to bring about a change in the environment either by alteration of residence or by explanations.

There are, however, certain complications only discovered through a profound understanding of the individual, which, when grasped, clarify the picture to an extraordinary degree.

There exists, for example, a fundamental difference in the psychic development of the first-born as contrasted with that of the second or last-born child. The individuality of an only child it is also simple to characterize. A family where there are either only boys or girls, either one girl among a number of boys or one boy among a number of girls, expresses itself in a definite psychic manner. It is from such facts and positions that children develop their attitude. Frequently it is possible to pick out the oldest or youngest child by his behaviour. I have always found that the first-born possesses a sort of conservative tendency. He takes the element of power always into consideration, comes to an understanding with it and exhibits a certain amount of sociability. Compare with this, for example, *Fontane's* biography where he states that he would give

x

much if anyone could explain to him why he always had a certain tendency to side with the stronger. I inferred from this and rightly, that he must have been a first-born child who regarded his superiority over his brothers and sisters as his inviolable possession.

The second-born always has before and behind him some one who can do more, of more importance, who generally possesses greater liberty of action and is superior to him. If a second-born child is capable of any development he will unquestionably live in a condition of continuous endeavour to surpass his elder brother. He will work restlessly as if under full steam. In fact, the restless neurotics are, to a preponderating degree, second-born children, the first-born rather unwillingly tolerating rivals.

In the attitude of the type perhaps most prominent found among *last born*, we find something infantile, a reserve and hesitation, as if not trusting oneself to perform praiseworthy acts that others are either seen to do or are assumed as doing. Such people easily infer that the whole question is one of stabilizing a situation originally existing. He is always surrounded by people who can do more, meets only people who are more important than himself. On the other hand, he is as a rule able to attract to himself all the love and tenderness of the environment without giving anything in return. There is no need of his developing his powers for he is automatically forced into the centre of his environment. It is easy enough to understand all the injury this entails to his whole psychic development, for he thus learns *to expect to have everything done for him by others.* A second type of last-born is the "Joseph type." Restlessly pushing forward, they surpass everyone by their initiative (Kunstadt) frequently transcending the normal and become path-finders. Both in the Bible and in fairy-tales, people's knowledge of mankind has generally given to the youngest with the greatest gifts, the possession of magic boots, etc.

The behaviour of an only girl among a number of boys is also important. Here so many tense situations develop that we may assume that an opportunity for abnormal attitudes to develop will arise; I am not speaking here of absolutely final results. It is made clear to the girl at an early age, that her nature is utterly different from that of the boy and that much will remain forbidden to her that is boy's right by nature, which he may claim as his privilege. It is not easy in such a case to have either praise or pampering serve as a substitute. For we are concerned here with emotional values that to the child represent something essential and irreplaceable. The girl is continually bothered, receives orders and instructions at every step. In such children we find a special sensitiveness to criticism, continual attempts to show the strong side, to appear free from all vices ; and at the same time a fear lest her unimportance be discovered. These girls frequently furnish the material for future neurotic diseases.

The same holds true in the case of an only boy among a number of girls. It is just here that the contrast seems even greater. The boy is generally provided with special privileges. In consequence the girls work in unison against their only brother. Such boys often suffer as if at the hands of an extensive conspiracy. Every word he utters is marked by the sisters ; he is never taken seriously ; his good traits are decried, his defects made prominent, and as a result the boy frequently loses his self-control and self-confidence and generally shows but poor progress in life. Then people speak of his indolence and laziness. However this is only an external manifestation which with its consequences is based upon a pathological abnormality of temperament, on a fear of facing life. The important point to remember is that we are dealing with people who have either lost their belief in themselves or are prone to lose it. Such boys will habitually recoil from action, are afraid of being made fun of, even when there is no reason for such an attitude. They soon give up all real work, devote themselves to killing time, and become demoralized. Difficulties of the same order are frequently encountered where an older brother is brought up together with a younger sister.

Another point to be taken up by the physician is the explanation of *sexual questions* to children. No single answer covering all cases can as yet be given because of the differences in various nurseries, of individuals and of the environment in which children grow up. One point should however be remembered, that it is an injustice that is very easily visited upon children, if they are kept in ignorance of their sex rôle longer than necessary.   Strangely enough this happens all too often.   Patients have not infrequently told me that even up to their tenth year they were not quite certain to which sex they belonged.   Throughout their development a feeling manifests itself as if they had not been born like other people as boys or girls and would not develop like them.   This gives these children a tremendous feeling of uncertainty noticeable in all their actions. The same is true of girls.   There are some who up to the eighth, ninth, tenth, twelfth and even fourteenth year grow up with considerable uncertainty as to their sex and who in phantasy always imagined that, in some fashion or other, they might still be transformed into men.   This fact is also supported by certain descriptions in the literature on the subject.

In all these cases the normally certain evolution is interfered with.   The years of childhood are spent in endeavouring to supplement their sex rôle artificially, to develop along masculine lines and to avoid making any decisions that might result in defeat.   An uncertainty of a fundamental character is either clearly shown or to be inferred from the pretentious and exaggerated actions in which they indulge.   Girls adopt a masculine attitude and force themselves preferably to a behaviour that seems to them and their whole environment as characteristic of boys.   They prefer to romp about, not merely in the wild harmless fashion which we gladly concede to children, but in an emphatic manner as if under some constraint, and do it so consistently that it very early impresses even their parents as of a pathological character.   Boys too show themselves as if possessed by some wild turmoil, but, taught by the obstacles they encounter, they generally soon desist and develop an hesitating attitude or turn their attention to girls.   The awakened eroticism then takes on in both sexes unnatural and frequently perverse traits that run parallel to their general attitude.

Let me now speak of certain manifestations that are commonly regarded as acts of defiance.   A large number of signs are assigned to *defiance* that the physician considers indications of illness.   As such are to be reckoned the frequently found form of *refusal to take nourishment* and even those types of rebellion connected with defaecation and micturition. All the pathological symptoms which in more pronounced forms we have found in enuresis, or in an inexplicable or unchangeable kind of constipation, are frequently based upon some deeply-rooted defiance in children, who would like to utilize every opportunity for escaping from the compulsion to which they are subjected, because they feel force, in any form, as an encroachment and humiliation. They derive a feeling of satisfaction from their refusal to adapt themselves easily to the demands of their environment as though this were a measure of their importance. We interpret it as a sign of revolt. It is simple enough to test the matter for we will always find other signs of defiance. The same is true for harmless bad habits like nose-picking, slobbering, and nail-biting. Bad habits clearly indicate a development in a direction antagonistic to the demands of the community. Someone with the rôle of an opponent is never absent. The symptom itself is almost always due to inferior functioning.

It is exceedingly interesting to follow the whole chain that is formed when we take into consideration the various transformations in the nature of a child's *choice of profession*, as, for example, in the case of a small girl passing successively from the rôle of princess, dancer, teacher and finally, somewhat resignedly, to that of the house-wife. We frequently find that the choice of profession in the case of grown-up children, is dictated by the desire to do the opposite of that suggested by the father. Naturally this opposition does not develop openly. The logical faculty is constrained by the pressure exerted by the nature of the final objective. The advantages of one profession will be especially emphasized and the disadvantages connected with another just as markedly underlined. In this way it is possible to argue both for and against every point. This attitude must likewise be definitely taken into consideration. But from another angle the physician is also concerned, both in regard to the advice he hazards about the *profession* as in regard to what he says about *the actual choice of a profession*. He must primarily be guided by his knowledge of the person's physical fitness; yet realize on the other hand, that the psychical factor is just as important and may, in some cases, be more fundamental.

It is, of course, an exceedingly disagreeable task to pursue every individual who has gone wrong or who is afflicted with a neurotic illness or a psychosis, in order to improve or heal him. That would constitute a tremendous waste of energy and it is about time that we seriously turn our attention more definitely to *prophylaxis*. There are already an ample number of secured points of vantage. We have for instance, constantly been trying to work toward the goal by educating both parents and physicians. Better results are, however, imperatively necessary in view of the tremendous increase of neurotic and psychotic phenomena in connection particularly with demoralization. Perhaps the first requirement would be to disseminate the ideas derived from a knowledge of men and the educational ideas obtained through individual-psychology; then to apply them so that all can aid us with their strength and in every possible manner. The psychic anomalies of development which at first seem but minor bad habits afterwards lead to the forms of neurotic disease and crime.

XXVII

The Individual-Psychology of Prostitution

I. *Premises and Standpoint of the Critical Observer*

IN life as in science we continually discover that the discussion of the simplest as well as of the most important questions frequently becomes futile because the selection and arrangement of the definitely emphasized reasons advanced for and against a position are based upon a biased and often untested stand-point. It is then not so much the acumen of an opponent as his differently oriented kind of interest which enables him either to advance criticisms or demolish them, to present data and statistics, to evaluate or to bring forward new points of view. No matter how great be the objectivity we ascribe to ourselves or which we would like to retain, it is the conscious and critical *stress upon the personal attitude* and the evaluation of every pro and con through this personal perspective that first gives us the scientific qualification for examination and discussion, just as it likewise furnishes us with the possibility of a systematic development of our premises. If we do not realize this then the whole spirit of inquiry turns in a circle to such an extent that it believes that that which at first it had merely presupposed represents in reality a conclusion. How all kinds of methods are tendentiously utilized for this purpose has been often enough commented upon in statistics.

In order to clearly delimit our scope of investigation I wish to state that by *prostitutes* I mean *individuals generally of the female sex, who use their sex for the purpose of making a living.* Looked at from the stand-point of man's feeling of kinship, prostitution is an occupation based upon the fact that *instead of insisting upon the manifold and fundamental responsibilities contained in sexual intercourse, it treats it on the analogy of trade as a monetary equivalent.*

From this conception there demonstrably follows a

further inference that society has, at least for some time to come, forced the intercourse of the sexes into definite forms, and brought them into association with certain responsibilities that have been tested and come to be regarded as necessary and useful for its survival. The duration of the marriage tie and courting seem to be forms that will endure. If we point out the freely-accepted compulsion that leads us to form friendships, to found a family and the demand that both personalities in such relations be respected, then we should easily be able to understand how all the consequences following simultaneously upon sexual intercourse should be regarded as self-evident demands of a society that is trying to safeguard its existence by just such methods.

Such an observation is in complete harmony with historical, juristic and sociological examinations. In fact it is, in addition, the only attitude that permits us to understand *the ethical problem* involved in prostitution, the old, hitherto unsolved question, why a society that *tolerates and facilitates this social phenomenon should nevertheless consistently stamp it as a disgrace or even punish it.* From our viewpoint we insist that society has in *prostitution, created a kind of outlet, a special exit and escape from difficulties besetting it; that numerous communities feel themselves condemned to accept this outlet, yet because it seems counter to certain of their goals that are differently oriented, they find it necessary to put it under a moral ban.*

II. *The Public and Prostitution*

As a compromise corresponding to our social structure —in the worst sense of the word, for two mutually antagonistic tendencies of society, condemnation and facilitation give prostitution both its form and contour —we shall find the psychology of public *prostitution* means a mass phenomena to many people as though it were a peculiar phenomenon and the attitude of individual people to the problem will be essentially conditioned by the position they take toward the preliminary one namely, to what extent such people affirm or deny certain consequences that inhere in our existing society. The position that a man takes toward prostitution will give us a better idea of his attitude toward the demands of society, will furnish us with clearer reflection of the degree of his social adjustment than, as a rule, he himself could give in words. For example, the well-fed, self-satisfied bourgeois will, in general, regard the *legitimate marriage tempered by prostitution* as a "self-evident" presupposition in his view of the universe. He who holds conservative views and is intent on maintaining the state of the family and, in particular, he who is aiming at strengthening and increasing the population will logically enough realize the disadvantages of prostitution. On the other hand, where there is a tendency toward breaking the ties of family, prostitution will be regarded, both as to its nature and importance, more sympathetically and possibly even furthered.

These various types of individual are difficult enough to keep apart or to understand and for that reason any bond they may have with society at large disappears if their attitude toward the problems of society is not consciously emphasized. We are, indeed, compelled in all investigations of this type, to determine the position taken by such persons toward the community, quite apart from any personal statements they may make. It is necessary to take their *attitude toward the opposite sex* into consideration to an even more marked degree, for their position toward the problem of prostitution is *directly* dependent upon the former.

So far our examination of the erroneous premises of all observers of prostitution has in the main disclosed three groups of prejudices, each of which when tested by their practical consequences have led to valueless, sterile or damaging attitudes.

The first group includes generally all those writers, observers and laymen who being inimically disposed to the world, in other words, pessimists, have ceased to concern themselves seriously with cultural progress. Corresponding to their attitude toward life, which they have never understood, and an attitude which in truth is expressed in their emotional carriage, they but see in prostitution another proof of the rottenness of existing things and they will mainly stress in what has been called the "necessary evil", the evil aspects of the question, insisting upon the inherited deficiencies of human nature, and they will stress in a hostile manner the uselessness of all human endeavour. Sometimes the sterility of this superstitious conception is replaced by a violent condemnation masquerading in the form of an ethical, moral or religious criticism.   But if we draw attention to the view we advanced before, that the position taken toward prostitution is dependent—*and based*—upon our solution of the antecedent question namely, the attitude toward society, then we shall find that all the paths expressed only serve a previously biased view-point and that all the moralizing in the world has not been able to do away with prostitution. Even force has not been able to do it.   We shall, however, be able to understand the reason for the uselessness of all the protesting tendencies as soon as we realize that human society needs *just this form of prostitution* and creates it from within itself and that certain elements exert a facilitating influence and others either obstruct or condemn.   The legal measures hitherto taken and the average morality of society correspond nicely to this policy of compromise.

However objectively we may view the nature of prostitution we shall always find that it can only have its roots in human circumstances which see no contradiction in the fact that *a woman is considered a means of gratifying sexual lust, or becomes a mere plaything and toy of man.*   In other words prostitution is only possible in a civilization whose goal is roughly that of giving gratification to men.   It is quite intelligible therefore why the feminists and suffragists regard prostitution as an indignity to woman, and attack it.   An unconscious presupposition inheres in the view-point, the view-point to which we take a sympathetic attitude and which we discussed above, namely, the purpose of revolting against and destroying the existing order of society with its masculine privileges.

Because of the indissoluble connection of two problems—prostitution and sexual disease—we must expect that those interested in public hygiene, in the lower classes, in nationalism, will make determined attacks upon the continuation of prostitution.   Such strivings are particularly noticeable in the case of small threatened nations, who are still expending tremendous energy towards increasing their population which has come to be regarded as a guarantee of their continued existence.   If we examine the relation of individuals in such a group to the existing circumstances, we shall unearth among them too, although to a lesser degree, corroborating tendencies of a striving towards a radical transformation of social life.

If one ask what may the history of that culture be which expresses itself as thoroughly satisfied with prostitution, we shall find the answer among those circles who hold the present condition of civilization to be useful and unchangeable. This is the circle composed of that large compact stratum that has rather romantically been called the Philistines. Since they form the larger part of the inhabitants of the city and country, their view-point becomes that of the authorities and governing bodies, who consequently deal with prostitution as if it were an unchangeable institution and only half-heartedly engage in the battle against venereal diseases. To this group also belong a large number of physicians and fathers who in the hope of sparing their children more intense emotions, and possessed of a kind of sexual fetishistic conviction of the necessity of youth indulging in habitual sexual intercourse, incite them to visit prostitutes.

But these supporters likewise show their contempt for prostitution. Indeed they go so far as to regard inhuman treatment of the prostitute's person as constituting a recommendation for sexual intercourse. They thus reflect most faithfully the psychology of a civilization not able to understand that this degrading prostitution supplements its purpose of putting difficulties in the way of the propagation of society.

Nevertheless there always exist a number of people whose psychic make-up calls for prostitution. We can disregard the above-mentioned physicians and those parents who think they are sparing their children greater conflicts in directing them to proceed *along the line of least resistance*. Just as barren do the attempts of those people appear to us, who, barely passed their boyhood, desire to attest the right of their tumultuous youth to frequent prostitutes. However in their psychic make-up we already discern elements more clearly found in *three distinct groups of men*, all of whom are in such intimate contact with prostitution that we shall only then be able to understand the psychological problem involved in it, when we have grasped the individual-psychology of these individuals.

III. *The Groups included in Prostitution*

The three categories of individuals we now wish to discuss are the following:

1. *Those in need of prostitutes.*—To this group belong that very large mass of people of a definite nervous type that I have described in detail in my work, *The Neurotic Constitution*, and also in the *Homo-sexual Problem* (cf. *Urologic and Cutaneous Review, technical suppl.* St Louis, 1914). I shall now give a schematic description.

The external attitude of these individuals is frequently quite similar. Among them are found individuals given to outbursts of rage and with a tendency to tyrannical lust of power, men, who, to a certain degree, exhibit great impatience and hyper-sensibility in making proper adjustments to society. They are also characterized by a noticeable kind of precaution; they generally select safe professions and are conspicuous for their boundless distrust and the fact that they really never can become friendly with any one. Their pathological condition and envy are quite marked. At times they feel themselves impelled to accept public offices, generally fulfilling their tasks by having frequent recourse to deception, intrigue and policies redounding to their personal prestige. Occasionally by mistake they succeed in founding a family. They generally treat their wives and children with the most inconsiderate severity, are continually bickering, always dissatisfied and finally find their way back to the prostitute. They may, on the other hand, treat their wives as prostitutes. *They either evade every difficulty or try to circumvent it by guile.* Their whole object and purpose in life seems to be the gaining of cheap triumphs and a willingness to be guided by a number of principles which always have as their purpose putting someone else in the wrong. Forever complaining and forever passing judgment upon others, their type approximates to the one we first described. Their rejection of society however and even of prostitution is more consistent than that of the first type. Their dissatisfaction extends to women in general whom they regard as a lower type of human being. To them as to the strict anti-feminists *woman becomes a means to an end.* They make use of her just there where, because of her inability to resist, they feel that *the superstition of masculine superiority* can best be demonstrated. It is this type of man who feels the need of the prostitute and maintains her. Among such individuals we find very prominent the conviction of the supremacy of the sexual instinct in human psychic life, although this is frequently disguised in rather bizarre or scientific dress. In reality the true although unrecognised motive for his view of life, the underlying supposition of his thoughts and actions, his masculine paroxysms, all merely slink around the really great difficulties of life in order to gain easy triumphs over persons either inherently powerless or made so. Closely related to this type are certain vice-crusaders who, through *fear of women*, erect difficult, often unfulfillable conditions for sexual intercourse, side-stepping at the same time all the real difficulties. Belonging to the group of unmistakable supporters of prostitution will be found children of good families often described rather superficially as " morally insane " and incurable, but who, according to our experience, really fall into the group mentioned above, *i.e.* into the group who, on account of a latent sensitive pride, evade the demands of life because of their own uncertainty, prefer to accept a moral condemnation to the chance of incurring possible defeat in the pursuit of honest tasks. How essentially related these people are to the public prostitutes toward whom they feel themselves impelled, will become more apparent later on. This same attraction for the prostitute is noticeable among people who fall easy victims to alcohol for they, like this whole group we have been discussing, desire to make easy compromises with life, gladly discover excuses for their non-fulfilment of duty and become expert in the art of pushing aside all serious responsibilities. People with criminal inclinations often show the same inclination for prostitution. *Criminal tendencies we shall find are at the bottom of their preference for evading the more difficult attempts that a solution of the important problems of life would involve and meeting them in their own way, which is to transgress the laws of society.* A peculiarly intimate connection exists between certain forms of neurosis and psychosis and prostitution. We may point out in addition that these individuals, as can be seen from their disease, possess *a feeling of inferiority, deficient self-confidence, a pathological desire to succeed, a tendency toward irresponsibility and a preference for psychic artifices and practices flattering to their self-esteem,* just as is the conquest of a woman although they pay for her. Psychically related to them are those individuals who seek wives of low culture or even prostitutes in order thus to still their fear of women and permanently satisfy a lust for domination.

Unquestionably included in the stream of visitors to houses of prostitution, others beyond these sharply defined types are found. We should remember that occasional and transcient attitudes may bring people of a different type into relations where an intensified inferiority feeling might then snatch at a quick, easy gratification. In the same way a girl who is not really adapted for this rôle may find her way into the ranks of prostitutes. The endeavour to make other social connections shows itself quite clearly in these cases. However, not these but the really large inexhaustible number of those who need prostitutes form the pillars of prostitution from its institutional side.

2. *Brothel Keepers.*—People will probably agree with us if we recognize as the basic psychic trait of brothel-keepers, the fact that these individuals prove the connection of prostitution with mass manifestations, for they possess *a deficient social feeling, an inclination to obtain easy successes, the idea of using woman as a means to an end and a tendency toward effortless gratification of their will to power.* The tremendous aid prostitution receives from this type of individual cannot be sufficiently estimated. The brothel-keeper has the function of a peace-maker and he or the pimp conduct the potential prostitute along the road of public prostitution, develop her secret inclinations and kill the last bit of feeling of responsibility in a girl who, if left to herself, might still waver and hesitate. The psychic relationship with the type who require prostitutes is quite clear. The personal strivings are all directed toward occupations demanding no work and the distance separating them from the criminal type is generally small. The tendency toward alcoholism and brutality represent paroxysms to be expected in individuals sensitive in regard to their feeling of weakness and are consequently to be regarded as compensatory acts of an ungratified desire for prestige. The attitude taken by the brothel-keeper towards society

certainly contains something in the nature of a critical, belligerent and revolutionary suggestion, and the insistence upon his important rôle as saviour and protector of the prostitute is an eloquent testimony to his desire to play the great man. Punishments inflicted by the court he bears as does a duellist his wounds, and he feels himself repaid and consoled by the increased respect and admiration he then receives from his own circle. He has thus gained and constructed for himself a fictive, subjective world far removed from a harsh reality and a world that will do justice to his pathological desire for importance. I hope we shall not be misunderstood if we emphasize his relationship with the "neurotic character." In conclusion, such an investigation casts a clear light upon the psychic constitution of those who, when placed before life's difficulties, seek an escape by turning their wives over to others as the price of their own promotion.

3. *The Prostitute.* — The ordinary views about the motives that lead to prostitution contain little psychological data of a helpful kind. The feeling that penury and misery are the decisive factors is untenable. For above all such an assumption tells us nothing about the manner of *selection* of those poor girls who *are liable* to fall victims to prostitution. Or will it be contended that this is merely dependent upon a lesser or greater degree of privation? If so I think we should certainly be under-estimating—I shall not speak of morals or character—the disinclination felt for that social humiliation *commonly* connected with the idea of prostitute. What is probably behind this erroneous analysis are those sad instances where, not infrequently, a girl under the pressure of worry and poverty sells her chastity temporarily or permanently, to the first one she meets, either without taking her inclinations into consideration at all or indeed often definitely in opposition to them. The difference between such girls and real prostitutes lies in *the continuous and industrious preoccupation of the latter with their profession* which goes so far that prostitutes who have become wealthy, continue to practise their occupation with the assiduity of trades people. What is it that binds these people with such firm shackles to their profession? *Is it not the same satisfaction that a business man obtains from performing his work?* Is it not

the *same need of prestige, the same " expansion tendency "* met with among all people, but particularly marked among those we are accustomed to call " neurotic characters "? In the preceding section we described the frantic attempts of some people either to visit prostitutes or become brothel-keepers, and were able to show that these *deceptive enthusiasms* represented evasions and borrowed illusions of power.   These unsocial manifestations reflect fear of the normal demands of society, which are consistently rejected, a deficient self-confidence in one's own ability to fulfil the expectations of society and finally an artifice for obtaining unobtrusively a subjective feeling of heightened personality by means of the sexual relationship.   That this self-enrichment is based upon a *heightened illusion of a perfect masculinity* has been already suggested. What if it were possible to find the same psychic motives in the make-up of the prostitute?   What if it is just these facts that render a girl amenable to prostitution and direct her to the path?

Before entering upon a discussion of the questions and the answers that have been advanced, let me mention another widely disseminated theory as to the psychic constitution of the prostitute and show its untenability.   It is, of course, pardonable if ignorant laymen who wish to remain true to their social obligations, picture the prostitute whose trade they condemn, as an abyss of lust, a permanently passion-inflamed individual.   Scientists, however, who come to such a conclusion can have done so only through carelessness or blindness.   But since this conception is frequently found in scientific monographs often interlarded *with Lombroso's impossible findings about the inherited nature of prostitution*, we must point out that the prostitute is utterly devoid of passion when plying her trade. Naturally this does not hold when she is indulging in a real love affair, in her relations with the brothel-keeper or in any homo-sexual relationship into which she may enter as she frequently does.   It may be said that it is only in this last type of relationship that her sexuality expresses itself, frequently enough in a perverted form sufficiently indicative of the prostitute's disinclination for her *feminine rôle*.   In her profession she plays the rôle of a woman only for an easily duped partner, for she herself is far removed from it, is simply a vender of her body and remains frigid. Thus while the man in need of the prostitute believes that he has demonstrated his superiority over woman, she is aware merely of her power of business attraction, the nature of her demand and *her monetary value,* and so degrades the man to the rôle of her means of subsistence. Both of them, consequently, come by means of a fiction to the illusory feeling of personal predominance.

By recognizing this we shall come considerably nearer to the cardinal point in the questions put above. The bold scheme of converting sexual intercourse into a monetary equivalent is as characteristic of prostitution as of the two groups described above. As in the case of men engaged in prostitution, this fiction of an achieved triumph, of an ever renewed importance, constitutes the reason for the permanence and unchangeability of the institution, just as it represents the principal incentive for all those concerned in it.

However, the ability to transmute a woman's body and soul—one of her inalienable functions—into money can only be possessed by an individual in whose psychic life *the presupposition of woman's inferiority* is firmly rooted. This is shown in the forms of social intercourse used and in the evolution of every prostitute. Corrupted generally early in life, these girls feel themselves to have been the *victims of the "superior man"*; he remains the respected assailant, she is condemned. It is not to be wondered at then that waiting for a man is estimated as weakness, as the enemy, as a fatal deception and that at the same time, it occurs to them to attempt *to imitate man,* to have a profession, to give up all feminine attitudes and morality. This will appeal all the more to the naïve mind, the more impossible it appears on account of the girl's previous history or the feeling of man's worthlessness, for the feminine rôle, marriage and motherhood, to become deepened and the expectations of society to be fulfilled. It is the persistent trait of every prostitute's career to obtain, by *prostitution, both an outlet* for herself and that prestige otherwise denied her. She takes up her career after fruitless or apparently fruitless attempts at work, be it as maid, governess, or working-woman. However, *the scheme of things* she dreams of is always that of *the "active"* man not that of the " passive " woman.

Y

Of fundamental significance in this developmental process is the universally disseminated *poison of a super-masculine view of life*. It permeates the family life of the prospective prostitute, permits fathers to exercise tyrannical arbitrary power and turns a wife and mother into a terrifying example of the nature of the woman's rôle to be expected. This then elevates the brother to an envied position and makes the girl feel that her femininity represents a stigma and a reproach. The belief in her own power decreases and the seducer, often himself immature, encounters a resistless, weak being who has grown up in the fear of man or in baffled rage at her feminine destiny, who probably for the same reasons—her revolt against the restrictions of her parents—cannot develop along normal lines, a course of evolution rendered still more unlikely by her seduction. The subsequent effects of her seduction are worthy of mention. The inferences she draws are not always made with the object of correcting the situation but merely to strengthen her inferiority feeling, her distrust of her own powers and her horror at the feminine rôle. The broad easy path of prostitution now opens before her, where, drunk with activity, *she may revolt against the demands of society*, escape from goals difficult of attainment, be brought nearer to the stress and turmoil of masculine activity ; a road that promises her prestige and saves her from a feeling of absolute nothingness. This explanation may not strike us as correct. But ask the prostitutes and the brothel-keepers !

IV. *Prostitution and Society*

The circle is now complete. To-day we still see human society unable to formulate its demands with any strictness or to render them possible of fulfilment. All this is further complicated by the presence of women who recoil in fear from the struggles of life and attempt to find easier outlets. To this is to be added a civilization that is more and more bringing all its ideals into harmony with its concept of world-market and trade. We see the victims of this civilization making a virtue of necessity, filling a gap in our normal social life and then perishing tolerated and at the same time spurned.

XXVIII

Demoralized Children

(*Lecture delivered April* 1920)

OF the "blessings" that came in the wake of the Great
War perhaps no one thing is of such importance as the
tremendous increase in the demoralization of youth.
Everyone has noticed it and many have taken cognizance
of it with horror. The published statistics were significant enough and their significance must become
greater to all who stopped to think that only a small
part of the damage inflicted comes to our knowledge
and that a large number of other cases are destined to
run their course in silence for months and years, until
finally we are confronted with individuals no longer to
be reckoned as among the demoralized but among the
criminals. The numbers are large and the number
that never finds its way into statistics, still greater. In
the early stages most of the demoralization takes place
within the family circle. An improvement is expected
from day to day and certain measures are applied. As
there are quite a number of transgressions that occur
among the demoralized youth that are not directly
punishable by law or juvenile courts, and although
they inflict extensive damage upon the family, they are
covered up without leading to any change in the nature
of the culprit. It is, of course, not at all necessary to
give up all hope about the mistakes and transgressions
of youth, but considering the remarkably deficient
knowledge and understanding with which these matters
are approached, optimism is not justified. Nevertheless
we should point out that in the developmental stages
of man, particularly during youth, not everything takes
its course along ideal lines, that deviations occur, and
if we were to transport ourselves back to our own
youth and our youthful companions, we would be able

to rake up a number of transgressions committed even by children, who subsequently became either tolerably efficient people or even distinguished men.   How extensively youthful transgressions spread, a cursory summary may perhaps show you.   I have occasionally attempted to make investigations in schools in such a tactful manner that no one could possibly be hurt.   On a sheet of paper on which no names appeared, answers were to be written to the following questions: Has anyone ever lied or stolen?   The general results showed that all the children confessed to petty thefts.   One of the interesting episodes was the participation of a female teacher in the answers and her recollection of having committed a theft in childhood.   But now let us call attention to the complicated nature of such a question! One child may have a kind and intelligent father who knows how to come to an understanding with him and in many cases may succeed.   Another child may have done the same thing but perhaps more clumsily, conspicuously or brazenly and he will then immediately feel the whole brunt of the family discipline descend upon him and the conviction impressed upon his mind that he is a criminal.   We should therefore not be surprised that the difference in the nature of the punishment is correlated with a difference in the subterfuges adopted.   It is the worst of all pedagogical principles to tell a child that he will never amount to anything, that he possesses a criminal nature ; conceptions that belong to the domain of superstition, although there are scientists who also speak of hereditary criminals.   We have thus reached that point at which current educational systems cease to have any method which they can apply for the control of the initial or later stages of demoralization.   That ought not to surprise us for we are here concerned with facts in the child's psychic life, whose understanding is as yet confined to an extraordinary small circle of people.

Generally when we speak of demoralization we think of the school years.   The expert observer will, however, be able to point out a number of cases where the demoralization began before the school days.   It is not always possible to attribute them to the bringing-up. Parents must be told that no matter how careful they are that part of the education of which they know or notice nothing and which emanates from other circles, influences the child more than their consciously superior education.

These extraneous influences that find their way into the nursery represent all the events and conditions of life and of the environment. The child is impressed by the difficulties with which he sees his father beset in order to make a living, and he realizes the hostility of life even if he does not speak of it. He will develop a conception with the inadequate means at his disposal, with childish interpretations and experiences. This view of the world then becomes for the child a measure of evaluation; he makes it the basis for his judgments in every position in which he finds himself and will draw the correspondingly necessary inferences. These are in large measure wrong because we are here dealing with an inexperienced child whose reasoning powers are undeveloped and who consequently is liable to make false deductions. But just visualize the tremendous impression made upon a child whose parents live in a poor dwelling under depressing social circumstances, and contrast it with that of a child who does not feel life's hostility so definitely. These two types are so distinct that it is possible to infer from every child's expression and manner of speaking to which group he belongs. How differently will this last-mentioned child's attitude toward life be, with his self-confidence and courage, and how markedly will this be reflected in his whole carriage. The second type makes friends with the world easily because he knows nothing of life's difficulties or can overcome them more easily. I have asked children among the proletariat of what they were most in fear and practically all answered—*of being struck* —in other words, of occurrences taking place in their own family. Children who grow up in fear of a strong father, stepfather or mother, retain this feeling of fear till puberty, and we must remember that on the average the proletarian does not give us the same world-satisfied impression as the average bourgeois who is more courageous. A good deal of this pitiable bearing can be traced back to the fact that he has grown up in an atmosphere of fear of life and punishment. This is the most venomous kind of poison for developing *pessimism* in children, for they retain this perspective throughout

life, have no self-confidence and are indecisive. To gain
a courageous attitude afterwards requires both time and
energy. The children of well-to-do parents generally
answered the question of what they feared most, by
saying school-work. This shows that neither individuals nor their own environment frighten them and
they feel themselves to be in the midst of life where
tasks and work exist of which they are afraid. This of
course makes us assume the existence of untenable
conditions in the schools, which instead of training them
to face life gladly and courageously merely filled them
with fear.

Let us now go back to the question of demoralization
before the school-days. We ought not to be surprised
to find, in view of the excitable state of the moods
called up by all the disturbing relations that create fear
of life, and in view of the envisaging of one's neighbour
as hostile, that children will make a persistent effort to
gain prestige and not to appear as the insignificant
personages to which people often try to reduce them.
It is one of the most important principles in any
educational system to take the child *seriously*, to regard
him as *an equal* and not to humiliate and make fun of
him ; for the child feels and must necessarily feel all
those expressions of his immediate surroundings as
oppressive, just as the weaker person possesses a sensibility different from that of an individual who finds
himself in an assured position of a mental and bodily
superiority. We are not even in a position to state
exactly how a child is affected by the fact that it cannot
do the things that he wonderingly sees his parents and
brothers perform daily. This should be remembered.
Everyone who has developed a capacity for reading
the child's soul, must have realized that every child
possesses *an extraordinary craving for power and importance*,
for increased self-consciousness ; that he wishes to exert
influence and appear important. The *young would-be hero*
represents but a special case of the power that all wish
to have.

Differences between them can be easily explained.
In one case the child may be living in harmony with
his parents, in another he may fall into a hostile attitude
and develop antagonism to the demands of society in
order not to utterly succumb to the feeling that he is

nothing, plays no rôle, is quite disregarded. If such a stage of development is actually reached, where children realize their insignificance and their loss of importance, *they set immediately to work to protect themselves* —all children do it—and then indications of demoralization may appear very early. I once met a five-year-old abomination who had killed three children. This somewhat mentally-retarded girl always resorted to the following method in her "crimes". She would look for girls smaller than herself—she lived in the country —take them along to play with her and then push them into the stream. It was only when the third child had been killed that the perpetrator was discovered. She was placed in a lunatic asylum. She did not show the slightest realization of the depravity of her actions. She cried, but passed easily over to other subjects, and it was only with the greatest difficulty that any information could be obtained about the nature of the whole situation and her motives. For four years she had been the youngest child among a number of boys and had been excessively petted. Then a younger sister had appeared upon the scene and the parents lavished all their attention upon the newcomer while she, the elder, was pushed into the background. This could not however endure and she developed a hatred of her younger sister that she was, under the circumstances, unable to gratify because the baby was very carefully guarded, and because she possibly realized that she could be easily detected. She thereupon generalized and transferred her hatred to younger girls, all of whom she regarded as potential enemies. In all of them she saw her own young sister on whose account she was no longer being petted. In this mood she now progressed to the point of even killing them. Attempts made to bring such children back to normal paths, within a short time, go awry, because these children are at times *mentally defective*, oftener than one believes. One must be prepared for a treatment of long duration, and by using infinite tact and a special kind of training, render the child capable of again taking part in the life of society. But these cases, which are exceedingly common, are of lesser interest to us because of their connexion with mental deficiency and we must, in a way, accept them as instances of biological sports, for they probably would never fit entirely into human society. But the great mass of our demoralized youth is free from any taint of mental inferiority. On the contrary we often find extraordinarily gifted children who for a time progress quite well and develop capabilities up to a certain point, but *once they have broken down they are utterly unable to prevent a catastrophe overtaking them along one of the main lines of life.* In every case we find the same regularly recurring traits :—*a marked development of ambition although not outwardly expressed ; sensitiveness to being pushed aside or ignored ; cowardice consisting not simply in running away but in sneaking away from life and its demands.* From these few traits we can draw a picture of the whole. Only an ambitious child is capable of being frightened away from a task that threatens to extend beyond its powers and of striking out along another path as though covering up its weakness. This is the ordinary course of demoralization found in schools. *This demoralization is connected with some failure* that either has taken place or is about to take place, and shows itself at first in absence from school. But as truancy must, of course, be concealed, we naturally find that at first notes of excuse are forged and then signatures. But what is the child to do with its free time ? An occupation must be found. *As a rule a union takes place of all children* who have gone along the same road, all who have been overtaken by the same fate. These children are, as a rule, all tremendously ambitious and desirous of playing a rôle, but do not trust themselves to attaining it along the main lines of human endeavour, and in consequence seek activities that will give them satisfaction. Some individual is always found to be best fitted for leadership and competition then ceases. Each one has some idea of what should be done. Imitating forms employed by their elders, they will develop a code of ethics applicable to a demoralized group. They try hard and with great ingenuity to think of deeds to perform that will enhance their importance in the eyes of their comrades. These are always carried out by deception, or hyper-deception, for they do not trust themselves to act openly—in consequence of their cowardice. Once on this road there is no turning back. Occasionally mentally defective boys join the group. They are made fun of, have tricks played on them and their pride, then incite them to exceptional efforts and actions. *Or it may be that being accustomed to a definite kind of treatment they are specially trained to obedience and their task becomes one of receiving orders and carrying them out.* It frequently happens that some one plans a specific transgression and the younger, inexperienced, inferior ones undertake it. I shall pass over other temptations although something might be said about them too, such as vicious books, the cinema, but they do not become directing forces until later. The cinema could never survive if it were not for the cleverness and the special skill displayed in selecting subject matter, whether criminal or detective, that stimulates the audience. In this overevaluation of guile and subterfuge, the cowardice to face life is manifested.

The formation of bands is so common that it is the first thing that comes to mind when thinking of demoralized youths. But the demoralization of an individual distinct from a group is quite frequent. Such a person's life is similar to that we have described above, though apparently the directly impelling motives are different. Let us keep before us the fact that in the cases of group demoralization described above, the fate of the individuals *is foreshadowed as soon as they have suffered some set-back or expect one.* The same is true of a single individual. The simple, almost unwitting, persons come under this rule to the same extent as the more complicated. It is always some offence to one's amour propre, the fear of making a fool of one's self, the feeling of some decline in power or the will to power, that becomes the occasion for a *deviation to some side-line of development.* It looks almost as if these children *were seeking for some subsidiary field of action.* Frequently demoralization shows itself in a special form of laziness, which must then be looked upon neither as hereditary nor as the acquisition of a bad habit, but rather as a method of preventing any of them being put to tests. A lazy child can always fall back upon laziness as an excuse. If he fails in an examination it is the fault of his laziness, and such a child prefers to attribute his failure to laziness than to inability. Thus, like an experienced criminal, he is forced *to prove an alibi ;* he must in each case demonstrate that his lack of success is due to laziness. And he succeeds. His laziness covers his failures, and from one point of view, that of sparing his conceit, his psychic situation has improved.

We know the demerits of our schools. The crowded classes, the insufficient training of many of the teachers, occasionally their lack of interest, for they suffer intensely from cramped economic conditions and more is hardly to be expected of them. Primarily, however, the greatest drawback of the school is *the prevailing ignorance about the psychic development of the child;* and that is the reason why hitherto the relations of the teacher and pupil have been so much more hopeless than those existing anywhere else in life. If the pupil makes a mistake he is either punished or given a poor mark. That is about the same as if a doctor called to treat someone who has broken a bone, saying: "You have a bone-fracture! Good-bye!" That assuredly is not the purpose of education! In the main the children take care of themselves under these horrible conditions and progress, but what of the gaps in their development? Children will proceed until they finally come to a point where their deficiencies assume such a form that a halt must be called. It is sad enough to realize how difficult it is even for the best child to progress, how under the weight of the accumulated difficulties he is afflicted with there emerges the painful feeling of being unable to perform the tasks others achieve, and finally to be a witness of his wounded and offended self-esteem! Many pass beyond this stage too, but many prefer to develop for themselves some subsidiary field of action.

Individual demoralization thus develops in the same manner as group demoralization. Here, likewise, the feeling of inferiority, of inadequacy and of humiliation tower above everything else. Let me quote the case of a boy, an only child, whose parents devoted great pains in educating him. At the age of five he already regarded the locking of chests, when the parents were absent, as a great insult and succeeded somehow in procuring a skeleton key and ransacking the chests. He was impelled to this conduct by his striving for independence, his will to power asserting itself in antagonism to his parents and the laws of society. Even to-day, at the age of eighteen, he indulges in household thefts unknown to his parents, although they believe they are aware of all of them. When his father tells him, "Of what use are these acts to you? As often as you steal I discover the fact," then the boy has the proud realization of knowing that his father does not know one in twenty and continues his thefts in the conviction that all that is necessary is to be clever enough to escape detection. Here we have an example of the frequent struggle between a child and its parents that induces the former to resort to acts contrary to the moral code of society. When fully grown-up this young man will undoubtedly provide himself with these psychic aids and supports that will enable him to transgress without feeling any pricks of conscience. His father is a business man, and even though the son is not permitted to visit his father's factories, he knows that the latter is engaged in the manufacture of chains, etc. When conversing with people he calls his father's attacks upon him unjust, because the latter is simply doing what he does, simply on a larger scale. So here again we have an example of the educative influence of the environment of which the parents are totally ignorant.

Let me now give one case from proletarian circles. An illegitimate six-year old boy is taken to the home of his mother who is married. His real father has disappeared and his step-father, a cranky old man, although not really interested in children, is very demonstrative to his own daughter, fondles her, brings her sweets while the boy is forced to look on. One day, a fairly large sum of money belonging to the mother disappears without a trace. Shortly after that, after further sums had disappeared, she discovered the culprit to be her son, and that he had spent the money in purchasing sweets, occasionally sharing it with his comrades with the object of showing off. So here we have another example of the secondary field of action, serving as usual the old main object of triumphing and gaining prestige at any cost. These thefts happened a number of times, whippings followed, and his step-father did not spare him. I saw the boy myself, covered with stripes, his whole body full of scratches and cicatrices. In spite of the punishments, however, the thefts, as might have been expected, did not cease. The mother, it is true, was rather clumsy, for she had made the thefts rather easy for the child. But how many mothers show

any intelligence in such cases?   The analysis showed
that the boy had been taken care of by an old peasant
woman who, when visiting the adjacent villages, had
always taken him with her and had given him some
sweets from time to time.   The child was then transferred to a new environment where he found himself at
a great disadvantage compared to his former home.
His little sister he sees petted and fondled, given sweets
denied him.   It is she, not he who attracts attention.
He was very good at school.   His transgression is
found exactly there where he would be expected *to look
for an enemy* and appeared almost as inevitable.   And
so it is in many cases.   Demoralization has the effect
of an act of revenge and brings to the child a psychic
relief.

Let me again emphasize the fact that the transgressions of demoralized people are not of an active,
courageous kind, except when they operate in large
numbers and this would again point to cowardice.
Their most frequent dereliction is theft, which is essentially the crime of cowardice.

If we wish to understand clearly both all the interrelations and the position of the children to society
we should bear two things in mind.   First that their
ambition and vanity are signs of their craving for power
and superiority so that in consequence they try to
obtain prestige along some side-path as soon as the
main-line of development is closed to them.   Secondly,
their relation to their fellows is somehow deficient ; they
are not good companions, they do not easily adjust
themselves to society, have something of the dog-in-
the-manger attitude and exhibit little contact with the
outer world.   At times, nothing but a meaningless
pretence or a mere habit is all that remains of their love
for their own people ; often even this is missing and
they may then even attack their own family.   They
play the rôle of people whose feeling for society is
defective, who have not discovered the point of contact
with their fellowmen and look upon them as hostile.
Traits of suspicion are very common among them ; they
are always on guard lest someone take advantage of
them and I have often heard these children exclaim that
it is necessary to be unscrupulous, *i.e.*, that superiority
must be attained.   Suspicion creeps into all their

relations and adds to the difficulties of living with them. Cowardly subterfuges develop automatically through this lack of trust in themselves.

The question now to decide is whether this craving for power, this deficient social consciousness is due to different causes? We can definitely answer in the negative for they do but represent two sides of the same psychic attitude. *The feeling of co-operation must suffer where the craving for power exists*, for a person possessed by the latter thinks only of himself, of his power, of his prestige, acts in utter disregard of others. If an individual succeeds in developing a feeling of co-operation the best guarantee against demoralization is given.

I am quite at sea as to what can be done in an age of intensified demoralization like ours. The correct and proper thing is clearly to act immediately. Even in times of complete peace our civilization was not able to gain effective control over demoralization and crime ; she could merely punish, revenge herself, frighten people, never solve the problem. She kept the demoralized at elbow distance. Visualize, if you can, the frightful fate of these people, whose loneliness must in itself drive them to crime ; people who are criminals only *because they have lost contact*. From that they develop into habitual criminals. It is a piece of utter stupidity, for instance, to herd together during examination, demoralized individuals with their own kind or with criminals.

We must reckon with about 40 per cent. of the crimes remaining undiscovered. Among the demoralized the percentage is even higher. A short time ago, a youthful murderer was convicted and his lawyer knew that this was the second murder for which he had been tried. When criminals meet they discuss the number of times they have not been caught and this naturally increases the difficulty of combating crime and constantly renews the criminal's courage.

Evils are also noticeable in the type of attitude taken by society. Both courts and police work to no purpose because they always centre their attention upon questions other than the really radical and determining ones. To improve the situation the first requirement is to have a different and a more humane personnel. Institutions ought to be erected for taking care of these demoralized children, for bringing them back to life ; not shutting them off from society, but, on the contrary, making them more adapted for it. That can only happen if we have a full understanding of their peculiarities. Nothing can be accomplished if any kind of person whatsoever (*e.g.* a retired officer or a subaltern) can be appointed director of an institution of this kind merely because he enjoys political protection. Only such people are to be considered for these posts who have a strongly developed community-sense and a full understanding of the people entrusted to their care. The essential point of my argument is this, that in a civilization where one man is the enemy of the other—for this is what our whole industrial system means—demoralization is ineradicable, for demoralization and crime are *by-products of the struggle for existence* as known to our industrialized civilization. The shadows of this struggle fall very early across the soul of the child, destroy its poise, facilitate its craving for greatness and render it craven and incapable of co-operation.

To limit and do away with this demoralization a chair of curative pedagogy should be established. It is indeed hard to understand why such a chair does not already exist. To-day a true understanding of the problem is exceedingly rare. All persons in any way connected with this problem should be compelled to take an active part. The institution itself should be in the nature of a central exchange bureau which would give information on all matters relating to the prevention and combating of demoralization.

In addition, county institutions of an advisory nature should exist for the lighter cases. For the more severe forms the relatives of the patients must suggest a method of treating them, for the patients themselves would never be able to find one.

In conclusion teachers should be made acquainted with individual-psychology and curative pedagogy, so that from the very beginning they might be in a position to recognize the signs of demoralization and to intervene helpfully themselves and nip the danger tactfully and lovingly in the bud. A model school for the practical education of the personnel should also be founded.

INDEX